I hope you enjoy
the story.
Thank-you.

DR. T

COVERED LIVES

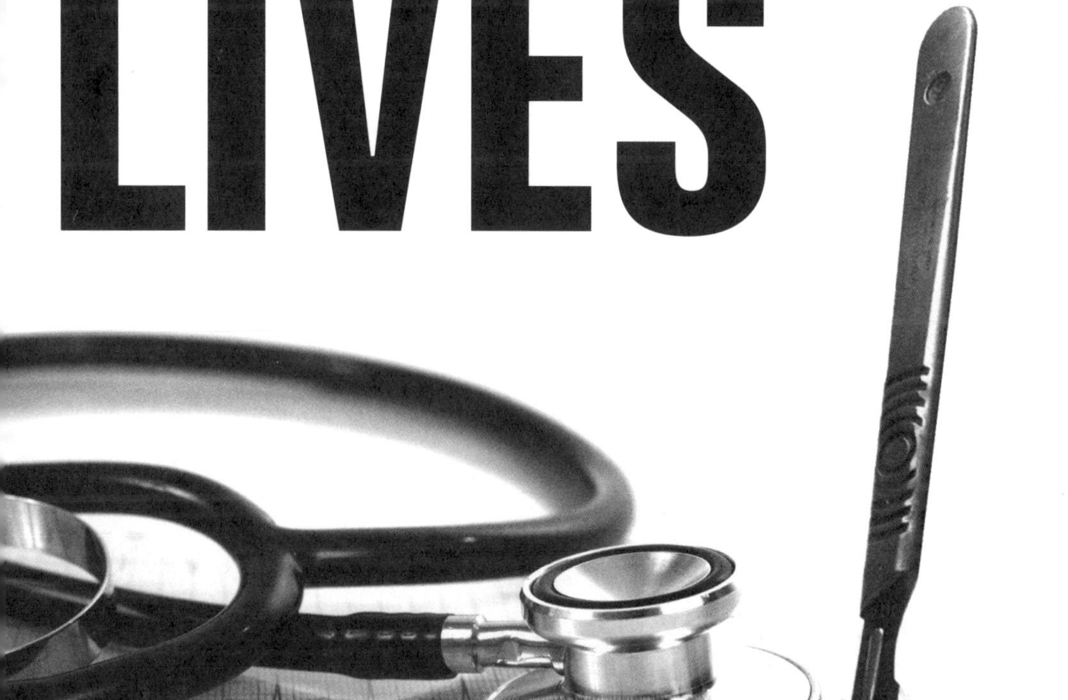

J. FREDERIC TEMPLEMAN, M.D.

Biosciences Publishing Inc.
1927 North 135 West
Orem, Utah, 84057

Printed in the United States of America.

In the health insurance industry, the term **'covered lives'** refers to those individuals who have been underwritten by an insurance firm. But, of course, we all live covered lives to one degree or another.

In order to suppress our primordial fear of the stranger and generate the courage to venture out into the world each day, we must believe that every human heart contains some measure of virtue. By projecting benevolence onto those we deal with everyday, we can feel safe from senseless random violence. We can live life in something other than a perpetual state of high arousal and vigilance. But the horror of reality always intrudes. And, when a madman with an assault rifle runs amok among people not unlike us, we are shocked and incredulous. Our essential illusions are shattered. Recovery, however, is quick. We trust again, almost immediately, because we have no other valid choice. We cannot constantly seek the psychopath behind every man's eyes. And thus, our lives are regularly catapulted into disarray by the eruption of the evil that incubates among us… waiting.

PROLOGUE

He lay motionless on his belly in the shadow of a hilltop oak. Below him, the light of the full moon projected the surrounding hills in crisp silhouettes upon the glimmering asphalt strip serpenting through the valley. Offshore, on the inky waters of Lake Blacksheer, its ivory image lay shattered into a million glittering facets.

A single pinpoint of light approached crawling down through the night from the western horizon, flickering on and off behind distant hills like a firefly.

The wind whipping over the windshield of the convertible flung her long hair up and back in a tumbling vortex. Reverberating from the stereo speakers, the cascading rhythms of Rachmaninoff's concerto in C-minor all but obscured the sound of a file folder snapping in the turbulence on the seat beside her. She was singing in wordless burst-lung accompaniment to the music she could feel vibrating up through the seat before it bounced off and into the night.

Her Mercedes flew along the blacktop straightaway, its speed reducing the dotted lane lines to a single ribbon of yellow unfurling endlessly in the beam of her headlights.

She glanced at the instrument panel. The tachometer needle was almost red-lining while the speedometer wavered around one hundred and thirty mph. The possibility that some state trooper might be lying in wait under a tree at a crossroad flashed into her mind and she interrupted her singing to laugh aloud at the image generated by the thought… 'H*ell, he'd never even catch me!*'

A heart-pounding high. Speed. Risk. Freedom.

So much of her life was confining, the expectations implicit in being the wife of a prominent physician, the emotional corset of motherhood cinched tightly by the ligaments of love... her stiff almost stifling law career where, as a woman, she had to be even more correct than any man. It was in this nest of obligations, years ago, that her disregard for rules, caution and restraint had been born and, on those nights like tonight when she raced death home, it still thrived.

She had a reputation, had been labeled when she began her midnight escapes into speed astride the Ducati racing cycle she'd purchased on her tenth wedding anniversary. The men who knew of her nocturnal habit were attracted and intrigued, puzzling over this enigmatic Celtic beauty who eclipsed them all in her audacious flirtation with danger. Women often reacted with disapproving envy as if her motorcycle were some lithe-limbed gigolo bursting with sexual ardor whom she kept hidden during the day.

And the riding had been almost sexual, her body molded to the machine, the power between her thighs, the massage of wind rippling over back and legs, the rush of the curves pulling her into them. The freedom she felt when riding was like running naked along a moonlit beach, surf thundering in, salt spray licking at her skin, the heady defiance of a world that would never approve of her adrenaline communion.

She had sold the motorcycle under duress. The pleas of her husband and children, like edicts from God, obliging her to part with a piece of herself for the sake of those who loved her, needed her.

The new Mercedes CLK63 was a compromise.

She knew this road. It was a familiar antagonist whose curves and hills she had tamed to the point where greater speed was the only challenge left. Tonight, she would top-end the speedometer along the scimitar curve of the road that ran atop the Blacksheer dam matching her skill against gravity and chance. Her faith in her mechanical accomplice was absolute.

She prepared mentally. Before the road began its dance along the spine of the dam, it warped to the right to accommodate the thrust of a small bay jutting like a sprained thumb away from the palm of the lake. To negotiate the approach to the dam at optimum speed, she would have to reach exactly one hundred mph at the top of the final hill. Any slower and she'd never reach top-end on the half-mile curve of the dam itself. Any faster and she risked losing control in the curve. She had done it many times before with the bike and, tonight, she would impose her will on the Mercedes and the road again.

As the hills whipped past she could feel her muscles tensing, her heart accelerating. She tightened her grip on the wheel more firmly and leaned into the seatbelt to more effectively feel the car beneath her. She would succeed. She knew it. Then, trembling with triumph, she would slide into bed beside her sleeping husband, stimulate him with kisses and caresses until she could consummate her arousal before slipping back into the narrow confines of her everyday life.

She often suspected that, when she sold the Ducati, the potential disappearance of these erotic denouements were why he had so readily agreed to her purchase of the powerful little Mercedes.

In the last valley before the hill she checked her speed, ninety-six mph and climbing. A mere moment later, she crested the rise and felt the wheels of the car barely tipple the pavement as it lifted off the road's surface, almost airborne, but at the requisite speed. She waited until she felt the automobile settle before easing the wheel to the right. Pebbles, deposited by past rains on the paved shoulder, ricocheted against the fenders like staccato gunshots as she hugged the edge of the pavement.

She was almost out of the curve when she felt it -- a jarring thump from beneath the vehicle loud enough to drown out the stone clatter and Rachmaninoff. The steering wheel jerked to the right, ripping out of her hands. A levitating blow against the floorboards so powerful that her foot was knocked from the brake pedal she had instinctively hit. A hiss of grinding steel. Sparks showering from the asphalt. The vehicle pivoting harshly to the right. A snarling implosion of molded metal as the front of the car rammed the reinforced roadside rails. The 'whump' of the airbags just as the windshield shattered spraying pellets of glass back into her face like blinding liquid fire.

The force of the impact and the vehicle's momentum catapulted the Mercedes trunk-first into the air over the guardrails. It twisted and spun twice end over end in the air like a mechanical gymnast executing a breath-holding dismount from a highbar before plowing its right front fender into the earth. A desperately awkward half-forward, half-sideways tumble followed as if in slow motion. Then, like a twirling figure skater drawing in her arms, the car accelerated into a tight spin whirling down the slope. It struck the lake water, wheels in the air, with a lash of liquid silver that blossomed skyward.

The vehicle rocked in place for a few seconds as if stunned by the impact, then it rolled lethargically upright, a drowning horn mewing mournfully. Slowly, it began to settle, the backend sliding under the water till it bobbed briefly like a silver buoy. A lone headlight searched the sky in a final forlorn plea before the mangled grill disappeared beneath the surface with a gush of bubbles.

A moment later, all that marked the watery grave was the muted glow of the wavering headlight disappearing into the depths.

Under the baton of instinct, an invisible orchestra of insects whose thrumming had been disrupted by the cacophony of the crash resumed its discordant harmony.

Arising from the grass where he lay, he passed a small object from his hand into his jacket pocket then folded a pair of binoculars and began his descent from the hill.

CH001

Amy Davis sat hunched over the steaming mug of hot chocolate, her nervous palms vainly begging comfort from the warm porcelain. As she reviewed the events that led her to be here in the restaurant waiting for her ex-husband to arrive, she began to question her decision to see him even one last time. Her apprehension, like blood seeping up from an unstaunched wound was rapidly staining the dressing of indifference with which she had bound up her lacerated emotions.

Since obtaining the restraining order five months ago, she'd had no contact with Riley Davis. So, when she'd heard his voice on the phone, it was like being poked on a forgotten bruise. Shocked at first by the rush of fear coursing involuntarily through her, she'd recovered quickly and become angry. She was angry at him for intruding once more into her life but she was even more angry at herself for reacting so elementally after all the therapy, after all the silent vows, after all the courage summoned to creep along the swaying footbridge to health that spanned the chasm where her terror of male anger churned and tumbled below.

As always, when he had wanted something and wasn't blasted with alcohol or high on drugs, her ex-husband had been charming. Seizing upon the startled silence after she answered the phone and recognized his voice, he'd begun spinning the silken sophistry that had made him Atlanta's premier defense attorney. It was the same web of deception he'd wound so effectively around her reason in the past until she'd been cocooned in self-doubt and impotence.

He only needed an hour of her time. Her choice of when and where. And then he'd leave her in peace. The restraining order would no longer be needed. They'd go their separate ways. Just one more time.

Her instinctive recoil at the mere sound of his voice had slapped at her hard-won self-confidence and her cheeks had burned with indignation and shame at the unwelcome reaction. Over the months they'd been apart, she'd convinced herself that he could never affect her in that way again. The proof that he could wasn't simply disconcerting, it identified a challenge she must face and vanquish if she ever hoped to be free. That's why she'd agreed to the meeting and chosen the *Trattoria Roma,* a busy Atlanta sidewalk café across from a police station.

The day was already hot and the air redolent with the aromas of cappuccino and tomato sauce. A bee, attracted by the odors emanating from the restaurant and the wash of bright spring colors on the patrons, hovered above the table next to her bouncing as if on an elastic tether. A fat man swiped at it in annoyance and it sped up and away.

Amy lost sight of the bee and dropped her eyes to survey the lunchtime crowd filtering in. At a nearby table, she saw a couple of starched and labeled Mormon missionaries with telltale pocket tags and military haircuts, diligently highlighting passages in their scriptures. She was grateful they didn't look up from their task because she knew making eye contact with them risked being misinterpreted as interest in their theology but she took comfort in presuming that they wouldn't ignore an argument or threat of violence to a woman sitting nearby, if it came to that. She might need their assistance if Riley Davis erupted in public as he'd done before.

Her therapist wouldn't have approved of her strategy, hiding from the threat of one man behind the strength of other men. Definitely a poor choice for an emancipated woman. Pepper spray, maybe. Better yet, a bullet in the brain of the abuser. But her therapist was extreme and Amy was still discovering what she was capable of in the face of male aggression. In the past, she'd already balked at murder. In fact, she'd repeatedly allowed herself to be beaten by her husband rather than kill him. Ironically, he had provided her with the means to eliminate him when he'd taught her to shoot a pistol then given her one *'to use for protection'*. What remained incomprehensible was his apparent ignorance of the risk he ran when he beat upon her in their bedroom with the revolver within her reach.

Later, during therapy when she'd thought through the abuse, she realized that there had never been anything rational about his savagery, or her passivity in the face of it. It had all been mutual madness.

But things were different now. She had changed. She would never allow him to harm her again and if that meant murder, so be it. However, she wasn't planning to kill him. She was here to confront his manipulations, his perverse logic and his intimidation. Face it all and, finally, walk away free. And so, she rationalized that she had come to the restaurant for herself and *not* because he had called and *that* view of things made all the difference in the world. She was choosing to challenge him and all that his wrath represented for her. It would be her acid test. She took in a deep breath and let it slowly escape from between pursed lips.

The buzz of conversation became louder as the tables in the café filled rapidly. Amy glanced at her watch, ten past twelve. She'd come early to the café to position herself advantageously but she knew Riley wouldn't be late. He never was.

A delivery van pulled away from the curb a dozen yards down the street and a silver Jaguar whipped into the empty parking space. The license plate read *'TOP DOG'*.

Her heart quickened. It was his car.

The windows were heavily tinted but she could already feel his eyes upon her and the skin prickled on the back of her neck despite her resolve.

She had become used to men looking at her and she no longer fled the experience. It had taken years but, gradually, her beauty had become a reliable source of power for her. She derived satisfaction from the knowledge that men couldn't ignore her, that she could turn their heads, that they would openly stare as she passed, or furtively glance her way if wives or girlfriends accompanied them. But, when Riley Davis turned his attention to her all she wanted to do was disappear. She clasped the mug a little tighter, her knuckles whitening with the effort.

Today, she had dressed to be ignored. Baggy sweatsuit and hair in a ponytail. Sunglasses and no make-up. Her choice of unaccustomed attire had been deliberate. She'd always believed that her beauty was the primary reason Riley Davis had married her. A powerful man needed to flaunt a beautiful woman on his arm but she was determined never to adorn his world again, not even momentarily.

The door of the Jag opened and a tall, imposingly handsome man got out and made his way across the patio toward her. He wore one of his trial suits, an Armani hand-stitched silk job. The red rosebud boutonniere that had become his trial trademark glinted like a bloodstain against the gray fabric. His face was tan and lean and he was smiling broadly the way he did whenever he wanted to disconcert an opponent. His eyes were locked on her face and never wavered even when he had to thread his way between tables. He was holding her with his gaze the way he monopolized the attention of a witness on the stand, shutting them off from everything and everyone else but him. She was being treated to the Riley Davis courtroom performance.

She needed to get in the first word to stamp the encounter with the tenor she'd decided upon. She called out to him sarcastically.

" Big case today, Riley?"

He sat down in the chair opposite her before answering.

" Most important I've ever had," he said, ignoring the sarcasm, "more preparation that I've ever put into a plea before. But, if you don't mind taking off the sunglasses, I'd like to see your eyes when I make my presentation. It's a lawyer thing."

"I'm sure you would, counselor, but I'll leave the glasses on anyway. *It's a victim thing.*"

An expression flashed across his face in a nanosecond and she recognized anger, but anger instantly stifled.

He looked down at the tabletop and raised a hand to massage his brow, hiding his face from her momentarily as a mime might do when changing expressions. She could sense him making a strategic shift from the ineffectual role of charmer to that of supplicant.

"Amy, please, don't make this any harder that it already is."

She interrupted him. "Harder on whom, counselor?... I don't give a damn how *you* feel, so cut the bogus charm and, if I hear the word 'sorry' dribble out of your lips even once, I'm out of here."

He looked up at her with brimming eyes and she recalled how he had once demonstrated to her, after winning a big case, that he could summon tears when it was strategically desirable. He'd told her he used to picture his dog, Dusty, lying in a puddle of blood under the wheels of the truck that had crushed him when Riley was five years old. Later, that long ago night, he'd celebrated a courtroom victory with five lines of cocaine and punched her in the face before raping her.

"Having visions of Dusty and the truck, counselor? Save the theatrics for the juries. You have ten minutes and then I leave." She was surprised by the jagged edge she heard in her own voice.

His tears evaporated and the anger flashed briefly again.

"Are you even going to listen to what I have to say?"

"Maybe... Make your case."

"Amy, I've examined our marriage over and over again and I know I was wrong."

"You weren't just wrong, Riley, you were criminal. That's why you were arrested and charged." She was scowling even as she spoke. " Don't waste your breath on apologies because there isn't anything you can say or do to change how I feel about you."

"Did you know I've been in treatment?" he asked.

"You mean you attended the court-ordered violence group, don't you?"

"More than that. I'm doing the AA and NA programs and I've been seeing a psychiatrist for the past five months as well."

"And?"

"And, I've learned something about what was wrong between us."

"You should have saved your money and just asked me," she interjected. "What was wrong was that you beat and you abused me... You are a drunk and a drug addict."

"I admit that I'm no longer under any illusions and I'm not proud of my flaws."

A waiter approached and he waved him away without a word before continuing. "I'm doing my best to understand why I was an addict."

"*Was*?"

"Right, you're right, *am* an addict. Anyway, I'm trying to get to the bottom of it all. Why I treated you like I did... Where my anger came from."

Amy could feel her discomfort growing at this uncharacteristic humility from the man who had abused her for twelve years and, quickly concluding that he didn't deserve even a moment of her discomfort, she blurted out.

"You're so full of crap, Riley, who scripted this tearjerker for you, your shrink?" She had leaned aggressively forward on the table and taken off her sunglasses.

His face tightened. Several seconds passed in silence as she watched his eyes to detect the anger she knew *had* to be there. Rumbling. Hiding. Crouching just beneath the surface. Ready to spring out. But, when he spoke, he used a neutral tone devoid of any identifiable emotion.

"Amy, have you had the courage to look at your role in our problems?"

"Are you asking me if I remember the cuts, the bruises, the pain and the terror? Absolutely!"

"I know there was all of that but there was more than that as well."

"What do you mean... *more than that*? Are you referring to the psychological abuse, the public insults, the sadistic mind games you played?"

"What I mean, Amy, is that you *expected* it from me… the abuse and the violence. Something inside of you knew that it existed in me. Knew how to smell it out. Knew how to ignite it. Knew that it would be directed at you and yet, you *chose* me as your husband. Perhaps, you chose me *because you knew it was there.*"

She felt a wave of nausea as the implication of his accusations registered and, choking back an acid sourness, she coughed once and took a sip of the now tepid chocolate. Then, with effort, she leveled her gaze and spoke almost menacingly. "Are you saying you believe I chose to marry you because I somehow knew that you would become a drug addict and beat the hell out of me?... *Are you completely out of your mind?*"

He shook his head and shrugged his shoulders in a gesture intended to display a degree of innocence incapable of malice.

"I'm not trying to downplay what I did... not for a minute, but I've researched our problems, talked a lot with my psychiatrist. There's good evidence, good scientific research that proves people like you and me play out unconscious roles that draw us together. Abusers and victims... We seek each other out."

A blur of emotions whirred like quail wings in her mind blotting out the lucidity she needed to answer. She squinted in disgust and shook her head from side to side as much to clear it as to signal her absolute rejection of what he'd just said.

"Think about it for a moment, Amy," he continued. "If you're being honest with yourself, you know you hid from me. You hid who you really are under an academy award performance that lasted our whole marriage. As for me, I got right into my role without pretense. You knew who I was, what I was, but *I never knew you*. In fact, I still don't know much about your past except that you hate your father. And, I'm convinced there's something real twisted hidden in your childhood that made you an accomplice in all this. Even if I was the abuser, *you* need to own up to some of the responsibility for what happened."

She had stopped shaking her head and just stared at him, still unable to respond.

He went on. "When people marry they agree to drop all pretenses. Secrets are revealed… If you can't be yourself with your spouse, chances are you can't be yourself anywhere."

He paused, but she still remained silent.

"In our marriage I *was* myself. You *never* were."

His voice trailed off and he shuffled his chair slightly sideways deliberately hiding his face from her. Amy speculated, even in the midst of her disarray, *'To hide his anger?'*

When at last she found her voice, she spoke deliberately. "I'm not going to sit and listen to you tell me why I'm to blame for being beaten and abused. So I'm leaving… Oh, and by the way, you're the last sick SOB on earth I would ever sit down with in therapy, so save your disgusting self-disclosure and your theorizing for your shrink. He gets paid to listen to it. I don't and I won't."

She'd been staring malignantly at the side of his head and now, she aggressively shoved her mug across the table to occupy the space where his hands had been before he'd turned away.

He turned to face her, flared the fingers of both hands and patted the air for emphasis. "Ok, just one last thing then, Amy. Straight from the hip. But you'd better listen carefully to what I have to say."

His face had transformed itself. Eyelids partially lowered. Eyes no more than slits under a thunderous brow. She knew absolutely now that his rage was tensed and crouching behind the obsidian bullets of his pupils. She had prodded it into betraying itself.

His words rang like footfalls in an empty marble corridor. "I will not risk disbarment… You will agree not to testify in the assault charges against me. If you refuse to be a witness, they have no case. If you know anything about me, you know that my profession is my whole life and I won't let you trash it!"

He paused for effect and then his face suddenly lightened and he shrugged his shoulders again. It was as if all the intensity had drained out of his voice in a single heartbeat.

"It's as simple as that and then we never see each other again," he said.

She smiled thinly.' *So that's what's at the bottom of all this. What this whole meeting is about… Let him avoid the consequences once more. And, in return, I'll be free of him*'.

"Well, you finally cough up the hairball, Riley. All that crap about flaws comes down to me letting you off. Nice strategy!... Intimidate the stupid little broad once more and watch her run scared like she always has."

She rolled her eyes in an expression of incredulity. "Do you really think that I haven't learned anything from what I've been through?"

As if he sensed what was coming, his tone became sarcastic and menacing. "Amy, you wouldn't recognize sincerity if it were etched in ten foot high neon letters in front of your eyes, so you think what you want. What I want... *what I will have at any price*, is my career, the means to earn a living and pay you alimony. It's not like there's nothing in it for you."

"Shove your alimony. Stick it way up there with your fake remorse and the rest of your lies."

She was almost hissing at him, both of them now leaning across the table, nose to nose. His eyes had ignited with the flare of yellow hatred she'd seen so often before but, this time, she was facing it down.

"You'll never abuse another woman again and I don't care if you have to clean toilets on your hands and knees in your Armani suits to earn your booze money."

His hands shot out and grasped her wrists like manacles where they lay on the tabletop. Her mug toppled off the table and smashed on the floor, spraying chocolate over their feet.

"Get your hands off me, now!" she shouted and stood up in a single motion, drawing back so that his grip on her wrists became clearly visible to the men at the surrounding tables.

The conversation around them was sliced off as abruptly as if a shot had been fired. Both Mormons were rising to their feet.

Riley glanced quickly around sizing up the threat. Slowly, he released her wrists while continuing to glare at her with the same murderous intensity she'd seen during the beatings.

Her heart was pounding in her throat. She wanted to run, to evaporate, but she forced herself to glare back at him. *He* would have to be the first to turn away.

"Are you ok, miss?" called the larger of the two Mormon missionaries, taking a step toward her table.

"Yes, I'm quite alright. Thank-you... The gentleman was just leaving."

There was no quaver in her voice. No echo of the terror of male anger she had lived with all of her life.

Something like elation stirred in her viscera and she felt herself almost smile.

CH002: ALBANY, GEORGIA

Dr. Jason Turner pulled his maroon BMW into the oil-stained parking stall below the black plaque bearing his name and began rummaging through the heap of mail and newspapers on the passenger seat for the day's appointment list his receptionist had handed him yesterday afternoon. He didn't know if it was there or not but he knew that it should be. He leaned further over to see if it had fallen into the space between seat and door but was pulled up short by his shoulder strap. He angrily snapped loose the seatbelt in a burst of irritation and heard the zipping hiss of the belt being sucked into the entrails of the door frame.

He searched the passenger compartment but the list was nowhere. He slapped at the pile of mail on the seat in frustration and turned to get out of the car, grabbing at his briefcase in the backseat. He knew the appointment list wasn't in his briefcase because he never opened it. He just carried it back and forth to the office occasionally for the appearance of organization it lent him.

It wasn't that he resented order or disliked neatness. On the contrary, he admired the order that both his wife and mother had imposed upon the chaos of homes filled with children. He even enjoyed finding his messy desk at the clinic clean and uncluttered after his receptionist's attention to it each Friday afternoon. It was just that he'd never felt any personal responsibility to be organized. In fact, he had always been secretly pleased with the dollop of entropy his own disorganization contributed to the universal equation of transformation and dynamics. He rationalized that his randomness sort of balanced out the anal retentiveness displayed by so many other physicians. But *this* morning, he was irritated with himself for misplacing the list.

The growing disarray in his life seemed to be just one more proof that the demons of insanity were honing their claws at the backdoor of his mind.

His world, which in recent years had been a reasonably comfortable place allowing him to live in benevolent disorganization, had suddenly and dramatically changed. The recent automobile accident which had killed his wife had also shattered his sense of self. Literally overnight, his existence had been reduced to smoldering rubble charred beyond repair by the flames of tragedy.

Each day, he awakened to a brutal fatigue that enveloped him like a paralyzing fog. Restorative sleep, appropriate appetite, adequate energy and even the desire to remain alive had been drained from him. It was as if some malevolent alien had appeared at his bedside while he slept, pried open his skull and sucked out all the vitality from his brain… Form left intact but without the ability to function.

He plodded through his days practicing medicine mechanically because his mind, like a dull scalpel, had become incapable of precision. All his difficult cases he now referred to colleagues. He was tottering on the brink of incompetence and TurnerWest Health Services Group, the company of which he was president and CEO, was suffering as a result.

And so were his children.

The effort of the charade he was putting on for the benefit of the kids was exhausting and yet he knew he had no choice but to continue. No matter how difficult it was for him, for the children it was worse. More than half their lives had vanished with their mother, and now, it was up to him to fill the vacuum, to somehow assuage their emptiness. And he was making a mess of it.

This morning, for example, breakfast had been an empty affair without conversation. Even his instincts were failing him with the children and he no longer knew what to say to them. When ten-year old Michael had been leaving to catch the school bus he had shaken the child's hand while saying goodbye at the door. Seeing the confusion in the boy's eyes at his bizarre behavior, Jason had stood in the doorway staring after him and feeling like a failure. His daughter Caroline had hugged him when he dropped her off at school but he suspected that she was nurturing *him* with the gesture rather than drawing solace from his embrace.

His thoughts had filled the minutes between car and office and he found himself automatically opening the door to his waiting room which was uncharacteristically empty.

He stood numbly on the threshold aware that he was forgetting something substantial but unable to summon up precisely what it was. Just at that moment, his receptionist, a petite attractive blonde who exuded efficiency and was always smiling, came into the room carrying a stack of patient files. He could tell from the look of compassion which flooded into her eyes when she saw him standing silently, that she knew he was confused again. He returned her gaze with a silent appeal for help.

"Dr. Turner", she said, agreeing not to embarrass him, "the meeting with the merger committee this morning is in the doctors' lounge, not here. If you go right down you'll still be on time."

* * *

Jason Turner tented his fingers against his temples and lowered his eyes to the table, pursing his lips. His face was a study in frustration. It had been forty-five minutes of the same old tired invective with no progress.

His partner, Dr. Mark West, was walking up and down the conference room while he spoke. His voice had an evangelical intensity to it and he gestured dramatically like a Baptist pulpit-banger lecturing wayward parishioners.

"Within two years not a single physician in this country will be self-employed. The writing is on the wall. Medicine as a cottage industry is over and if we refuse Cumberland's offer, it'll be the end of TurnerWest."

He stopped talking and was staring at the floor as he paced, as if he were somehow drawing inspiration from the weave of the carpet. Then, raising his eyes, he locked them onto his partner's face.

"Do you realize you're presiding over the destruction of what we've worked so hard to create, Jason?… Are you prepared to sink us on a point of pride?"

Jason felt like crap. The last thing he needed this morning was more of Mark West. He had to force himself to answer.

"It's principle not pride, Mark. My objections to the merger aren't just trivialities I've dreamed up to spoil the deal. It's all about our responsibility to our patients, not what we can get out of a deal with Cumberland.… Haven't you been able to grasp that simple fact yet?"

As soon as he'd spoken, Jason knew he should have just shut up if he wanted the meeting to be over. His pulse was thudding like a jackhammer in his temples and he felt like pounding his forehead on the table just to alter the sensation even momentarily.

"We're in committee here, guys. Let's keep the insults out of it. There are sixteen of us to think about, not just you two."

The voice belonged to Roger Atkins, one of the two other physicians at the committee meeting. The anesthetist was a bear of a man with the top-heavy body of a weight lifter, a square-jawed face with bushy red eyebrows and a bronze beard. He looked like a Viking time-warped into the room in an ill-fitting suit.

Despite his aggressive appearance, Atkins' intense dislike of conflict had led him to a career as an anesthetist where he presided over screens and dials and never had to argue with anyone. In the numerous heated discussions between Jason Turner and Mark West over the takeover bid by Cumberland Healthcare Corporation, he'd played the role of mediator.

"If you've got something new to add, Mark, we're here to listen but no one is going to be stampeded into signing with Cumberland through scare tactics. We know managed care is a fact of life. Our decision is whether to get into bed with Cumberland or wait for a better opportunity."

"In bed is right!"

It was Dr. Cal Mellows speaking. "Cumberland's looking for an easy lay. Their track record shows how they deal with physicians. Anyone who crawls into bed with them is asking to get screwed!"

Mellows was the fourth MD and the only surgeon on the committee. His views were typically surgical. Sharp lines of distinction, no imprecision... cut and discard the devitalized. He supported Turner's resistance to Cumberland's attempt to swallow TurnerWest but he couldn't be counted on to bring logic or compromise to any argument.

West answered. "Cal, the horror stories you've heard can't be confirmed, and, even if some docs have had problems, Cumberland hasn't become the second largest HMO in America by riding roughshod over their physicians. Give them some credit for smarts."

West had no use for Mellows and was attempting to sound reasonable only in order to keep Atkins uncommitted. He would have loved to hack at the surgeon with sarcasm but he held back. He'd known for months now that neither Turner nor Mellows would budge on their positions but Atkins was still a potential ally. If he won him over, the merger committee would be split down the middle.

"You'd sell us all down the river to get into the Cumberland boardroom… You read their best offer… two weeks vacation and we'd need a note from some administrator to go to the bathroom! We'd be lackeys in white coats ordered around by idiots who don't know a stethoscope from a toilet plunger," snapped Mellows.

The surgeon's face was pinched white around his mouth and eyes with emotion. He continued. "We'd get our medical education allowance *only if they approve the courses*… I left that kind of crap back in residency and I'll be damned if I'm going back to it!"

West looked away to hide his disgust. In the past six months, Mellows had become the toilet in his life that wouldn't flush. He'd agreed to allow him a position on the committee at Turner's request and had regretted it everyday since.

Jason, fearing that Mellows might become completely unhinged, interrupted.

"Cal's points about lost autonomy are valid but there's more to it. This is a moral decision that we can't ignore.... Who'll care for the uninsured and the poor?"

"Who cares for them now?" shot back West.

"We've got Medicaid yet for a while. But no one knows what'll happen down the road," Atkins ventured, a conciliatory note evident in his voice.

"C'mon Roger, we *do* know what will happen," said Jason.

" Cumberland has already scooped up Medicaid contracts in ten states and they're salivating over Georgia as we speak."

"And just how is cutting out the fraud and abuse from Medicaid making their management of the program a bad thing?" asked West, still deliberately avoiding eye contact with Mellows who seethed silently at being ignored.

"That's not the point… There's no argument about cleaning up fraud… The problem arises when you put a private bureaucracy in charge of public welfare..."

Jason's head continued to ache. This wrangling was taking its toll on him physically and West's image began to blur in and out of focus in his vision. He knuckled his right eye with the back of his hand and paused.

West was shaking his head.

"So you're telling me Cumberland is less efficient than the government? I don't buy that. They have a bottom line and shareholders they answer to regularly. Government answers to no one.... I'd rather trust the Mafia than the government."

Turner decided his head would never clear and his mouth now felt like it was full of raw dough.

"Dammit, Mark, government has a contract with the people. It's in the constitution. The` *right to life'* means protection from disease and access to medical help when prevention fails. If government were to say to the uninsured: *'You're on your own'*, it would be a violation of a fundamental moral agreement... reneging on a basic promise and.."

West broke in.

"What's this got to do with Cumberland's offer… Get to the point."

Mellows was half out of his chair and looked like he was ready to mix it up physically with West but Turner raised his hand to hold him back.

"The point is that government is bound in its dealings with the public by the constitution. Big business isn't."

He continued.

" If Cumberland, or any other private enterprise entity, refuses *to transact business with someone who can't pay for a service offered in the market place. There is no moral conundrum.* It becomes nothing more than a financial problem that will be solved like every other financial problem in the free enterprise system... You don't get what you can't pay for. When government steps out of the healthcare business, the poor will have no recourse left open to them. Big business will do the dirty work of refusing healthcare... something government can't do morally."

"Don't lose any sleep over it, Jason. The *poor*, as you bleeding hearts love to call them, will always find a way to suck tit on the system. Anyone who wants to work in this country can find a job. People are poor by choice. They're importing Mexicans to Maine to tend chickens because your '*poor folk*' can't stand the smell of real work…. But we're here to decide about Cumberland, not to get into philosophical hand wringing about the welfare system. We need an answer by Friday when Kleinberg gets here. We've got three days and no more!"

West surveyed the faces of the other men. Mellows glared back at him, his eyes hard black marbles. Atkins inhaled deeply and tousled the hair on the back of his head while his breath escaped like a breeze sighing through a knothole but his face was empty and West couldn't read it.

However, something was definitely happening to Turner even as he watched. His partner looked exhausted, almost dazed. Feeling a grin tugging at the corner of his lips, West quickly tightened them into a button to conceal his satisfaction at Turner's obvious plight. If he could just keep the pressure on, Turner would collapse completely and West knew that he could deal with Mellows, one on one, if that happened.

After several moments of taut silence, Turner spoke. His eyes seemed to be focused inward as if he were reading from some stuttering script on a defective teleprompter in his brain.

"I'll put together a position paper. I'll try to sum up what could be agreed to by all of us, by Thursday morning… We'll vote on it Thursday afternoon… We're done here…."

His voice trailed off and he was already to his feet as he finished speaking. He almost staggered as he left the room. A whistling sound, like air rushing through a confined space hummed in his ears and, behind the hiss and the pounding in his temples, he could hear her voice...

"Jason… Jason… "

Annette's voice, his dead wife calling him from beneath the dark waters that had entombed her. His eyes went blank for a moment, then winked back ...full of pain. He made his way along the hallway supporting himself with one hand against the wall while tears rolled silently down his cheeks.

Jason Turner was a bough bent to the point of breaking.

CH003

Five miles into the Georgia mountains past Morganton, the pavement came to an abrupt end and the Mustang bucked as the mesmerizing murmur of tires on asphalt shattered into stone clatter. A sudden impulse to stop, turn and flee rather than go back to the house where she was raised suddenly seized her but Amy had to go on. She needed answers. Desperately.

Without answers to understand herself, she risked blundering through the hereditary underbrush of her life, just like her mother had done before her. If some loathsome chain of abuse had come snaking down to her through generations of her female ancestors and she didn't know why or how to protect herself, she risked being dragged by its damning weight into the fathoms of despair that she sensed lay bottomless below her.

But the search itself wasn't without danger. She had to protect herself not only from her father's violence but from the riot of her own emotions as well. In order to do so, she had decided that she would come searching for her answers like a dispassionate archeologist methodically sifting the debris of the past, probing the sediment of her childhood, seeking clues to explain herself and her genome. At least, that was her plan. But, as she got closer to the house and the memories, the sharpened tip of doubt like a splinter under a nail jabbed menacingly.

Unruly thoughts began to proliferate in her mind like rumors whispered in a crowd.

'He'll be there and he'll kill me... She'll never tell me the truth... I'll learn nothing...'

Amy quickly made the decision to tamp down the menacing emotions her thoughts were spawning. She knew, that left unchecked, her emotions had the power to toss her about like a mouse terrorized by a cat. She had already lived that hellish scenario too often and remembering the experiences galvanized her determination to curtail them.

To escape the automatic train of her ruminations, she opened the car window and began studying the sky and the mountains.

A storm was approaching and the wind that had begun to thrash the foliage on the ridge above the road was laden with the musty scent of summer rain. Thunder grumbled in the next valley and slate-gray clouds churned into sight above the ridge, roiling like mud in the stream water of the sky.

She remembered the suddenness of the mountain thunderstorms of her childhood... Remembered how they used to bunch for the attack behind a forested peak before bounding down the mountainside hurling leaves and pellets of stinging rain. She'd reveled in the freedom she'd discovered confronting their fury. The freedom that came from screaming in chest-rending defiance. From standing in an open field, arms above her head, fists clenched against the potent forces of the storm. Daring the lightning gods to char her into oblivion... into the welcome release of nothingness.

The needle stabs of the driven drops on her face, bare arms and legs, had never exacted any physical concession from her but closed eyelids. She had stood her ground, exhilarated by the liberating intensity of her own screams and the rampaging fury of the storm crashing on the slopes around her patch of valley field, destroying century old trees, yet leaving the child unscathed.

The ultimate triumph of innocence confirmed.

Those times had been moments of pure but essential insanity. They had restored her sense of existence, provided the strength to endure the life of an abused child held prisoner in a hostile world at which she could only look up and out... powerless.

Oh, how she had loved the affirmation of those storms… their promise of survival and escape!

As she mused, the storm struck. Skeletal fingers of lightning slashed greedily at the trees on the ridge so close that a pungent whiff of ozone reached Amy's nostrils at the same moment the crash of thunder caused the Mustang to shudder. Daylight was in full retreat before the forces of the storm. A curling wave of cloud shadow surged across the valley breaking over the road and dragging an undulating curtain of liquid silver behind it.

A few fat sentinel drops struck first and then the sudden din of a million more slamming into the metal and glass of her vehicle obliterated the stone sounds of the road. Before her, the sharp edges and angles of the world distorted, then dissolved into amorphous grayness. She slowed to a stop.

It wouldn't last long but the mental map of the curves of the road had been tucked away in the recesses of her memory too long to be accurately resurrected in an instant. Better to sit the storm out rather than risk sliding off a sodden shoulder into the swollen waters of one of the countless streams with which nature had highlighted each crease in the mountain's flank.

Amy used the humdrumming of the rain and the solace of the storm to marshal her courage. Her right hand, after cutting the ignition, went to the glove compartment and opened it. The .38 caliber Smith and Wesson that Riley Davis had given her lay cold-blue under the pin-spot of the minuscule bulb. It was heavy and familiar and she knew how to use it.

Confidence seemed to leach from the pistol's grip. She passed the gun repeatedly from hand to hand, almost caressing it, and even held it to her cheek while she waited for the rain to pass which it did in only a few minutes.

As the light returned, she could see the storm's leading edge still battering an advance far up the slope of the mountain on the opposite side of the valley. Mist, like smoke rising from a silent battlefield, gathered in silver-gray wreaths under the emerald canopies of nearby oaks. In front of her car, a light rain dimpled the mirror surface of a large puddle reflecting a sky with only a few scudding clouds left to struggle against the returning sunlight. She rolled down the window and drew a deep breath. The air was fresh with the scent of renewal, of leaves and blossoms scrubbed clean by the rain.

She smiled. After all these years, it seemed that the alchemy of the storm still worked for her.

CH004: ALBANY, GEORGIA

The TurnerWest boardroom was an easy marriage of quality and beauty. Conceived in the mind of Dr. Mark West and nourished with the attention to detail that characterized all of his creations, it had been faithfully translated into tangible reality.

The sixteen foot Saaman wood table that dominated the center of the room had been hand-polished with a secret formula of tropical oils that holographed the rich grain of the hardwood above its flawless surface. West had brought two tradesmen from Trinidad to spend a full week assembling it and administering one last secret massage. Either the oils or the wood itself contained aromatic elements that perfumed the room with a delicate scent of fruit-spice exoticism.

Sixteen chairs, with graceful arching backs carved from the hearts of long-dead tropical giants, stood in formal attendance along the sides of the table. High above, gently stirring the air, five antique ceiling fans purloined from Hemingway's Key West retreat turned lazily.

The blond oak flooring, pegged in with hand-fitted dowels, rivaled the luster of the tabletop when it reflected the light from the cathedral windows. The Virginian artisan, who specialized in the restoration of historical buildings, had taken nearly a full month to finish it.

No one entered the boardroom unimpressed and few could withhold their compliments.

Dr. Mark West constantly sought to impress and, from clothes and automobiles to real estate and beautiful women, his taste was impeccable. He was, in that regard, without equal in all of South Georgia where elegance and refinement were the cultural hallmarks of the `Planter' society. This traditional upper class had transitioned itself in the last half century from a dependency upon agribusiness to a heterogeneous domination of all economic pursuits.

As a prominent physician-entrepreneur and master of the family's West Winds plantation, Mark West was the archetypal scion of southern aristocracy and well aware of the fact.

Today, as the four men walked toward the boardroom, Mark West was resplendent in a navy blazer with a gilded crest on the pocket bearing the same 'West Winds' monogram that had been tastefully engraved on the gold buckle of his slim belt. He wore a light blue silk shirt, open at the neck, which transitioned into expensive gray slacks with knife edge creases. A gold Rolex glinted at his left wrist.

In comparison, Jason Turner looked distinctly nondescript.A plain gray sport's jacket with worn suede patches on the elbows clashed with his snap-collar white shirt and French cuffs. His pants were wrinkled and baggy at the knees. Without Annette to coordinate his apparel, he looked as if he dressed in a dark room selecting his clothing at random from a closet. He appeared unconcerned, probably because he was unaware of the impropriety of his appearance.

Milton Kleinberg, the vice president of Cumberland Health Care, was a study in intensity. No more than five foot eight inches tall, he was lithe and compact with the flat-bellied, narrow-waisted body of an aging fitness buff who hadn't yet figured out that the ten years his vigorous exercise added to his life would all be spent jogging. His tanned face was narrow and cheerless with a hyphen of a mouth that had hooked downward at the corners for so long that permanent vertical creases had formed in the skin at the sides of his lips like two negative exclamation marks. Dark, almost black, adversarial eyes that roved in a continual sweeping motion over his surroundings like radar, matched his close-cropped hair that was only flecked with gray despite his age. He wore an expensive silk double-breasted suit cut in a European taper.

Behind the other three men, trailing like a petulant child being compelled to attend some adult function, was Cal Mellows, the surgeon. Perhaps in spiteful symbolism, he was dressed in casual slacks and a golf shirt. Roger Atkins, the fourth member of the TurnerWest merger committee was absent having been taken ill the previous day.

The men paused upon entering the boardroom and Milton Kleinberg, a man not easily moved to compliments, spoke in admiring tones almost as if he'd been cued by West.

"Well, gentlemen, you've been holding out on me... at last, a setting worthy of our discussions. I feel a little ashamed of the venues I chose for our previous meetings."

Mark West beamed and even Jason Turner felt a squirm of satisfaction at one-upping a vice president of the second largest HMO in the nation.

"We're pleased y' all like it, Mistah Kleinberg," said West deliberately affecting a southern drawl, as he imagined his grandfather might have done while entertaining an important Yankee senator.

"We haven't the resources of CHC here at TurnerWest but we do ah best... Please be seated."

Mark West was the public relations face of TurnerWest and he reveled in the role.

Jason Turner, in contrast, was soft-spoken and almost self-effacing in business encounters. More than one executive, meeting them both for the first time, had presumed that Dr. Mark West and not Dr. Jason Turner was the CEO. It was a reasonable mistake to make and one that had often provided Turner with the opportunity to size up a new face while the newcomer pitched his interests to West. In the past twelve years, he and West had made a good team and the growth of TurnerWest had been the natural product of that compatibility.

However, all that was now over.

Kleinberg chose the chair at the head of the table where four places had been set with copies of TurnerWest's four page position paper and notepads. It didn't even occur to the CHC vice-president that there were meetings anywhere over which he shouldn't preside.

Despite the psychological malaise caused by his awareness of his depression, Jason almost smiled at the man's innate arrogance. It reassured him that the battle he'd been locked in with West to stave off CHC's attempts to absorb TurnerWest was worth the high cost of the conflict. '*The CHC board is probably packed with pompous pricks like this guy who assume destiny has conferred upon them the right of hegemony in the healthcare industry,*' he thought.

For Jason, CHC represented all that was wrong with health management organizations. For Mark West, a merger with CHC was his opportunity to accede to godhood.

Kleinberg sat down, and without further preamble beyond, "Ahh, here's the document", began to read.

West and Turner who knew its contents thoroughly were watching intently... Turner watching Kleinberg's face and West watching Turner's.

The fourth member of the group, Cal Mellows, vice president of surgery at TurnerWest, stared out the window at the magnificent June morning and wished he were golfing. In his opinion, a meeting that didn't occur around an anesthetized body was wasted time. It rankled him that the morning of his day off was being sacrificed on the altar of corporate affairs.

The position paper was the end product of a bitter and protracted struggle among the partners and associates of TurnerWest. Over West's vehement objections, it represented Turner's latest attempt to render his little organization unpalatable to the predator HMO by puffing it up like a blowfish with spiny demands that would prove fatal to the takeover proposal. It was designed to stick in the throat of the deal and strangle it.

The strength backing Turner's position of resistance to the merger had been drawn from the innate fear and dislike that most physicians had of HMO's. For them, HMO domination was only marginally better than outright government control of their profession. West had fought an uphill battle, when, at each stage of the conflict, he had opposed Turner's attempts to make physician's rights the centerpiece of their response to CHC's offer.

Both men knew full well that CHC regarded physicians as mere employees, better remunerated and requiring more attention from their handlers, but in essence, no different than secretaries or janitors for that matter. It hadn't been a hard sell for Turner to convince the majority of the sixteen physicians of TurnerWest that failure to obtain wholesale concessions from CHC on all points of objection concerning physicians' autonomy rendered any change in management unacceptable.

West still hoped for further negotiations. For him, merger with Cumberland simply meant that he would be rising to the levels of power for which he'd been born. Cumberland would be his Mazerati out of provincial South Georgia to become a player on the national scene.

In another era, Mark West would have been a city prince in Machiavelli's medieval Italy. He was clever and tenacious with a studied appreciation for intrigue and he knew that, despite present appearances and the unfavorable document on the table, secret machinations still rendered his position tenable.

While the rupture of his longtime friendship with Turner over their disagreements had troubled him initially, he had rapidly moved past regret to less noble sentiments. He smoldered with the indignation of the privileged for whom things had suddenly and uncharacteristically ceased to work out.

For West, all the sharp edges of life had been hammered blunt with the golden mallet of affluence. The waters of opposition had always parted miraculously at his approach. He was unaccustomed to having his aspirations thwarted and, now that his partner had become the infected thorn in his paw, hatred had rooted out the last vestige of friendship from his heart.

For months, West had been focused on winning the struggle. Now that he hadn't succeeded, today's meeting with Kleinberg was a formality, an important formality, but nonetheless a formality. What counted in the long run was how successful he was at consolidating his personal connection with Kleinberg during this visit. If the matter of the merger didn't die today, as Turner intended, time would be on his side.

Studying Turner's face he could see the tint of torment in his eyes. Someone less well acquainted with the man, might have presumed a headache or some other minor distress but Mark West knew the depth to which his wife's death had ravaged Turner's life. He had watched the steep decline in Turner's performance since the funeral and he knew the mental devastation that still lay ahead.

In fact, he was counting on it.

Kleinberg was a quick study and in five minutes had digested the document. When he spoke his face and voice betrayed little emotion.

"Mr. West, Mr. Turner, I'm surprised at the tenor of this reply. If I'm not mistaken, there's more than a hint of animosity in it. Could you enlighten me on what may be written between the lines before we consider its actual contents?"

He leaned back in the chair and crossed his arms, his body language in clear contrast with the apparent sincerity of his offer to listen and attempt to understand.

Mark West began.

"Mr. Kleinberg, I'm sure you realize that TurnerWest has partners and associates with a variety of opinions. It isn't uncommon that we disagree. Even Jason and I, despite our long association and work relationship, often come out on opposite sides of an issue as we have on this one. In my opinion, the paper is a reflection of things as they are at the present moment. If there is a message between the lines I suppose it is that our physicians' concerns about being employees have not been fully alleviated by CHC's proposals to date."

His tone was conciliatory and he had bracketed his remarks with warm smiles.

Beside him, Jason Turner was cursing inwardly, not particularly at what West had said, but rather at his own paralyzing dull-wittedness. His depression was a tangible handicap that hampered his thinking processes like thick gear oil would foul the mechanism of a fine watch. Although he knew his position well, he hesitated to speak fearing that he would literally stumble over his words. It had been happening to him lately. A word like '*salary*', formulated at the cortex, would be delivered as '*celery*' or '*salivary*' at the lips. Appearing as the village idiot, at this point, would play right into West's hands. He'd made sure that Mellows had attended the meeting for just this eventuality.

Cal Mellows was a surgeon, a known quantity. A blunt, confused or rash response in his mouth wouldn't shock Kleinberg like some blooper would if it came from TurnerWest's CEO.

Turner spoke, indicating Cal with a nod of his head.

"Although you've asked for Mark's and my opinion, perhaps Cal has something to add as well. He represents our surgeons."

Mellows had been following the events in the room with the second string of his intellect. His starting line-up had been mentally analyzing bunker shot technique as he stared out the window. He startled almost visibly at Turner's invitation and blurted.

"We don't like it because we'd become peons in an organization that can grind up any single doctor, or for that matter, any group of doctors, who disagree with CHC's policies..." and he broke off without closure to his intonation, like an actor who had suddenly forgotten the rest of his lines.

'*Not bad, Cal*,' thought Jason, '*crude but to the point*.'

He had other more sophisticated and principled objections to offer, if he'd been capable of doing so, but at least Cal's input addressed the most strategically important issue.

Kleinberg continued looking in Mellows's direction as if he expected more but Cal obviously had nothing to add. Perhaps the realization of how he'd said what he had registered in his mind as embarrassment because he blushed deeply suffusing with a crimson glow even the expanse of bare scalp fenced in by his Friar Tuck fringe of graying hair.

After a moment's pause, Kleinberg dismissed him by not commenting on what he'd said and turned slowly back to Turner. Mellows flushed even more violently, the skin of his bald head literally swelling with rage at the obvious put-down. He switched from his golf daydream and began mulling through a fantasy of performing surgery on Kleinberg... perhaps a hemorrhoidectomy... perhaps without anesthesia.

Turner knew he'd have to say something but he was determined to keep it simple and succinct in order to reduce the chance of appearing befuddled.

"Mr. Kleinberg, TurnerWest is flattered by CHC's interest in our little group but as is always the case in the south, newcomers are regarded with suspicion. We've only seen you in action for a little over a year since you purchased PalmGrove hospital. Things change slowly here in Dixie and the message between the lines, in my opinion, is *'we'll keep you in mind'*. But, for now, our decision is firm."

Jason sighed inwardly. He had pulled it off but he hoped for an abrupt end to the meeting. He was feeling suffocated, almost claustrophobic, despite the walls of ceiling- high windows and the significant expanse of the conference room.

A dew of nervous perspiration, which he prayed would pass unnoticed, was condensing on his brow. West was watching him and Jason thought he saw the handsome features of his estranged partner crinkle in an inappropriate half-smile.

Kleinberg scanned all three of the doctors, unfolded his arms and chuffed twice in his throat in the manner of pompous men no longer permitted a herald to announce that they were about to hold forth.

"I see," he said, as he assumed an aggressive posture leaning onto the table.

His hands were clasped in a fist and his forearms outstretched not unlike the battering ram on the prow of a Roman galley.

" We obviously didn't succeed in selling you on our goodwill. I'll accept the blame for that miscalculation. However, there are other more objective realities that I feel compelled to draw to your attention."

He fixed his gaze first on Mellows.

"CHC is here to stay in Albany. We've waded into this market to the tune of twenty-six million dollars with Palm Grove hospital and that's just the beginning. We intend to become a real presence here and, of course, we'll be glad to share our state of the art surgery suites at Palm Grove with all surgeons as long as market realities will permit it."

His words constituted a veiled threat since all neurosurgery was now done at Palm Grove and TurnerWest's two neurosurgeons worked there exclusively. He could have saved his breath as Mellows, still stinging from the earlier snub, just stacked the threat like so much cordwood onto the pyre of anger in his mind. He stared back balefully at Kleinberg. In his mind's eye, he could see the CHC VP's butt cheeks being stretched open by his retractors.

Like a tank turret shifting to a new target, Kleinberg swiveled his arms and face slightly to the left to confront Turner who sat opposite Mellows and beside West.

He continued in measured tones.

"Our insurance subsidiary, CareDixie, is already actively offering a superior product to your area employers. In just over ten months, I've been told that we've acquired over 36,000 covered lives, a substantial base from which to work. To date, during negotiations with employers, we've left local providers in the service loop to care for these patients. But," and he paused for emphasis, "that situation may have to change."

This threat was even blunter than the one delivered to Cal and simply confirmed for Turner that his assessment of CHC as a ruthless raider was exactly on the mark.

Despite his growing distress, which had little to do with the presence of Kleinberg and everything to do with the stirring of an internal chemical enemy moiling away, acquiring a slow but inexorable control over his brain cells, he had to say something.

With effort, he spoke levelly, implying the existence of some undisclosed strategy adequate to meet Kleinberg's aggression.

"If you're suggesting that you'd seduce away our partners or import competitors, Mr. Kleinberg, you need to know that we've considered those possibilities and discussed them frankly".

He struggled to maintain his composure but he could feel the internal pressure building and he needed to escape the confrontation. He didn't have another lunge left in him no matter where the discussion led them.

Kleinberg remained leaning on the table for several moments during which the two men fenced silently with their eyes and then he slowly sat upright unclasping and withdrawing the battering ram.

"Mr. Turner, permit me to suggest that I detect a whiff of paranoia in your comment. Please, let me reassure you. CHC is here to work *with* you, if at all possible. We recognize that your group of physicians represents a rare collection of superior talents. You've acquired the community's confidence and goodwill with your impeccable standards of practice. We could hardly fulfill our mission here without you. That's why I'm here in person to negotiate our differences."

'*Must get out of here*,' thought Turner whose visual field was suddenly being pockmarked with minuscule explosions of light. '*This conversation doesn't matter... I need fresh air or I'm going to lose it.*'

He swallowed twice to moisten his dry mouth, tried to twist his lips inward unobtrusively to moisten them as well and said.

"No doubt you are, sir... but our position is clear and, for the moment, we haven't anything to add to it, so if you'll permit, I must excuse myself."

He bared his teeth in a forced smile as he pushed his chair back and got to his feet. "Mr. West is taking you to lunch at our finest watering hole. I trust your meal will be enjoyable."

Kleinberg watched Turner as he got up while still speaking. Something was very, very wrong. He knew Turner had booked off the rest of the morning to discuss CHC's proposal with him but he sensed that nothing would be gained by resisting his premature departure. Besides, West seemed to be staying put and the surgeon, Mellows, was an inconsequential idiot anyway.

Cal could hear the siren call of the links and hardly believe his good fortune at the abrupt termination of what he had feared would be a marathon session. Continuing to glare aggressively, he was up and giving Kleinberg's hand a perfunctory shake, even before Turner got to the VP.

Kleinberg had noticed Turner surreptitiously wipe his palm against his pant leg as he approached him for the closure handshake. This wasn't the same self-assured entrepreneur he'd met with in Chicago last January. Like all predators, the CHC vice president had a nose for weakness and he was picking up the spoor of Turner's vulnerability as efficiently as a hyena on the blood trail of a wounded antelope.

TurnerWest's physicians did have the Albany community in a love embrace. Kleinberg hadn't exaggerated on that point. What he'd left unspoken, however, was the fact that CareDixie, the newly-formed health insurance arm of CHC that was being aggressively flexed in every market south of Virginia, was lying in their sales pitch. On his authority, they were promising employers that care would continue to be provided through the same physicians the firms now used. This implied that TurnerWest was already a CHC provider. It also meant that today's refusal couldn't end matters.

Either TurnerWest had to come on side or be destroyed and its physicians assimilated. There were no other possibilities. Kleinberg knew it and he suspected that Mark West, who still sat expectantly to his left, knew it too.

Jason finally burst out of the boardroom door brushing past Cal Mellows who seemed to want to spend a moment together cursing Kleinberg. Mumbling an apology about needing to get to a bathroom, he almost sprinted across the hallway to the stairs. Alone in the stairwell, he took the stairs down two at a time. For him to enter the claustrophobic confines of the elevator would have been tantamount to Jonah stepping willingly into the fetid maw of the whale. In his current distress, only a direct unequivocal command from God could have exacted that from him.

He reached the ground floor in less than a minute. Rushing out the side exit with such force that he slammed his shoulder in haste against the door when the release bar didn't click open fast enough, he gulped in mouthfuls of fresh air like a drowning man breaking the surface of a pond.

His heart was fluttering in his chest like a desperate bird trapped behind a window and seemed incapable of supplying adequate blood flow to his brain or muscles. Invisible bands seemed to bind his chest so that his best efforts at breathing were rendered ineffectual. He tried to run but managed only to stagger forward like a drunk as he headed toward the empty picnic tables provided for the TurnerWest staff under the umbrella branches of two nearby pecan trees.

He was shaking both inside and out. His vision alternately accelerated to a blinding white then dwindled to a blue-gray blur as if some evil goblin were holding him by the hair and dunking his face in water and then yanking it out to hold his eyes to the blazing sun. Death *seemed* imminent... but he *knew* it wasn't.

Sequestered deep in his brain in a still functioning nidus of intact neurons, was the doctor's savvy and it was actively diagnosing a panic attack. That same command module gave him permission to stagger toward the tables with the assurance that he *would* survive... and the surprise that he still *wanted* to.

He flopped on his back in the soft grass beside the tables. Above him the leafy canopy of the pecan tree oscillated so wildly that he grasped handfuls of grass to secure himself should the earth suddenly flip over and spill everything off it into the emptiness of space. Perspiration poured off him like fat from a suckling pig on a spit.

Although it was no moment for rational thought, Jason Turner, in the midst of his turmoil, was making decisions.

Secretly, he'd been taking Prozac, the green and white mind-mellowing anti-depressant, but now he suspected that in some quixotic turn of events the drug's side effects may have precipitated the panic attack. Even if he stopped it today, it would remain in his system for eight more weeks.

He had to leave. Flee. Run faster than the madness pursuing him. And he needed to go immediately.

He was rapidly becoming a danger to his patients, a burden to his children and a liability to TurnerWest's management. The sooner he left, the better for all concerned. No one would suspect he was disabled if he took a leave of absence. Annette had died three months ago to the day and he hadn't mourned her publicly yet. Now was the time.

The unconscious concentration on his overall plight had been serendipitously beneficial. While he'd been planning he'd defocused on the effects of the anxiety and, as a result, he could feel its poison draining away from him, perhaps seeping into the earth to drive the worms mad with visions of ten foot tall robins pecking murderously after them.

Even if the cause of the panic's decline was as obscure as its precipitant, he was grateful to see it go.

The treetops slowed their whirling. The viscous oxygen-poor air he had been breathing with so much effort thinned into acceptability. He began to catch his breath again. His heart decrescendoed and gradually became efficient once more. After several minutes, he felt well enough to stand and scan his surroundings to reassure himself that no faces were crowding the windows of his building mocking his temporary madness. He saw no one.

It was decided. He'd scrape his wits together and plan for an early departure to the St. Lucian spa to which he'd directed several of his patients when the tissue of their lives had begun to unravel in the raging winds of depression.

CH005

With the abrupt exit of Turner and Mellows from the conference room, Kleinberg and West were left without an agenda to guide their conversation. Kleinberg spoke first.

"Well, I had anticipated more of a discussion than we had."

It was an invitation that West didn't miss.

"Jason is having a tough time with personal problems right now. He's really not himself."

"So I noticed. He's not very realistic about the options open to TurnerWest," Kleinberg said, carefully searching Mark West's face to gauge the man's sentiments.

"I agree with you and there is no sense pretending that I'm not firmly opposed to the position Jason has ramrodded through our merger committee."

Kleinberg's eyes brightened and he crimped his lips, nodded his head and began to tap the eraser of his pencil on the table rhythmically.

"How much disagreement really exists between you two?" he asked cautiously.

Mark West turned to establish firm eye contact before he spoke. "We're polar opposites on this merger. I couldn't overemphasize the breadth or depth of our disagreement, Mr. Kleinberg."

Kleinberg smiled, "Milton... if you don't mind, I'd prefer less formality. It's Mark isn't it?"

"Yes, it is," said West, returning the smile.

"Well, if we're going to discuss things openly, I'd like to be assured that we're alone," said Kleinberg.

West looked a little puzzled and cast his eyes briefly around the empty conference room.

"I'm referring to any recording devices, Mark. Is it safe to talk in here?"

"Oh, yes... of course," said West mildly embarrassed that he hadn't understood immediately the intent of the question.

"The microphones are controlled from my office," he lied, attempting to repair the damage of appearing less than prudent in the security measures of the conference room.

"The system's off. Jason's a little difficult when it comes to surveillance. He agreed to placing the mikes but he never uses them and so we didn't record today's proceedings."

"I'm not surprised," said the CHC executive. "He's not really aware of what's at stake here, is he?"

"Not at all," replied West before adding hastily, "but I certainly am, Milton."

"*Are you really, Mark*?"

Kleinberg got up from his chair at the head of the table to take the one next to West which he pulled conspiratorially close to West's own chair. He spoke in a lower tone, almost as if he doubted West's reassurance about monitoring devices.

"What do you think CHC is willing to do here in Albany?"

West recognized the question as the trap that it was.

"Well, I assume that when CHC decides on controlling a market, they do it only after research and planning. I'm convinced that you know a lot more about TurnerWest than you pretend. The warning about neurosurgery suites, for example, wouldn't have had any bite at all if you hadn't known that our neurosurgeons had flatly announced to us they wouldn't operate anywhere in town but at the new suites at Palm Grove."

Kleinberg pursed his lips and nodded again. "That's correct Mark... anything more?"

"Is this a test, Milton? Are you probing to see what we know of your methods?"

West's tone of voice was devoid of offense or aggression. He needed Kleinberg to be well disposed toward him.

Kleinberg straightened up a bit in the chair and let a chuckle escape his throat.

"Yes, it is a test of sorts... No sense pretending otherwise. I came here today to get something substantial accomplished. Our formal meeting got us nowhere so, I'm sort of testing the waters with you. I need proof of your collaboration in order to decide to proceed."

"Proof of my collaboration." repeated West slowly. "Well, I hope you don't think me unreasonable if I want to know what Cumberland is prepared to promise me before I provide the proof you're looking for."

Kleinberg chuckled again and actually leaned back in his chair with his arms crossed. "Straight to the point. I like that."

"That's the way I like things, too," replied West.

"I'm not in a position to promise, Mark, but I'll lay out for you our overall strategy for the South and you can see where you might fit in. How's that?" said Kleinberg.

"I'm all ears."

"Albany and area is a key element in our plan to dominate the South. Managed care, in general, has made a lot of mistakes in California and the West and we've made our share of them too. I'm sure you've heard about the doctors' unions we're battling in Arizona. We need an uncontaminated area to try to do things differently."

"And your competitors aren't all here yet, is that the point?" interjected West.

"Exactly," said Kleinberg, "but it won't be long. They're already in Tallahassee and we have a real battle on our hands there and in the rest of Florida. A lot of small hospital systems are very effectively playing us off against each other and that's counter productive."

"How's Albany going to be different?" asked West.

"What we want to do here is solidly nail down the provider network first. In the past, we've used other strategies and, I'll be frank, we've stirred up a storm for ourselves when physicians turned on us after we bought up hospitals. We weren't prepared for what happened."

"Where does TurnerWest fit into that plan?"

Kleinberg moistened his lips with the tip of his tongue and pinched the end of his nose between thumb and forefinger as if he were deciding something before he continued.

"If TurnerWest, or its physicians... because we really don't care if we take TurnerWest whole or dismantle it and assimilate its assets... is secured quickly and efficiently, we intend to establish a new paradigm for HMO-physician relationships. We have some ideas but we're still working on exactly how we'd set it up."

"And my part in all of this?" asked West.

"We need someone on the physician side to orchestrate things. As TurnerWest goes, so go the other physician groups in the region. Believe me, these merger talks are being watched closely by Tifton, Thomasville and Columbus."

"So, I bring TurnerWest on board and what next?"

"You're ambitious, Mark. You talk like the TurnerWest tussle was already a thing of the past," said Kleinberg, raising his eyebrows.

"With respect, Milton, you don't know what I've already done to assure my success. I'm in this for whatever it takes, but it would be easier with your...," he hesitated momentarily, "backing, shall we say?"

"You mean our money?" asked Kleinberg flatly.

"And your manpower," added West. "I need to know how committed CHC is?"

Kleinberg sat back and interlaced his fingers with the index fingers steepling together and setting just under his chin.

West could tell he'd pushed him to the point of commitment and he was deciding which path to chose. Kleinberg seemed to be literally chewing over his options as a small knot of muscle was visible clenching and unclenching at his jaw angle. It was a long minute before he finally spoke and his face had taken on an air of cautious hesitation.

"This is a bit fast, Mark. After all, I really don't know you."

"Nor I you, Milton but what's the old adage... he who hesitates is lost?"

West had already spoken to a dozen CHC people but none with the power of decision Kleinberg possessed. He believed what he had just said.

"We're prepared to bring down manpower if we work with you," said Kleinberg.

"To do what, Milton?" replied West without allowing even a few moments for reflection.

Kleinberg's eyes took on a steely glint. He'd decided.

"Whatever it takes," he said firmly. "Isn't that what you said you'd be doing as well?"

"This won't be any cakewalk. Turner is no pushover. I've been battling him for over a year but we can't dick around with him much longer."

"I guess you need to know this, Mark, so listen carefully. I'll send down my point man. I've used him before. He's a bit eccentric but he's efficient. Work through him as much as possible. You and I will communicate directly only in emergencies... that's best for both of us... deniability."

"And the bottom line for me, Milton? If we succeed, what do I get?"

West was now leaning forward as well.

"You're asking for promises, Mark?"

"Yes, I am," said West flatly.

"VP at CHC for Physician Relations... *senior* VP," said Kleinberg. "I can't promise more than that on my own authority."

West nodded and straightened up in the chair, nodded again and extended his hand.

"It's a deal, Milton, but I need to know one more thing..." and he continued holding Kleinberg's hand so he could better judge the man's reaction to what he was about to ask. He needed to know whether Kleinberg was prepared to do everything that might be necessary.

"What if things get rough, and say... someone dies....?"

He felt the VP's hand become even firmer in his grip.

"We're in the healthcare business, people die everyday, don't they, Mark?"

"Yes, Milton... unfortunately, they do."

CH006

The Mustang was climbing the last grade before the 'homestead' appeared. The rocky slopes of Appalachia absorbed little water and miniature torrents scoured down each side of the road. Small boulders, reluctant refugees from the rockslides which dotted the roadside, were being hustled downhill in sprays of angry red-brown water as the millennial process of the blunting of the mountain peaks continued.

The car's tires crunched and bumped through a temporary stream that had chosen the path of least resistance across the graveled surface of the road, its erosive flow dissolving the hard-packed earth beneath it.

Amy could feel her heart beating faster. She swallowed audibly when she saw the rusty contours of the barn roof appear among the trees. Hunkered on the top of a hill like a wounded bear, the ancient structure's original lines had been warped into tired curves as the stout hewn timbers of its walls sagged forlornly where the stonework had crumbled beneath them.

Brush and bushes rose well above the dilapidated fence of the barnyard testifying that hogs hadn't frequented it for years.

The house itself was set further into the flank of the mountain and was not yet visible except for the occasional silvered glint of weather-worn board that flashed between the pine trunks as she approached the driveway. When she turned off the road its silhouette emerged from the greenery.

The omnipresent Appalachian porch ran the full length of the dwelling, its dilapidated roof teetering on whimsical supports of rotting cedar that threatened imminent collapse. The darkness beneath the warped floor of the porch glared out, undoubtedly hiding the presence of an aged hound too old to rouse itself at the approach of a vehicle. There had always been at least one dog. It was the only thing upon which her mother had insisted.

In the heat of the summer nights when the alcohol raged and the blows fell, Amy had often sought refuge under the porch with the dogs till he passed out and her mother had stopped sobbing. She would then emerge slowly and rinse off the dust of hiding from her knees and arms in the water of the small stream that still ran beside the driveway before she would sneak into the house and her bed.

The windows of two dormers, set like blind eyes in the building's face, had been boarded over giving the impression of the scarred sockets of a medieval torture victim. It was as if the owner of the house had determined that the value of light from without was outweighed by the need to keep the prying world from glimpsing the misshapen soul of the family that dwelt within.

Amy remembered that the ancient tin roof had always leaked, but now whole patches of rusted metal dotted the sloping surface like so many ulcers. Even the metal had been slowly consumed by the same force that eroded the mountains, grinding down the creations of both men and nature.

A gentle rain had begun falling, feeding rivulets of rust-stained water that wavered off the roof's seams and were fractured by gravity into glistening shards that shattered against the ground. '*Even momentary contact with the place contaminates everything pure*,' thought Amy as her Mustang rolled to a stop ten yards from the open door of her childhood home.

Still no dog. She could see no figure strained by the screen of the door either. Nothing but the rain.

She turned off the wipers and watched as raindrop prisms on the windshield slowly disassembled the house and its porch into an impressionist's mosaic. When the weight of the accumulating droplets coalesced until vertical tear streaks altered the view again, she reached for the ignition key and killed the engine.

Her mouth was dry but her palms were wet. Her pulse drummed against her temples, unpleasant echo of her thudding heart. She shouldn't be here. This place was cursed... a lair of evil still capable of swallowing her into its belly, to be trapped again.

She forced herself to draw a deep shuddering breath against the clutch of her fear.

It seemed as if she were suddenly a child again. She half expected to begin to shrink bodily, to drop below the height of the windshield, to find the steering wheel looping above her, her legs too short to touch the floor. Unable to escape.

From the depths of her mind she heard herself... her other self.... ordering her out of the car: *'Don't be a fool... get out and go in... it's only a house. Hell, it isn't even a house anymore... it's a shack... a forlorn, pitiful shack almost in ruins and if he is in there you can deal with him.'*

Her right hand, after cutting the ignition, had automatically gone to the glove compartment and opened it. The .38 caliber Smith and Wesson revolver lay cold blue under the pin spot of the minuscule bulb. It was heavy but familiarly comfortable and she knew how to use it. Confidence seemed to leach from the pistol's grip into her hand and slowly to her heart.

She opened her handbag, dropped the gun in and slipped the strap of the bag over her shoulder. Reaching behind her to the back seat she grasped one strap of the knapsack, her only luggage, and swung it forward beside her.

One more glance at the screen door revealed that no one was there although the inner door stood open behind it.

She scanned the yard craning her neck to the right to verify that no vehicle was tucked in beside the house. He was gone. As she straightened, the handbag bumped comfortingly against her flank. In one movement of resolve she pushed open the door and stepped out then turned to drag the knapsack across the seat and out as well. She thrust her hip against the Mustang's door which thudded shut.

Still no dog.

She was facing east now and off into the distance could see the storm clouds, their bellies still pregnant with rain, bunched against the distant mountain peaks, crouching in preparation for their assault on the next valley. Their billowing rearguard, sprayed by the rays of the westerly sun perched like a red wafer on the opposite rim of the valley, had been bleached of its darkness, alchemized from evil to good by some mysterious force stronger and more powerful than the storm.

"Perspective," she said aloud as if to reassure herself in the midst of reborn doubts.

The rain had transformed the red clay of the yard into a cloying goo that the child in her imagined was conspiring with the evil of the house to grasp her ankles like hardening cement and hold her fast, preventing all escape. She began to survey the area to the right and the left searching for some less intimidating place to cross before she remembered that she had come to face her fears, not avoid them. She stepped defiantly into the muck and strode resolutely to the base of the steps.

The light of the setting sun illuminated the porch highlighting the uneven contours of its well-worn planking. Knots, that had stubbornly resisted the erosive forces which had worn down the wood around them, jutted menacingly above the plane like obstacles planted on beaches to resist invaders. Two windows which flanked the doorway on either side stared balefully onto the porch, their murk successfully resisting the efforts of the sun to dispel the menace of the place. Below one window a single amputated willow branch wilted against the edge of the galvanized bucket in which it sat like some blighted biblical stalk. Undoubtedly plucked to be transplanted, it had died neglected, its leaves now shriveled and brittle.

Amy climbed the steps and abruptly dropped the knapsack in an automatic gesture of hesitation. The house-smell wafting through the screen of the door had stopped her. A potent melange of mildewed neglect and accumulated grime, it caught in her throat like a cocklebur and reminded her how much she didn't belong here anymore.

Odors were powerful stimulants for her compelling memories and emotions that often threatened her self-control. In her apartment in Atlanta she opened the windows even on the coolest winter mornings to exorcise any and all odors. She scrubbed obsessively behind furniture and appliances as if some scent spore from her childhood might have magically found its way into the shadows and germinated there threatening to reproduce one of the smells from her past.

An involuntary tremor of revulsion caused a tightening of her throat muscles. She forced a swallow to reassert control.

The well-worn handle of the screen door gleamed darkly against an even darker swatch of frame stained by skin oil from a thousand palms and a hundred thousand fingers. If she touched it, she would cross her Rubicon, for the door marked the threshold of both the house and her past. She realized with muted foreboding that reentering what had been sealed for so long held the potential for catastrophe.

Her mother was in there. Amy knew it; sensed it just like she was certain a dog was under the porch even though it gave no sign of life to betray its presence.

Her mother's note, scrawled in response to Amy's letter in which she'd explained why she was returning to talk, had been succinct.

'I'll be here when you come... Love, Ma.'

Amy could feel her presence inside the house. Knew she was waiting, watching, studying her daughter through the screen but, like the dog lying in the shadows under the porch, she hadn't moved.

Mary Tyler would be fearing this meeting even more than her estranged child.

'But Amy had requested it. I didn't. If the girl suddenly turned, bolted down the steps and drove off to the silence into which she'd slipped fifteen years ago. Well... I've already learned to live with that loss.'

Her mother's thoughts were being read in Amy's own mind, conjured from the copy of the woman that existed in there... that had been inserted piecemeal and unconsciously by the child over her developmental years. Internalized as all mothers are. Good or bad. Comforting or fearsome.

Amy's gut wrenched and she flinched from the sensation. The skin of her scalp prickled and a chill slithered through her bones. Her vision began to blur and she could feel herself detaching from reality, depersonalizing from the stress of the imminent encounter. Only action could abort the process. She put her hand out and grasped the handle.

The hinges of the door protested with a protracted squeak as it opened. She stepped into the blue-black gloom squinting to focus on the shadowy angles of the furniture inside.

"Ma..?"

A moment's pause.

Then, "I'm here..."

The voice came from deep within the room. Amy focused her efforts to see in that direction and a woman's form began to coalesce from the molecules of darkness like a tele-transported being arriving from the center of another universe. Amy's eyes were adjusting to the penumbra.

Her mother's silhouette was sitting in a tall-backed chair on the far side of the only table in the kitchen. She had been facing the door.

Amy's mind was afrenzy with thoughts and questions she'd rehearsed but nothing coherent enough to be spoken emerged from the hubbub in her brain, and so, she said nothing. Moving cautiously across the room, she placed the knapsack she had retrieved before entering on one chair and felt for the seat of another with her hand.

She could see more clearly now... well enough to detect that her mother's blank gaze continued to focus on the screened rectangle of light at the door even as the woman spoke.

"How are you?"

Blind folks did that sometimes. Stared where a person had been while listening for some clue as to where they might be now before shifting their faces to a new focus of attention.

A sudden pang of guilt... could she be blind? Blind for years and all alone because her only child had burrowed an escape into exile and had never chosen to look back until now?

Speaking softly she said, "Ma, can you see me?"

Without turning her eyes toward Amy, she responded, "Yes."

A flush of relief in Amy's mind was pursued immediately by a surge of irritation at the woman's fathomless indifference to her only daughter's presence.

Amy crimped her lips in frustration. In her opinion, her mother's passive indifference to personal interactions had always been detestable. She realized that indifference may have been the sole defensive strategy in the woman's psychological arsenal but she resented how her mother deployed it with damaging skill.

Attempting to overcome a defense of passive indifference was like flailing vainly at a ghost, doing battle with a shadow, for nothing seemed capable of penetrating... nothing except physical blows like her father delivered as virtually his only interaction with his wife.

Odious as he was, as revolted as she'd been by his brutality, his method of connecting with Mary Tyler made hideous sense to her. After all, here she was, back home for the first time in fifteen years... flesh of the woman's flesh... blood of her blood, and yet her mother stared past her as if she possessed no more substance than a gossamer silhouette. The refusal to fully acknowledge her presence seemed almost like an attack to Amy but she knew she could do nothing against it, and therefore, she chose to ignore it.

"I came to talk, ma, but I'm well. Best I've been, maybe. How are you?"

"Oh, nothin' changes, I reckon." And she continued looking at the door, her eyes unblinking, her face empty.

A non-answer.

'*She was still not engaging*', thought Amy. '*Does she think, perhaps, I'll just get up and leave?*'

She had never understood her mother and the bitter mixture of sadness and anger that had tainted her sentiments for her mother began to well up in her throat. '*I'll ask about him. Maybe that will jolt her into a substantive response.*'

"And Pa, what of him?"

"Him... he's mostly gone."

Amy listened saying nothing for more than a minute, employing silence as a lever to pry more information from her mother's lips but the woman's eyes remained silently locked on the door and she said nothing.

"Dammit, Ma why won't you talk?... Why didn't you ever talk?" she blurted in frustration.

"What fer?" was the flat reply, the woman's face expressionless as she continued to evade the challenge in her daughter's words.

Amy's thoughts were like snapping dogs inside her head. '*What had she expected? Why would anything have changed? She would learn nothing. She was on a fool's errand.*'

Her nose was prickling, a soft stinging prelude to the tears she could feel coming. Rebelling at this unwelcome evidence of her own emotional fragility, she squeezed her thighs tightly with white-knuckled fingers.

Amy pursed her lips into a bud of pensive reflection and dwelt momentarily on her outburst and the ease with which she had abandoned her calm. She found it distressing that she so often failed to control her own behavior more effectively.

Most of the time, Amy believed self-control wasn't just desirable but essential. Passions and strong emotion, however animating they might be, had rarely proven to be trustworthy guides. Almost all her regrets in adult life arose from unguarded moments of intense emotion... but, then again, she never felt so much alive as when she experienced the pounding exhilaration that dropping all restraints allowed.

Today, however, she was convinced that what was needed was caution and restraint. Her mother, like a frightened animal, might retreat into total silence. After all, the woman's whole existence had been a religious devotion to the discipline of non-engagement. Push excessively and she could lose her entirely and learn nothing. She told herself that she *could* deal with her mother dispassionately. As she strategized, she appraised her subject physically.

Mary Tyler had always been a small woman but the distillation of a lifetime of abuse, like some jungle potion, seemed to have shrunk her to the size of a large child.

Amy's chair was positioned so that she could see the woman's premature dowager's hump, the pernicious deformity by which nature literally grinds down the bones of the physically inactive. In her mother's case, a lifetime of staring at floors had accelerated the compression of her vertebrae, so that, at fifty-five, she looked twenty years older. Her hair, never robust, fell in stringy gray meshes upon her thin shoulders and across her face, effectively blocking eye contact with others the way window curtains ward off the intrusive gaze of strangers.

Her eyes themselves were pale gray and furtive; lackluster portals taking everything in but allowing nothing out to connect with others. Beneath them, almost like bruises, were large dark smudges of weariness. Her wizened face was too small for her head. Its features were sharp, rodent-like, with lips too thin to speak with... incapable of kissing. The waxy bleakness of her complexion seemed borrowed from a face in a morgue. A shapeless gray frock hung from her rounded shoulders, her body's form giving no hint of her gender.

All in all, she was a pitiful creature which was exactly the impression Amy had always believed her mother had sought to convey. Compassion was a rare human quality, hence, those whose appearance and manners evoked pity could count on a life virtually devoid of interaction with others. Such a life suited people like Mary Tyler whose ultimate goal was not to be loved... *but to be left alone...*

Amy was, now, resolved to pursue the purpose of her mission. She would begin by ignoring the woman's powerful body language. If necessary, she would proceed as if she were addressing a disembodied spirit called forth by a medium. She needed information and she would obtain it no matter how often a question required repeating. She *would* pierce the carapace of Mary Tyler's passivity by drilling relentlessly with her questions until the knowledge she was seeking seeped out.

"Pa's gone?"

"Yup."

"Where?"

"To town. He spends most of his time thar, now. Bin that-a-way since you left."

"When does he come back?"

A tremor of anxiety shimmered in Amy's voice since she really didn't want to see him… She was afraid of what he might do... of what she might do, if they met. Automatically, her hand closed over the bulge in her handbag grasping to dispel the discomfort that even talking about him summoned forth in her.

"Never know really. Ah jist hears the truck and he's here."

"Does he know I was coming?"

"No."

Amy's hand relaxed its grip on the bag.

"When he comes, ma, does he still beat you?"

"If he's bin into the likker, he do, but he don't drink so much sinct he mashed the truck up and spent two weeks in jail last summa. Ain't got a license no mo' but they'uns in town won't tell the sheriff if'n he only drives the nightime."

"Ma, if they can put him in jail for drunk driving, they can jail him for beating on you, too. Do you know that?"

"Heared that onest." Her tone was still flat and expressionless. Her eyes empty.

"So why don't you call the sheriff?"

"If you think Jeb Stayner's gonna listen to me, gal, you forgit wher' we is." A tinge of bitterness, almost sarcasm, leached from her words, but it gave Amy hope as it was the first sign of *any* emotion.

Amy hesitated persisting with this line of questioning lest her mother, threatened by her own feelings, lapse back into non-communication. However, the reason her mother did nothing to stop the ritualistic persecution by her alcoholic mate was germane to Amy's quest. After all, Amy had lived with an abusive man for twelve years herself.

Until she'd been in therapy with Julie Klein, the feminist counselor who hated all men because one man had abused her, she hadn't known what questions to ask even of herself. Klein had taught her how to hate her father which Amy recognized as a corrosive emotion but it was so much better than fear. Now, the twin sentiments, fear and hate, yoked as a team, had pulled her back into her past to search for answers about herself and her mother... and, more ominously... to face the possibility of a reckoning with him. She decided to resume by following a tangent back to the same theme.

"What was it like while he was in jail?"

"They shut off the electric."

"Did you tell them not to?"

"Didn't know they was up to it. They'uns come to check the bill box, I thought, then they jist up and shet it off."

"What'd you do?"

"Waited till he got out. He gived 'em some money and they'uns come by and put it on agin."

"And you sat in the dark saying nothing?"

The unguarded edge of incredulity in her tone seemed to flick a switch in the old woman who let the question pass unanswered. Amy retreated to a position of flattened affect vowing to screen all inflection from her questions and get to the basics.

"Why did you ever marry him. Ma?"

"Ma daddy tol'me to."

"How old were you?"

"Past thirty, I reckon."

"But, Ma, I was born when you were twenty three."

"Maybe it were sooner. Don't remember much."

"So your daddy chose him for you?"

"Pretty much did... yup."

"Did you ever love him?"

There was a pause before she gave another toneless response despite the apparent deliberation. However, this time her hands moved, clasped first and then clenched. Emotion was there; not yet in the voice, but already in the body.

"Don't reckon I evah did. No."

"Did your daddy want you to marry him for money?"

Her mother laughed suddenly, just a brief bitter chirp of sarcasm, but it startled Amy who had never before seen anything resembling anger in the woman.

"No, Billy Joe Tyler was trash! All them Tyler's is and always was trash. He didn't even own a hound to hunt with."

She had responded with almost palpable disdain, before continuing.

"Mah daddy give him this farm when we was married. 'Twas the only thing he ever owned 'ceptin that truck... He's a sorrowful piece of work Billy Joe Tyler... Jist lookit the farm now."

She was talking almost freely and even if her voice was far from awash in emotion, she seemed to be feeling something. Amy's hopes lifted. Perhaps the shroud of silent passivity would fall and she'd see some element of her mother never before revealed.

"So why do you stay ma? Why did you stay when he beat you so often long ago... You could have gone back to your folks."

"Oh, chil'. Ah already tol you... mah daddy sent me out to him."

Amy sensed there was some enigmatic clue in this answer but it eluded her.

Mary Tyler's hands were now kneading the material of her dress in her lap and one leg jittered in a nervous dance beneath her hands.

Afraid, lest the momentum be lost, Amy pushed again.

"But did your daddy know he was beating on you?"

"Yup."

"And he did nothing?"

"Chil', mah daddy beat on your gramma 'bout worse than Billy Joe evah beat on me... Beat on us young'uns too. What would I evah say to him?" and the woman began to shake her head slowly from side to side.

It was Amy's turn to sit in stunned silence. Her worst fears had been confirmed as another generation's length of the damning chain of domestic violence came sucking out of the muck in which the history of her female ancestors lay buried.

'Her grandmother had been a battered woman as well'.

Amy shuddered involuntarily in her distress. And then it happened. It was as if the mother sensed the daughter's turmoil for the first time and she spoke without a question being asked. This time, Amy clearly heard the emotion in her voice, fleshing out the words, giving them substance. Now, however, her quivering had spread from her leg and her whole body was quaking. She was paying a price in the heavy coin of anxiety even as she spoke.

"Oh chil', yuh need to unnerstan an accept. *You must accept.* Mah daddy drank, too. He loved his shine like his father befo' him. Our blood is cursed from forevah. Only God knows what crime made it so. But it's like that, chil'. Our men drinks an' they beats an' they..."

Her voice cut off abruptly.

Amy had recovered enough to jump on the clue.

"And they what ma, *what*?"

"It's jist that way chil'... an' we cain't nothin' agin it... I cain't no more than yer gramma could... an' you cain't neither... They drinks an' they beats on us an' they pester our young'uns..."

Amy's heart sank. Her mother had known about her father's abuse. She couldn't hold back. She blurted out words bursting with emotion.

"You knew, ma?... You knew what he was doing to me?"

Her mother made no response except to let her head wilt down into her hands. A soft wail pushed its way out through her thin lips. A mournful choked-off sound that crescendoed until it seemed like the moaning of the dammed was rising up through the earth from the depths of purgatory.

Amy was devastated by the loathsome revelation. She sat in silence, her hands clutched against her chest where a grinding pain had arisen like an auger boring into her heart.

The two women seemed to be stranded on a ledge of melting ice overhanging a chasm of bitter memories, from which they both could plunge into the depths of chaos together.

The minutes passed with Amy staring in stunned silence and her mother wailing. Then, Mary Tyler began to rock slowly back and forth, face still buried in her hands. The eerie sound of her mother's despair quavered with her body's motion, unsettling the younger woman even more.

Amy was seized with the impulse to flee from this Dantesque scene, from this house and its palpable aura of evil. Horrified by her mother's travail, she, nonetheless, tried to retain control of her own heaving emotions but could manage only the compromise of paralysis.

Ten more minutes passed before Mary Tyler managed to partially escape her demons. The moaning decrescendoed to a whimper. Her upper body remained folded upon her own lap, face hidden from sight, but she spoke. Her voice was childlike, high in timbre and fragile. She seemed to be speaking, not to Amy but to some unseen listener.

"Ah cain't do this... oh, God! Ah cain't do it... Cain't... Please leave me alone... No more! Please! No more!"

Amy remained paralyzed with indecision, her inner turmoil etched on her features. Her eyes were open wide and staring as if, somehow, clarity of vision could lead to clarity of understanding. Her mother had ceased rocking and wailing but remained with her head buried in her hands.

The younger woman's instincts were pushing her to approach and cradle Mary Tyler's shuddering form in her arms. She wanted to whisper soft reassurances but, in her whole life, she had never hugged her mother and more than a little of her feared being rebuffed. She was surrendering to her impulse to touch the woman's shoulders when she heard it and froze half out of her chair

Tire sounds.

A vehicle splashing through mud and puddles.

Close!

An instant later, she heard the shoulders of the hound bump against the floorboards across the room as he moved out from his hiding place and a muffled howl, like a cry from deep within a tomb, issued from beneath the house.

The dog had been there all along.

CH007

Jason distractedly rolled a piece of scrambled egg across the plate with his fork. He'd eaten only a single mouthful and that, because Caroline had made breakfast for them.

Forced to recognize that he was depressed, Jason still could not accept the loss of physical power and mental competence that were the hallmarks of the disease. It was as if satanic worms had silently mined all the vitality of his brain and heart until he was no more than a husk. A disfiguring slash across the face would have been easier to explain, to accept. But his debility was internal, hidden from observers who didn't look deeply into his eyes.

What would he say to the children? How could he make them understand?

It was Saturday morning and he hadn't slept... again. Over the past months, sleep had been an elusive, faithless companion. Promises whispered to him each dawn were broken each night when it failed to appear. And, when Jason did close his eyes and trade the emptiness of reality for the teeming realm of dreams, he'd been jerked regularly to wakefulness, chased from slumber by nightmares. Heart pounding, sheets wet, throat dry, breath coming in labored gasps, he'd find himself staring frantically at the dream altered shapes of his room. Quavering walls. Distorted furnishings. And then, as he oriented himself, sleep would flee completely. His heart would beat more slowly as sorrow welled up in his wounds and he'd lie numbly on his bed until another dawn shouldered aside the shambling remnants of the night.

He'd become accustomed to functioning without the repose of regular restorative sleep but he paid an awful price.

"Are the eggs too cold, dad? I can nuke them for you... I didn't know they'd get cold while I made the toast," said Caroline apologetically.

It was as if she wanted to shoulder the blame for his lost appetite, to remove a little weight from her struggling father... just enough to see his shoulders rise in relief.

He looked up, and seeing the concern on her face, did his best to smile. "Sweetheart, the eggs are great. Good taste and not cold... It's just that, well... I'm not hungry."

"I'll eat them, dad, if you don't want them. I got soccer this morning and I need the energy." Michael quickly stuffed the last forkful of his own food into his mouth and was pushing his empty plate across to his father's side of the table.

"Mikey, you don't need them. Dad does. He doesn't hardly eat anything and you're already getting a beer belly."

Caroline's tone was mixed, half solicitous wife/mother, half rival sister/older sibling ready to mix it up with her brother... perhaps to distract herself from her father's dour countenance. She grabbed her brother's plate and tugged it toward her.

"Look who's talking Miss chubsey. I don't eat half what you do..." and he pulled back on the plate.

"Hold it. Hold it before you guys break something."

Jason's voice, in transition from morbid introspection to something else, was devoid of anger or irritation. The kids' tiff provided a welcome respite from his somber ponderings and he reached out to grab the plate as well.

The game was on. It had an element of desperation to it as if all three of them had tacitly agreed that the slightest pretext for even forced levity must be seized and exploited in a home from which all laughter had long since disappeared.

Michael had risen from his chair as had his father. He let go of the plate suddenly, which caused Jason to topple toward Caroline across the table. Michael made a grab for his father's eggs with his open hand. Caroline, too, let go of the plate and seized her brother's wrist as he tried to get the handful of egg to his mouth. Both were now laughing.

"You pig"... she giggled. "You'll wear those eggs before I let you eat them." And she threw herself at Michael who sat down suddenly under the force of her rush when the chair caught him behind the knees and they both fell backward to the floor.

Jason dropped the plate which he now held alone and it clattered off the table and disappeared. He scooped up the two slices of ham and what was left of the eggs on Caroline's plate into his hands and knelt beside the struggling children.

"Hey, why don't we all share the food," he shouted and wiped one hand onto his daughter's hair and the other on his son's forehead. They paused in their struggle in surprise.

"You're so gross, dad..."

Caroline was fingering the food caught up in her hair, actually extracting what she could of it, surreptitiously. In an instant, she leapt onto her father pushing him off his knees and onto the rug.

"You need the food not me..." and she smeared egg and grease across his cheek as he raised his arms to cover his head and rolled face down on the floor, hiding and laughing.

"Food fight!" yelled Michael who had picked up two pieces of buttered toast from the table and joined his sister to attack their father.

For a good three minutes they rolled, wrestled and laughed. The kids struggled to force food onto Jason's face while he fought them off by holding their wrists, feigning revulsion when one or the other crumbled toast against his lips or pushed egg into his nostrils.

Shortly thereafter, by unspoken but mutual consent with her father, Caroline relaxed her attack and Jason quickly climbed astride Michael, who, like any ten year old boy, never knew when to quit. If he'd had the choice he would have gotten jam, syrup and anything else he could get off the table to use in the fray but, at this point, his dad had pinned him to the floor on his back.

Caroline laid her face against her father's back, feeling his muscles working against her cheek. Her arms were clasped around his chest relishing the physical connection with a parent once again. She was panting and laughing.

The standoff between Jason and Michael went on for a few more minutes, Jason holding fast to the struggling boy's wrists.

"I'll let you go if you promise it's over..."

"I promise, dad... I promise."

And then, as soon as his hand was freed, Michael would try again to smear food on his father's face.

"Well, I guess we'll just have to stay like this all day, Mikey. I'm not working today so I've got nowhere to go," said Jason, teasing his son.

From behind his ear, almost in a whisper, Caroline said, "I'd like that, dad... just stay like this... all day." And he felt her head snuggle against his neck as her arms tightened ever so slightly around his chest.

Emotion surged into his throat so that he couldn't speak but, in the same moment, welcome relief flooded throughout his body. He let go of Michael's wrists and half-sat up on the boy's legs so he could twist about and take one of his daughter's hands in his own.

The impact of his father's sudden rush of emotion wasn't lost on Michael who stopped struggling and held up a strand of his hair busying himself removing fragments of food while his father and sister shared the serendipitous moment of respite from grief .

The three remained on the floor looking like some comic statue. There was no real movement, but the paralyzing tension which had invested their lives since Annette's death had been shattered for the first time, and now, it lay with the bits of food scattered on the floor around them.

Several minutes passed. The healing and the physical touching pulled them closer, hinting that something truly might be left of the family.

Jason spoke first.

"I need to talk to you guys... something important. Can we do it now?"

Caroline released her grip on his chest. She sensed bad news was coming since there was no more good news in life anymore.

"Can I get a quick shower, dad? Five minutes, no more."

"Sure sweetheart."

He knew she wanted to prolong the good feeling they had discovered by accident in the last ten minutes. She deserved more.

"Take your time. Mikey and I'll wash up too."

"I'm ok," piped up Michael, "I'm just going to soccer. Nobody cares what I look like and I already washed once today."

Duty prodded Jason to oppose his son's suggestion but he didn't want to risk conflict.

"Mikey will let the dog lick him off, Caroline. You and I'll have showers."

"Gross, Mikey... Super gross", she said as she disappeared up the stairs.

* * *

Jason was sitting uncomfortably on the only straight-backed chair in the room. It seemed appropriate for the unwelcome task that lay ahead. He'd been mentally rehearsing his lines for almost ten minutes when his daughter came downstairs her hair wrapped turban-like in a towel and wearing a bathrobe. The skin of her face glowed rose-petal pink where she had scrubbed it. He immediately saw the mother in the child and something in his chest snapped with a stab of pain. Caroline forced a smile not knowing how to interpret the look on her father's face.

"Dad..." she asked quizzically, cocking her head to one side… "You're staring... are you ok?"

He cleared his throat and averted his eyes.

"Not exactly, sweetheart. That's why I need to talk to you kids. Could you get your brother to shut off the cartoons and I'll be right back. I... um... just need a drink of milk."

On his way to the kitchen, he stopped in front of the hallway mirror to study how he could change his expression. He forced himself to smile for the kids, but try as he might, he couldn't do anything with his eyes. They opened directly into his soul and were beyond effective camouflage. He'd just have to avoid eye contact as much as possible.

He opened the fridge door, clicked bottles audibly about and, without drinking anything, screwed up his courage and returned to face his children.

They were sitting side by side, ramrod stiff, on the sofa. Caroline had obviously briefed her younger brother on the solemnity required because his hands were clasped in his lap and his lips were pursed nervously into a button. Four foot five inches of humming apprehension... a taut wire.

Jason sat down on the straight-backed chair and fixed his eyes on a point on the wall just above Caroline's head to which he spoke.

"I guess you kids know that I've been pretty down since Mom died."

He paused but they said nothing.

"Well, these real sad feelings I've been having are supposed to get better as time passes but mine aren't. I'm in what a doctor calls depression. Do either of you know what depression is?"

After a moment's silence Caroline answered.

"I do, dad," but she volunteered no definition of the word.

"Do you know Mikey?" Jason asked.

Hesitantly. "I'm not sure... Maybe it's like so much sadness that your heart breaks."

His brown eyes were brimming but he remained erect and unmoving.

"Yes. Mikey... that's exactly what it's like. And, when you're depressed, you can't think properly either, so I've been making mistakes at work. I'm afraid I might hurt someone and it's not fair to my patients."

"Dad..." it was Michael's voice quavering even with his single spoken word.

He tried again to speak but his lower lip trembled uncontrollably and his own sadness ran in glistening streaks down both cheeks. He tried again.

"Dad... if your heart is attacked by depression and gets broken... does that mean you'll die too?"

Jason rose from the chair and went to the sofa, knelt before his son and took the boy into his arms. He felt the tension melt away as the child's arms closed around his neck with a strength born of desperation and fear. He summoned up a reassuring tone and prayed to God that his voice would not betray him.

"No, Mikey. I'm not going to die and my heart is hurting but not breaking. I'm never going to leave you by dying. That's a promise."

His son's arms tightened even more and the child sighed deeply and whispered, "Good..."

They continued hugging each other and Caroline leaned over and began to run her fingers through her brother's hair to comfort him.

'*So much of her mother in her.*'

After a long minute, Jason cleared his throat and heard his two children attempt to do likewise. He released Michael from the hug but held him at arm's length by the shoulders and repeated.

"I won't die from my sorrow, Mikey," then he added, "but I do need to see a doctor about my depression so I can get well."

"Which doctor, dad?" said Caroline.

Jason turned to face her, let go of Michael's shoulders and took one of each of their hands in his own.

"Not one close by, sweetheart. I've got to go away. If I stay here people will still call on me. You know what it's like. People want their doctor and if he's anywhere around, they'll find him."

"Yes," said Michael brightening at the recollection, "Remember when that man slept in your car all night so you'd have to see him in the morning and then Mom saw him first and thought he was dead… that was funny."

"Yes, it was Mikey, and it shows why I have to go far away to get well."

"When will you go, dad? Will Mrs. Quinteras look after us?"

"No, Caroline. I may be gone a month, perhaps two. I've got to do everything it takes to get well and that's too long for both of you to be with Mrs. Quinteras. Besides, she has her own family to care for. Don't forget she's an old lady. She even looked after me sometimes, when I was your age!"

Michael became suddenly animated and slid forward on the sofa exclaiming, "So we get to go with you!"

"No, Mikey", said Jason somberly. "You can't come with me... I'm going to a hospital and no children are allowed. They don't even let people call us on the phone while we're there, except for emergencies."

"Sounds more like a prison than a hospital," volunteered Caroline, her voice laced with apprehension.

She knew that some decision to which she'd had no input had been made and was about to be announced.

"Then where do we go, dad?" his son's brow was furled in puzzlement.

"I'd like you to go and stay with grandma and grandpa McLean while I'm gone."

Jason paused to let them digest the news, then added.

"What do you think of that as a solution?"

Caroline had begun to fumble with the towel holding her hair and she turned her face away from him. Michael blinked once or twice, then asked excitedly.

"Do we get to stay at the castle?"

"I'm not sure, son. It's summer vacation but grandpa Angus was still in Grosse Pointe when I called him yesterday. He usually goes to the island for most of the summer and he probably will this summer, too."

"Wow! That'd be great, dad," and the child flung his arms around his father's neck again, this time enthusiastically.

Jason touched Caroline's shoulder.

"No comment, sweetheart?"

Her reply was partially muffled by her work with her hair.

"Would it matter if I didn't want to go... if I just wanted to stay here with my friends?"

"Of course it would. Whatever you think matters to me, darling."

At his response, she turned to face him, her tresses falling upon her shoulders as she stopped working with them. She looked into his eyes.

"So I could say no?"

"Yes. I hope you know you could."

"What would you do if I did say no?"

He managed a smile remembering what he'd practiced in front of the mirror. "Well, sweetheart, it would be back to the drawing board and I'd try to figure out something else."

She looked him straight in the eye. He tried in vain to camouflage what he knew she would see there but he couldn't bring himself to turn away from her searching gaze.

She leaned forward suddenly and kissed him on both cheeks, the way she'd seen her mother do so many times in the past, then snuggled her face into the crook of his neck and spoke.

"I want you back un-depressed, daddy, and whatever is necessary, I'll do it. I love you. Do you know that?"

"Me too," chimed in Michael who had slipped down onto his knees to join his father on the floor.

Jason tried to speak but his heart had ballooned up into his throat. He pulled Caroline down to him and all three of them hugged tightly.

CH008: DETROIT, MICHIGAN

Angus and Mary McLean had been devastated by their daughter's death, following as it had the senseless murder of their only son two years before. The doyenne of Grosse Pointe society had collapsed physically following the funeral and had retreated for a month to the sanctuary of a Carmelite convent sequestered in the forests of the upper Michigan peninsula. Like a Greek heroine, her mourning took on mythic proportions that spilled beyond the boundaries of the faith she had inherited from pious ancestors. She was inconsolable and could find no refuge from her agony in contemplation or prayer. In truth, during her retreat, she had railed at the God who had allowed her children to precede her in death.

The old judge, unlike his wife, had fled from his pain not into philosophic turmoil, but into action... bitter, unuttered recriminations and dry-eyed machinations. Before his daughter's body had been laid to rest beside her brother in the family crypt, he had begun to plot for the return of her two children to the influence of the McLean clan. They were his only surviving progeny... his only heirs.

Like a shaft driven by the force of despair, this sudden obsession had been embedded deep within his soul.

Angus McLean loved his grandchildren with a passion that knew no equal in his life except his disdain for their father. Each summer, since his granddaughter Caroline had been five years old, he had left the bench for the full month that their mother Annette had brought them to the granite greathouse on Mackinac island.

As the clan patriarch, he felt it was his duty to instill in them an attachment to their ancestral kin who lay interred in the walls of the small stone chapel that was the exact replica of the chapel standing in the shadows of the McLean greathouse in Glencairn, Scotland. He had assumed his responsibility with a religious zeal.

Each evening at sunset, weather permitting, he would sit on the chapel steps with his arms round their shoulders. Together, they would watch the rays of the setting sun torch the pyre of clouds piled on the horizon into incendiary billows of crimson and orange as the remains of the day were consumed.

Such scenes, he knew, would mark their impressionable young minds forever. The old Scot chose his teaching moments well as he extolled the family legends and the past glories of the McLean's in riveting tales framed indelibly in the children's memories by the splendor of nature. Their roots would be anchored deep in McLean soil even if they didn't bear the revered surname.

He would regret eternally that he had performed the same daily ritual, in years past, only with his son, Colin, and not with his daughter, Annette. Had he tended to her loyalties to the clan as he had done with his beloved son, she could never have eloped with that upstart southerner as she had done, shaming the family in the process. Had he spent the time with her that he had lavished on Colin, she might never have preceded her parents in death to lay stone cold beside her defunct brother. Both his dear children cut short in the flower of youth, ripping the bloom from their parents' lives with their sudden and tragic passing.

He felt cursed, a son laid low by the hand of an unknown assassin in an act of senseless violence and a daughter, running wild without the restraining hand of a powerful husband, recklessly destroyed in a high speed accident.

And now, his dear wife Mary was drifting rudderless toward the shoals of madness… broken on the rack of maternal grief.

As he descended the stairway a half step at a time, concentrating upon a task younger men perform unconsciously, Angus McLean's bent frame seemed bowed under a mountain's load of sadness. His chin had wattled into his neck long ago at about the time his shoulders and chest had begun to slump toward his waist and his belly had assumed a crouching position upon his belt. Hands that shook ever so slightly were blotched with liver spots but still retained thickness and strength. His hair was pure white and remained thick, although his forehead, like a beach at low tide, extended backward beyond its natural bounds. While the features of his face had also surrendered in their struggle with gravity and the weight of the years, his eyes with their ice-blue pupils had not changed since his youth. Because of their electric intensity and his habit of locking gaze with those he encountered, as if he were peering through their eyes and into their souls, he had become know as 'hawkeye' during his years on the bench. It was a designation he had found flattering.

His body lent him the appearance of doddering senescence, a disarming camouflage for a rapier intellect and iron will that remained untouched by the infirmities of his flesh. He had always lived more in his mind than in his body and, therefore, his physical limitations were perceived by him as mere annoyances. Inside, he was vigorously alive... but bitterly wounded by his losses... and outraged at the hand dealt to him by fate.

Crossing the large reception room with its chandeliers, dark paneling and portraits of his parents and grandparents staring down in a timeless vigil from the walls, he searched for Mary.

She had become silent of late. The effervescent hostess, brimming with charm and graceful wit, had cocooned herself in sorrow. In his daily searches, he'd discover her sitting in chairs never meant for sitting, staring at walls or out windows or wandering aimlessly on the sprawling grounds of the mansion that overlooked the blue waters of lake Michigan.

Today, he found her on an antique settee in a hallway opposite a wall of windows, one leg drawn up under the other as she examined her nails. Even in her distraught state, she was always physically impeccable. The hairdresser and manicurist visited every few days and her face was always made up before she appeared in the morning with not a hair out of place.

Mary Mclean was the perfect physical counterpoint to her husband in every regard except her arthritis. Erect and poised, she possessed a regal presence that had always dominated any group she'd frequented and, even now, she looked the part of the heroine in a Nathaniel Hawthorne tale. Her face had been spared the ravages of age and, aided by the complicit dexterity of a plastic surgeon, she appeared at least twenty years younger than she was.

An eternal beauty.

He adored her. Always had. And thus her affliction sat as heavily upon him as it did upon her.

He approached her silently and touched her hair before bending to kiss her forehead.

She looked up at him, her eyes smiling through the sadness that had settled like a permanent veil over them.

"Angus, darling, have you eaten this morning?"

"Roger brought me kippers and hash to my room... Do I look malnourished to you?"

His tendency to overeat had been a subject of gentle jesting between them for decades, so it was quite natural that she should begin their conversation with such a question. Perhaps she would be more lucid today, he silently hoped.

"Oatmeal would have been more suitable… but you know that, don't you?" and her eyes, for just a brief moment, took on the mischievous light they always possessed when she scolded him. Patting the settee beside her, she shifted to make room for him.

She looked better this morning and his heart rose at the prospect that she had perhaps found a pathway back from her despair. He took her hand in his.

"What were you studying so intently, Mary?" he asked as he examined her fingers.

"The rings, Angus. Grandmother's rings. Who will wear them now, when I am gone?" and her voice quavered slightly as she looked down at the diamonds she wore.

His voice was firm and intended to be reassuring enough to banish her apprehension. "Why, Caroline will, of course, Mary. She's next in line and almost as beautiful as you, my love. She'll do them great honor."

He paused then added.

"But you aren't leaving yet, so keep them securely on your lovely fingers," and he raised her hand to his mouth caressing the back of it with his lips.

"Angus, we never know what will happen… I may be gone tomorrow and never see Caroline again." She sighed and looked wistfully out the window at the breeze tossing the tresses of the willows by the lake.

"Well, if you don't die tomorrow morning, you shall see her again because she and Michael will be here tomorrow evening."

She startled at his words and turned to look at him, eyes wide in disbelief.

"Here?... Tomorrow?"

"Yes, darling. *He* called just a few moments ago. He's become ill with some nebulous affliction and will be leaving the country for two months to recuperate. The children will stay with us."

Her face suffused suddenly with delight. She took him by both hands, drew him toward her in an excited embrace and spoke over his shoulder.

"How wonderful... Oh, how wonderful... The dear children with us for two whole months!.. What extraordinary news, Angus, and you state it flatly as if you were announcing that the gardeners planned to spray the back lawn... You naughty fellow, you should have run down the stairs and through the hallway shouting out the good news."

She had pushed back from him and resumed her scolding expression, but her eyes were radiant.

His heart melted within him to see her so animated again. He suspected then that the children might be the key to her re-opening the door on life. "You know that I run nowhere any longer, Mary. I shuffle. And were I to shuffle along our hallways shouting at the top of my lungs, I'd be prepared to sign my own commitment papers."

"Don't be so silly," she scolded and gave him a mock slap on the cheek followed by a kiss.

"I must prepare for the children... so much to do," and she sat upright, straightened her blouse and patted her hair before she arose and left him.

He watched her leave and his throat was thick with emotion, his vision slightly blurred by a tear perching on his lower lid.

'*Her salvation is the children*' he thought, '*and as I love her, I will secure her happiness whatever it takes*'.

CH009

He was here... just outside the house!

With that realization, Amy's pulse rocketed to stroke level and her breathing suddenly became rapid and labored as if the air had somehow become inexplicably viscous, almost impossible to breathe. Her nostrils flared in sympathetic spasm with the muscles of her chest.

She reached for her handbag fumbling in haste to find the revolver.

A truck door slammed and, a moment later, she heard a second howl from the hound, much louder than the first, that transitioned into a low-pitched growl of aggressive menace. A sudden shotgun blast rattled the windows obliterating the growl and sending Amy stumbling against the table. A stab of pain in her side made her grab to see if she'd been shot, but her hand closed on intact flesh.

She pushed off the table, the .38 now in her right hand. Her eyes darted in a split second assessment of the room before she sprang toward an open closet door. The musty spore-sodden odor of ancient cloth and dust enveloped her as she burrowed hurriedly inside. A spider web, like an evil widow's veil, clung to her face and a strand of the repulsive silk fell between her lips. With a quiver of revulsion she spat it out fully expecting to feel the web spinner itself descend on spiny legs from her hair onto the skin of her face. She shook her head violently in an attempt to convince any arachnid hitchhiker that flight into the clothes was the better part of valor.

Squinting out through the crack between door and wall, she had an unobstructed view of the front doorway, a rectangle of fading yellow dusk light sifted by the screen of the exterior door. Her heart began a pounding march up her throat as an adrenaline surge sucked the moisture from her mouth as effectively as the desert sun parches the sands of the Mojave. She could feel her tongue thicken and it seemed that all the purloined moisture was pouring out through her palms where her grip on the Smith & Wesson was becoming disconcertingly clammy.

Footsteps sounded on the stairs. Then silence. A board creaked and a shadow leapt in and then, a moment later, back out of a window.

'*He's trying to see inside...*' she thought with a clarity that she found surprisingly reassuring.

She knew who it was without needing to see him. She could feel the same ice-cold clutch of apprehension she had known as a child hearing him coming up the stairs to her room. But she was no longer a helpless child, and... she had a gun. She hoped she had the courage to kill the prick if it came to that. In her nightmares, she'd felt the kick of the .38 many times as his face had exploded under the impact of her hollow points, only to awaken and know that he still breathed... somewhere... unscathed and unpunished.

As she huddled watching the door, a new rush joined her fear. It was a foreign, yet welcome exhilaration that actually hoped for an attack vicious enough to frame her patricide with legitimacy. Instinctively, she knew she needed only a feeble excuse to avenge her shame and satiate her rage. Despite her earlier apprehension about encountering her father, it now occurred to her that perhaps this moment of ambush and not her need for information had been the unconscious but real motivation behind her quest. Somehow, that explanation seemed more dignified and acceptable than the plight of a battered woman seeking out her battered mother.

If she killed him, Julie Klein would surely approve.

The shadow leapt again into the room smothering the dwindling sunlight on the floor. She could see his silhouette peering through the screen, left hand shadowing his eyes. The ominous thrust of a shotgun, barrel to the floor, hung from his right hand.

'*He's as stupid as he is evil...*' she thought, the sight of him stimulating sufficient disgust to replace her fear in a welcome exchange.

Whatever he could see appeared to satisfy him, because he stepped back from the screen and reached for the handle. He came in with the shotgun at the ready. She could see that he was unsteady and drunk. He stood swaying, his feet planted wide apart and bellowed...

"Who the hell's here, woman?"

Her mother stayed folded double as he swung the gun in a wobbly arc across the room, his eyes searching the murk of every shadow.

"Kilt yer damn dawg, woman, and I'll blow yer guts onter the wall too iff'n I hev to... I said, who the hell's here?"

He pointed the gun toward the closet inside which Amy had dropped to her knees beneath the hanging clothes in a modified shooter's stance, the gun held firmly in both hands before her. She was all but invisible in the twilight leaking in from the doorway and the windows. What little of it penetrated to her hiding place was deflected by the closet door. She wouldn't shoot from that position unless she had to as he was between her and the old woman.

He didn't see her and turned back to his wife still doubled over in her chair. With a broad-based gait to compensate for the alcohol's effect, he tottered toward her.

"Damn yer eyes, woman. Who's here?" he shouted punctuating his demand with a jab of the gun's barrel into the woman's shoulder causing her to rock back and cry out.

"You prick!" muttered Amy almost audibly.

As she stood up, the foul-smelling clothing caught on her hair before sliding down her back but her fear of spiders and Billy Joe Tyler was gone. In its place, hatred and anger infused her muscles with energy, charging them for what she now knew lay ahead.

He raised the barrel to strike at his wife and Mary Tyler cried out in anticipated pain. She lifted her arm to fend off the blow which struck her hand knocking it aside before it landed with a meaty thud on her left shoulder. She cringed with pain but didn't cry out again.

"You bitch! Who's here?" he bellowed as he raised the shotgun again.

Amy was behind him cat-quick and quiet. He remained intent on his beating. With all the force she could muster she brought down the underside of her revolver onto the back of his skull. She felt the jolt of the blow snap her wrist back and the gun skittered sideways striking his shoulder with enough force to turn him, in a half step, to the right.

His shotgun hit the floor and discharged, the blast obliterating his scream. A chair launched itself toward the wall behind the table shattering in mid-air and spewing splinters in a prickly shower under the force of the buckshot. The old woman screamed reducing her face to white eyes and dark throat.

Billy Joe Tyler folded more than he fell, bending sideways with enough instinct left to stretch out an arm toward the floor rushing to meet him. He hit and lay face down, a hand fumbling to locate the spot on the back of his skull from which the lightning had flashed. Groaning, he rolled partially onto his side and his torso heaved convulsively. A harsh protracted retch thickened the air with the acid odor of vomit.

Amy was in transition, a malevolent empowering metamorphosis. Like clay in the hands of some mad deity, she was being molded into a distortion of humanity... capable of violence... capable of murder. She began to tremble, a profound visceral vibration that escalated rapidly recruiting every muscle in her body until she was shaking violently with rage. Flashbacks of childhood horrors perpetrated by the man lying at her feet strobed in her mind's eye with convulsing force.

She spat her words when she spoke.

"You bastard! You stinking lousy bastard!"

She launched a right-legged kick into his belly with sufficient force to flip him onto his back.

His eyes were jammed open in incomprehension and terror. His tongue protruded, bleeding where his teeth had snapped shut on it with the force of the kick. Vomit drooled out of the side of his mouth and hung in gluey slathers on his chin whiskers.

"Amy..." he croaked. "Amy..."

"Yes, Amy, you piece of garbage! Amy the daughter you violated! Amy, the daughter you raped!"

She dropped her knees onto his belly with the full weight of her body and he buckled at the waist under the impact, his knees jerking upwards. The breath exploded out of his mouth and strings of vomit-beaded mucous splattered against Amy's left shoulder and the side of her face. She palmed frantically at her cheek in disgust and swung the gun blindly at his face.

"You son of a bitch..."

When she spoke, her voice was a guttering rasp so deformed that she did not recognize it as her own.

Rage pulsed through her with every hammering heartbeat and her eyes narrowed to slits, the pupils appearing almost elliptical and reptilian. She felt possessed but had no inclination to resist the shadowy control that slid across her will like an eclipse across the face of the moon. She spat into the crimson depth of the ragged gash the revolver's barrel had flayed open in the flesh of his left cheek. She could smell the sour taint of his fear in her nostrils as she straddled him. His arms came up to cover his face as he cried...

"No more! Please no more..."

"You bet no more, you scumbag… No more… No more just like you listened to me and ma!"

She struck him with the gun again, two full force blows, first from the left then back from the right, knocking his arms from his face.

He seemed ridiculously small and impotent lying beneath her quivering in terror. The face which she had remembered as monstrous, oversized and distorted from a child's perspective, now appeared shriveled, almost shrunken. His eyes were rheumy and bloodshot, his skin a jaundiced parchment testifying to the ravages of a life steeped in alcohol. He breathed a mist of vomit, beer and putrefaction. As she jerked her head back involuntarily when the stench hit her nostrils, it struck her that he was already dead, rotting from the liver outwards. A shell of carrion appropriately housing a ghoulish spirit that had gorged itself on the innocence of childhood... without a twinge of regret or remorse. Now, the shadow of the fiend he'd been would have to pay for his sins.

"I came for answers you scumbag and you'll answer or you'll die here in your own puke..."

"Okay... Anything... Okay," he choked.

"Why did you rape me?... I was your own flesh and blood! Your own daughter, you animal..."

He cringed in anticipation of further punishment and blurted out his words in panic. They landed like acid in her ears.

"Not my daughter… not mine… I ain't yer father… ask her!" and one arm sprang out to point towards her mother...

"Ask her! Please ask her… You was in her belly when I got her from her pa… I ain't yer daddy… Never was!"

The impact of the message had the effect of a dose of curare. Amy's hands dropped to her sides and, for almost a minute, she stared blankly not even breathing.

"How could it be..." she stammered aloud finally, "How?... How?"

Then the incestuous logic of it all flashed clearly.

A wave of nausea and horror tapped at the back of her throat. She reeled in stunned disbelief at the conclusion being thrust into her awareness, his confession violating her mind as effectively as he had raped her child's body. When the outrage of denial and revulsion poured over her, her fury returned more strongly than before.

"You lying scum!" she erupted. "I'll blow your lying mouth out of your lying face!"

She began to pummel him viciously with both fists, the gun in one and madness in the other. He screamed without stopping as she ripped again at his arms, with a ferocity he couldn't resist, to get at his face.

His sparse yellowed teeth came into view and she rammed the gun's barrel into his mouth dislodging two of them, a fine arterial spray pulsing onto her fingers.

"I'll shut up your lying once and for all."

Her tone had suddenly become steady and deliberate as she spoke through clenched teeth.

His arms flared up in total surrender and he gurgled an unintelligible protest. She was almost calm as she worked her thumb over the hammer and cocked the revolver.

'I'm going to do it,' she realized. *'I'm going to blow his head off.'*

She heard herself laugh and, for the second time, didn't recognize her own voice.

Her finger was tightening on the trigger when, without warning, she felt arms around her neck pulling her backwards. Her mother's voice was insistent in her ear.

"No chil', not you… it aint fer you to do... git off'n him and give me the gun!"

She recognized her mother's voice but it had no whine to it, no sniveling undertone.

She startled out of her trance and looked to her side where the woman was kneeling. Even in the dimness of the rapidly darkening room she could see that her mother's face had been transformed. Her eyes were alive, intent and piercing. No hair hung across her face obscuring her features.

Mary Tyler's hand slid down her daughter's arm and closed over Amy's hand with a force she'd never felt in her mother before.

"Gimme the gun chil'… now!"

Amy relaxed her grip on the gun and slumped backwards. She watched in mute astonishment as the old woman took the revolver in her hand then raised her skeletal arm and drove the weapon butt first into her husband's forehead with such force that the air escaped his lungs with the prolonged hiss of a slashed tire. His pupils rolled up into his forehead and his body melted beneath her into the flaccidity of unconsciousness..

"Git up chil'..."

It was an order spoken in gentleness. A stranger's words rigid with emotion in her mother's mouth.

The two women rose together slowly and stood facing each other beside the body of their tormentor. Her mother's eyes were limpid, her gaze now connecting and warm. There was a presence, an authenticity to the woman that Amy had never experienced before. Her face, so recently a barren, expressionless mask, now radiated concern and affection. Her arms came up and she pulled her unresisting daughter down to her bent frame...

"Oh chil'… How ah luv ya… Ah've always luvd ya..."

Her voice cracked with emotion.

"Couldn't never tell yuh that… Ah were a wounded animal... bin thet way sinct I were jist a girl... Ah hid wher' ya could never find me… Ah'm so sorry, so sorry… Please chil', forgive me."

Amy was dumbstruck, her throat garroted with the same force of emotion that had unleashed a fountain of tears in her head.

"They'uns wanted me to give ya up to the same rich folks from Atlanta… like they made me do with my first little girl, but ah couldn't, ah wouldn't… so I runned away inside mah head… hid from everyone, everything, but ah got lost, couldn't escape… until now."

"Maw, I have a sister… a sister?"

"Hush! Chil', hush, now," Mary Tyler continued "yuh'll learn it all… I promise, but now ya must leave and nevah return. Ah don't know how longkin ah stay here… but ah gots tings needs tending to thet ah cain't leave undone no mo'and ya gotta leave this place."

Amy's body shook with the force of her wordless sobs. Her mind was spinning. She offered no resistance as her mother picked up her knapsack and handbag and led her by the arm across the room into the evening's cool freshness. Stepping over the hound's blood-soaked carcass, she helped her into the Mustang.

Before she realized it, Amy was seated behind the steering wheel, her knapsack on the seat beside her.

The old woman bent to kiss her cheek then cupped her hands around her daughter's face speaking to her eyes with an intensity that commanded Amy's shattered attention.

"Go now chil'… forgive me… and don't come back no matter what… I need ya to promise me thet."

Her hands tightened and pulled the girl's face closer to her own, her grey eyes bright with electric energy.

"Promise me, chil'… promise me!"

"I promise ma, but..."

The old woman cut her short with a finger laid gently but firmly on her protesting lips..." No buts chil', no buts!... Now go!"

And then she herself was gone and kneeling beside the hound stroking its gory flank.

"Go!" She commanded once more without turning her head to the car.

Amy twisted the key in the ignition and the engine roared into life. Automatically, she switched on the lights which bore a tunnel into the gathering gloom of the night for her to follow.

A moment after she had turned from the yard into the lane way, she heard a shot ring out. Her foot came off the accelerator and the Mustang staggered. She opened the door and leapt from the rolling car to stumble and fall from her forward momentum before she remembered her promise. She got to her feet and stood searching the silence that had swallowed the echo of the shot.

Suddenly, some winged thing began thrashing frantically about in the branches of a nearby tree seeking to flee the commotion.

Her breath was coming in shallow rapid gulps. A twist of evil foreboding knotted her throat and she could feel her terror churning below it trying to force its way out in a scream. She picked her feet up and down rapidly in a jittery dance of anxiety and clenched her fists so tightly that her nails bit into her palms. Part of her wanted to race to her mother's side but a larger part was terrified of learning any more in this day already too full of sordid revelations.

She wanted to scream '*time out*' like in a schoolyard game of tag in which she was being run down without hope of escape. She wanted to stop the world, but she couldn't even control her own body.

Two more shots rang out... four seconds apart.

As if from a distance, she heard someone scream, the sound more animal than human... A ghostly echo rebounding off the mountain carried the sound back to her ear and *this time*, she recognized her own voice.

She spun around as if being pursued by Lucifer himself and half fell, half stumbled into the car. Stomping on the accelerator she spun gravel and mud in twin plumes behind her as the Mustang leapt forward barely negotiating the turn at the end of the lane way before it fishtailed away into the night.

CH010: ST.LUCIA

The BWIA 727 banked easily to the left and tufted green hilltops, as if in response to some magical '*open sesame*', swiveled sideways to reveal a ribbon of asphalt shimmering with the absorbed energy of the tropical sun. Miniature automobiles, like shiny beetles feeding upon an abandoned hoagy sandwich, nudged around an elongated white building that had to be the terminal of Castries International Airport.

In the distance, the sea in deepening hues of blue, stretched placidly to the horizon. Several small motorboats, black specks with white tails, penned a nonsensical message in disappearing script on an azure page.

The pinging signal for seatbelts pulled his attention back to the cabin where a brown-skinned beauty, the exquisite product of the marriage of Africa and India was checking passenger compliance with landing procedures. At the row before his, her radiant smile transformed momentarily into a sultry pout as she waggled her finger in mock admonishment at a male passenger, old enough to be her father, who was delinquent in some detail of his preparation. Jason imagined the fellow beaming in feigned ignorance as she leaned over to buckle him in, her bronze cleavage inviting a wishful glimpse.

On impulse, he decided to fumble helplessly with his own belt in hopes of becoming the transient object of her attention but she was on him too quickly and when she said 'Belt, sir?' he simply held up both ends for inspection like a smitten schoolboy trying to please. His reward was a wink that caused him to blush as if he'd been exposed in a pubescent fantasy peeking at her breasts.

Many women could read men's minds in things sexual but only a rare few were able to do so without intimidation or disgust. Those few understood that most male imaginings were harmless tributes to beauty, more compliment than threat. Occasionally, they might even offer soft encouragement to their admirers, as this flight attendant had done with her wink. She trailed her fingers lightly over his shoulder as she passed and he knew immediately that he would fly BWIA again.

The flight from Miami had been routine. There were only a few passengers, mostly islanders with a smattering of Americans and two Cuban-American couples who had chattered and laughed so loudly that it seemed someone's 'cumpleanos' celebration was being held in the rear of the passenger cabin.

Jason had been assigned a window seat but, after takeoff, he had moved to the aisle seat in an empty row. Opposite him across the aisle, another American woman had done the same.

Jason normally read fiction while flying, but reading while depressed was as discouraging as swimming against a brisk current, and so he had stuffed his novel into the elasticized pocket in the seatback before him and willed himself to slide into the nether world of daydreams. After ten minutes, however, he was still preoccupied with thoughts of the children and affairs at work. He made a determined effort to meditate, closing his eyes and emptying his mind by focusing on the mental image of a tree with branches stretching to the sky and roots probing serenely into the nurturing earth. But birds intruded, perching on the branches distractingly, and earthworms mined noisily through the earth with sucking, slithering sounds as they churned soil into humus. He abandoned the attempt.

His gaze strayed to the young woman across the aisle from him. She seemed engrossed in a paperback. He'd studied her surreptitiously several times during the flight and decided she wasn't a tourist.

She wore a tasteful two piece suit of light tropical material that she had left unbuttoned at the neck just far enough to hint at the rise of her breasts. Her waist was trim and, from the definition of the muscles in her calves and the line of her thighs under the short skirt, he guessed she had power-stepped her way to the upper end of the fitness curve.

In profile, her face was sketched in easy graceful curves that nature had benevolently proportioned between brow, nose, mouth and chin. Thick luxuriant hair fountained up against the seat and tumbled onto her shoulders in nonchalant disarray. Its color was a struggle between red and blonde, slightly darker than the burnt honey hue of her cheek. The one hand he could see had tastefully long well-manicured nails with conservative polish.

He had begun looking at her as an incidental activity but, as his appraisal continued, he became curious about why she was traveling to St. Lucia. She wasn't dressed like a tourist visiting an exotic island. In fact, despite the plane's bumpy maneuvering for the imminent landing, she hadn't even looked up from her book. She seemed to be passing time and not much interested in her surroundings or her destination.

Jason had always appreciated female beauty. In marrying Annette he had pursued and won such beauty and now, as he studied the woman across from him, he experienced surge of guilt realizing how much she reminded him of his dead wife. His guilt was linked to some amorphous sexual stirrings that his ever vigilant superego was condemning as inappropriate so soon after Annette's death. And yet, he was pleased that he could feel aroused. It was so much closer to life than remaining mired in the morbid sentiments of the past several months. Those somber emotions, like grim faced pall-bearers, had ferried him down to the depths of depression from which he was now actively seeking to escape.

The engine noise lulled momentarily as the plane seemed to float for two or three seconds and then thumped heavily, twice in rapid succession, onto the runway. The jolt of the landing caused the luggage in the overhead bins to rattle. Startled passengers chirped in alarm and one of the Cubans in the rear swore loudly in tainted English. A hum of nervous excitement and relief arose among the passengers. The flight attendants were up almost immediately flashing company-issued smiles down the aisle in efficient reassurance.

The cockpit voice announced in a lazy southern drawl, "Ladies and Gentlemen we just *hit* Castries, St. Lucia… I apologize for the landing and assure you that we aren't asleep up here…"

A nervous twitter, punctuated by a few laughs, rippled through the ranks and the Cuban, obviously not mollified by the apology, swore again, this time expansively and in Spanish.

Jason glanced over at the woman across the aisle. She was donning a pair of sunglasses and appeared unconcerned by events. He found her composure in the midst of the anxious effervescence, intriguing.

Debarcation was uncomplicated as only a dozen or so passengers had chosen Castries as a final destination. The woman from across the aisle preceded him as the plane emptied and he lagged several steps behind her, experiencing a mixture of guilt and voyeuristic titillation as he watched the enchanting twitch of her hips moving under the thin cloth of her skirt.

When he stepped through the exit from the plane onto the stairs, a wallop of tropical heat and fragrance buffeted him, stimulating a quiet flutter of excitement in his chest. He had visited the islands of the Caribbean often and always experienced an invigorating surge of anticipation upon arriving, as if the plane had carried him not simply over distance but also across the intangible frontier of another dimension. For him, the exotic ambiance of the tropics had always been kinder and more forgiving than the exacting reality of his life elsewhere. Despite his depression, he experienced a welcome fizz of energy. He almost smiled.

Inside the terminal, his passage through immigration and customs had been facilitated by the ten dollar bill, folded behind his tourist card, that he had passed to the inspectors. He smiled as he walked past his fellow passengers whose bags and passports were being ravished by frustrated custom's agents unlucky enough to have clients, who either ignored the unofficial practice of petty bribery, or who were returning locals laden down with foreign purchases.

A small hair dryer slipped from the grasp of an inspector onto a metal-covered custom's bench. With the spring of something animate, it popped into the air and landed on the cement floor just ahead of him with a snap of ruptured plastic. The apparent owner, an enormously obese black woman with the face of a manatee, clasped her hands to her temples and began to wail as loudly as if an infant's skull had just been shattered upon the concrete. Jason stepped over the fractured treasure and made his way toward the crush of porters and taxi drivers jamming the exit from the terminal.

He permitted his bags to be snatched from his grasp by an energetic teenager who tried to capture his document case as well.

"I'll keep this. Take the bags to a clean taxi," Jason said authoritatively.

"Yes sir... This way. Please follow me."

And the fellow waded into the wedge of humanity behind him shouldering open a brief passage for his white patron that was slammed shut with black bodies as soon as the American had passed.

Jason had learned long ago that resisting the horde of porters at third world airports was an exercise in futility, so he always passed his bags to the first one who appeared strong enough to carry them and still fray a passage through the melee. It was the only effective solution. Much like the bribes.

As he stooped to slide into the back seat of a red Corolla, Jason caught a glimpse of a white woman standing next to the taxi behind his. She was in the periphery of his vision, that distorted half-conscious zone of perception where the inanimate stirs and a shadow becomes a person to either startle or soothe. His heart leapt instinctively and his breath caught in his throat. He swung to focus fully upon her but saw only a leg and a flash of tawny hair as she disappeared into the vehicle.

His reaction startled him, for it had been weeks now since he had glimpsed his dearest Annette in a crowd, or walking across a park, or sitting in a dimly-lit theater as if she were unaware of his presence. A ghost. A spiritual echo clothed in flesh, but always elusive. And now, here she was again... behind him... perhaps watching him this time.

Turning to peer through the rear window, he knew he would see her only indistinctly. He resisted the mad impulse to leap from the cab and rush back to pull open her vehicle's door. He'd already succumbed too often to that futile temptation in the past, for each time he'd pursued her, she'd metamorphosed into someone else and he'd felt foolish and dejected.

With deliberate effort, he turned his head away from her shade sitting in the other cab. When he did, he saw the driver of his cab and the teenaged porter on the sidewalk haggling over the five dollar bill he'd passed to the boy. Feeling suddenly irritated, he rolled down the window and barked at the driver.

"There'll be no tip if you don't get us moving."

The driver was galvanized into action by the threat and soon they were hustling through the traffic around the airport and on the way into Castries.

"To dee Holiday Inn, sir?" queried the driver, his disembodied eyes staring from the glint of the rearview mirror.

"No. I'm going to the Renaissance Center."

He saw the mirror's eyes widen, then immediately squint, as if to study him better.

"To dee 'head hospital'?... Dat's what we calls it here."

Jason ignored the cheeky interrogation and replied flatly.

"To the Renaissance Center without conversation or comment... You know where it is?"

"Yessir.... Ah do."

As the taxi sped along, Jason stared absently out the window while lush greenery, punctuated by occasional dashes of cleared land, flowed past. The image of his own face flashed faintly on the glass with each pulse of verdant background. His eyes were solemn. He was remembering the copper-haired woman.

His thoughts sidled uneasily closer to his memories of Annette. Knowing in advance the gentle aching pain and longing he would experience, he rubbed his brow in an ambivalent effort to erase the image of her face which was already insinuating itself into his awareness. But it wasn't really a conscious choice. Annette came because she chose to come. Because more than a little of him wished her to. Wanted her. Still needed her.

He saw her tawney hair lit with golden highlights, tumbling onto her shoulders. Her eyes, bright as blue silk and sparkling with the impish pleasure she took in teasing him. Lashes that flared like doves wings lifting into the morning light. Generous lips drawn back in an open-mouthed smile at his perplexity. Her smile had never failed to raise his spirits, to dilute his sadness, to cause his heart to swell with elation at the realization that this extraordinary woman belonged to him and, he to her.

Annette had been his greatest admirer. Had always seen him as being more than he knew he was. She had loved him without restraint. Unconditionally. In her devotion, she had given him what his whole life, until her arrival, had been unable to provide. A sense of belonging. Fulfillment.

His wife had seen the world and life uniquely. Armed with a liberating awareness of her own insignificance in the grand scheme of the universe, she had neither feared death, nor believed it was the worst thing that could befall her. Thus, freed from the common angst, she had dared to test the limits of experience. She had inhaled sensation like other mortals breathed air. She had taught him that life was meant to be a dynamic adventure, full of risk and exhilarating rewards, and not the tedious passage he had come to accept as his lot. She had, with her presence, filled the numerous voids that had pockmarked his life. Living with her, drawn into her existence, he had become alive for the first time since the death of his mother.

Lying with her after lovemaking, his ear pressed to her breast and soothed by the steady rhythm of her heart as she caressed his hair, he had discovered a shared oneness; escaped solitude; found solace.

She had become the center *and* the circumference of his life.

And now, she was gone.

Jason felt palpable despair clutch at his heart and marveled at how quickly the superficial exultation he had experienced upon arrival had dissipated. Would he ever love again? Could the void Annette's death had excavated in his existence ever be filled? Would he ever regain the freedom from fear and despair that she had shown him?

Full of tears he could not give himself permission to shed, he ached to the very marrow of his soul.

"We's here, sir."

The voice of the cabby intruded obliquely into his awareness, as if it emanated from a vent connected to another existence. Jason stirred himself and noticed that they had stopped in the palm-shadowed yard of an imposing villa.

A young East Indian man, in white shirt and shorts, had emerged from an archway constructed of salmon-tinted coral blocks and was proceeding with militaristic intensity toward the car. He snapped open the car door holding on to it as if it were one jaw of a trap set to snap shut with bone-rending force should he falter in restraining it. Jason paid the fare and stepped into the brilliant sunshine of the courtyard.

"I'll fetch your bags, sir", volunteered the young man as he shut the door and sprang to the Corolla's trunk with energy Jason couldn't remember seeing before in the tropics.

Shading his eyes against the glare, Jason surveyed his surroundings. Magnificent royal palms, like palace guards, stood at rigid attention around a cobblestone courtyard. A blush of brilliant bougainvillea bushes burst from the earth on both sides of the archway leading to the villa in a twin splay of color and fragrance. In the distance, he could hear what sounded like a dozen parakeets squabbling over fruit in the canopies of several mango trees that dotted the green carpet of manicured lawn. A yellow brick pathway led through the archway and up several steps to two massive mahogany doors hung on black iron hinges as long and thick as a man's arm.

'A trip to Oz', thought Jason, wryly... amazed again at the hairpin turn his emotions had just negotiated. Being able to joke, if only with himself, after the emotional tumult he'd experienced in the cab just minutes ago, seemed quite incredible. His moods were pitching and yawing like a cheap carnival ride.

"Depression," he mused aloud flatly in an undertone.

"I'm sorry, sir?" It was the young man with his bags.

"Oh, nothing... Just talking to myself," said Jason and then realized how incriminating such an admission could be in a mental health facility.

"Of course, sir. Very healthy, sir. Dr. Landry always says, 'Internal discourse clarifies our conflicts."

Jason glanced in surprise at the youth who apparently listened at keyholes with the curiosity of an aspiring therapist.

"Do you talk with yourself often?" he asked with a grin.

The young man turned to look at him. An ebony face glistening with perspiration was surmounted by two huge white eyes that fairly jutted from his features, as if he suffered from an overactive thyroid. He spoke with the forced sincerity of an underling seeking to please or to avoid blame.

"Oh, no sir, I'm not that advanced yet, but I hope to be able to do so with great purpose, one day."

Jason widened his grin and said nothing more.

"Please sir, watch your step sir. These stairs are deceptive," his guide said, nimbly scampering up the three yellow steps sideways, with the two suitcases swinging as he went.

Jason concluded that the Renaissance Center's astronomical rates guaranteed that most of the clientele were geriatric, if these three simple steps truly posed a hazard. He took them in a single hop, then bowed for the approval of his guide.

"Very nicely done, sir. I can see that you are very athletic… You must surely play tennis."

"I do… badly, I admit, but I do..."

Jason could feel his mood lifting perceptibly as he bantered with the youth.

They were at the doors and Jason pulled on a huge wrought-iron ring before the young man could set down the cases and reach it. When he opened the door for them, he saw genuine consternation in the fellow's ample eyes. Obviously, he was comfortable only when everyone remained strictly within their appointed roles.

"I shall follow you in, sir. That would be proper, sir, if you will permit it."

Jason shrugged and stepped into an icy thermoclime obviously maintained by air-conditioning despite the ceiling fans turning lazily above the large reception area.

The yellow brick of the 'Oz' walkway had given way to rough-cast Mexican-style tiles, of the same hue, that glistened in the light spilling into the room through ceiling-high windows that composed the complete right wall of the room. Rattan furniture, upholstered with button-studded green pillows, was scattered about the room.

Incongruously, like a diamond lying amidst paste jewelry, a mat-black grand piano dominated the center of the room and Jason's eyes instinctively lingered on its elegant lines. His fingers hadn't touched a keyboard in years and he experienced a pulse of yearning that he quickly dismissed.

Four large round pillars of the salmon-colored coral rose to buttress a ceiling laid on rough-hewn beams that spanned the considerable expanse of the room. They appeared to be centuries old and hinted at a more luxurious past for the villa. Jason could imagine a colonial governor's retinue, in starched linen and button-festooned livery, scurrying about busily in preparation for a gala reception.

In reality, only one young black woman with a multi-colored scarf knotted about her head was present. She was cleaning the already invisible glass of a set of French doors which led through the wall of windows to a broad coral block balcony, overlooking the sea.

"Sir, we can proceed directly to your quarters, if you wish. Dr. Landry counsels all afternoon in private sessions and will meet you in the evening for dinner."

"As you wish... Do you have a name? I'm Jason Turner."

"Oh, yes sir, indeed sir, I do have a name. It is Mohammed, sir... and I am totally disposed to your service, Mr. Turner, sir."

"And very ably Mohammed, it's a pleasure to meet you."

"And I, most likewise, sir," replied Mohammed, bobbing his head deferentially and gesturing, at the same time, to a corridor which led off the room to the right. "This way, please."

They followed the corridor, for only a moment, before they passed through glass doors and emerged in a covered walkway open to the sea on the south and separated from what seemed to be a garden, on the other side, by a wall of red round hollow tiles through which the fragrance of tropical blooms drifted pleasantly.

Below them, some fifty yards away, stretched a black sand beach and a turquoise expanse of empty sea. The beach was hemmed by several huge flamboyant trees on the extreme right. Far to the left, an expanse of black volcanic rock, with the texture of petrified sponge, rose from the sea to form low cliffs approximately a quarter mile off at the other edge of a small bay.

Two black men, barefoot and clad only in shorts, were sweeping the sand around a number of unoccupied beach chairs on the nearest stretch of beach using large palm-whisk brooms with crooked, knotted handles polished with sweat. They chattered quietly as they worked.

Below the balcony to his left, he could see an open-air dining area with several round tables, bare now except for large crystal bowls in their centers that were filled with floating hibiscus blooms. There was a peaceful, almost deserted quality to the place, and Jason's first impression was favorable. There was solace in solitude, when anxiety could be excluded.

Mohammed had come to a set of stairs leading down to yet another yellow-brick pathway that disappeared under the shadows of palms and overarching flamboyants. An olive-hued lizard, larger than a cat, waddled across the pathway, paused to study them for a moment with a pair of dysconjugate googly eyes, then disappeared unhurriedly under the leaves of a low slung palmetto.

"That's Horace. He's Dr. Landry's iguana. He tolerates the rest of us, sir, but he will only eat from Dr. Landry's fingers."

"Fine, by me," ventured Jason who had no natural affection for any reptiles larger than one of his fingers.

As they passed under the first flamboyant, Jason could see five small thatched cabins constructed of the same coral blocks as the villa. Each was situated at the end of narrow yellow brick paths which spread out from the main walkway like the spidery fingers of a giant hand. The cabins were set at angles that provided a view of the bay, yet preserved the privacy of small balconies set just a few feet off the ground, at the sea face of each building. Hedges of hibiscus and crotons ran between them and hanging baskets of orchids marked their doorways .

"Your cabin is at the far end sir, just as you specified," said Mohammed beaming and showing a set of crooked teeth that seemed to be competing for position in his mouth like spectators on a Mardi-Gras balcony.

The youth had obviously learned that if nature hadn't favored you with good looks, and Mohammed's face was clearly a biological mishap, you had to compensate with an aggressive willingness to please, if you sought acceptance in life.

"I take the reservations personally and I remember that you had said 'I would prefer privacy over luxury, if that becomes a choice,' and so, I chose this cabin for you, Mr. Jason Turner, sir... I'm hoping that it will be pleasing to you in all regards."

Jason liked the lilt of East Indian English almost as much as he enjoyed the Scottish renditions of the same tongue. Mohammed's presence here on a West Indian island was a pleasant surprise.

"Mohammed," he replied, imitating the fellow's overuse of names and stilted formality in conversation, "I'm certain that I shall find it pleasing in all regards and I congratulate you on your excellent memory and your diligence in heeding my request..."

The boy's face was almost bisected by an even broader grin that exposed more crowded teeth. He bobbed his head again in pleasure and Jason found himself bobbing his own head, in reply.

The cabin's interior was simple with bare coral walls, more rattan furniture, a television hung from a fixture high up in a corner, and a couple of woven sisal throw rugs on the tile floor. It had indeed been a real choice between luxury or privacy.

A large bathroom was furbished with a jetted Jacuzzi tub, an expensive pink toilet with a side flush action, and a spacious sink of the same color with gold faucets. The bathroom's ostentatious furnishings clashed with the simplicity of the rest of the living quarters and Jason wondered how much time Dr. Landry spent in the bathroom.

Mohamed fussed about, opening closets and even drawers in his enthusiasm to please.

"It's lovely, Mohammed and I'm very satisfied."

"Do look at the sea, sir. Notice how close it is. You can hear all of the waves easily. Awakening here each morning, sir, will be pleasurable for you, I am certain."

Jason stepped to the little balcony and looked out. Indeed, the quiet lapping of small waves could be heard clearly and, from the balcony, all other buildings were hidden from view by foliage. He could pretend he was on a desert island, if he chose to do so.

Together, they admired the view in approving silence, for a few moments.

"I must go now, Mr. Jason Turner, sir, for I am also responsible for your meals and I need to supervise the cooks."

Then, touching Jason's arm in a gesture of familiarity that was probably uncommon for the man, he added.

"These West Indians do not work well without supervision... They can be slow and careless, too, at times... I am often experiencing much frustration with them, but Dr. Landry and my dear mother trust me, and so, I am alright with it all."

"You seem to have numerous duties Mohammed... How did you get this job?"

"Two years ago my mother invested and became the partner of Dr. Landry. My family used to own a hotel in Karachi but, when my father was killed by Musharif's rascals, we came here, sir. No one troubles us here and life is good. I am happy to be a part of Dr. Landry's clinic and someday I have the hope of going to university to become a psychiatrist. Many of my countrymen are psychiatrists in the United States of America, sir."

"Yes, I have noticed that," said Jason. "Sometimes, I wonder who's left to do psychiatry in your own country."

"Oh, we do not have much need for psychiatry, sir. Our lives are in many ways simpler than those of Americans. I have noticed, that as a people, you seem to be bothered by many things that you cannot change. We do not concern ourselves about such matters. We expect life to be somewhat difficult and accepting that fact makes it easier for us..."

He was speaking so sincerely, and with such lack of guile, that Jason couldn't hold back a smile.

"Am I amusing you, sir?" said Mohammed with a look of perplexed concern on his face.

"No, Mohammed... not amusing me... I am smiling because what you say makes a lot of sense. You may be more of a therapist than you suspect."

"Oh, you are most kind, Mr. Jason Turner, sir." And if a blush could have been seen on his dark features, Jason felt that it would have been profuse.

"I will be leaving you, now until dinnertime."

Jason riffled through the contents of his pocket for a bill as a tip, but he saw the youth's face cloud over.

"Mr. Jason Turner, sir, I do not need money from you, sir. This is my mother's establishment and I am here to serve you as a host, if you please."

It was Jason's turn to blush slightly.

"I apologize, Mohammed, I didn't understand... I meant no offense..."

"No offense was taken, Mr. Jason Turner."

Mohammed smiled, bowed his head again and took Jason's proffered hand in both of his.

"I will see you at dinner."

And he was gone.

CH011

Her first night in St. Lucia, Amy had been serenaded into restorative slumber by the chorus of chirping tree frogs but, tonight, she lay on her bed oblivious to the nocturnal trilling that wafted in through the slatted shutters. Sleep had ignored even her most desperate entreaties, floating like a phantom just out of reach. Although her body was numb with fatigue from a long afternoon walk in the hills and her eyelids leaden, anxious thoughts animated by the menacing prospect of tomorrow's group therapy session bounced along the ceiling of her mind like frenzied mosquitoes.

Amy Davis, first and foremost, was self-contained. Like a sealed amphora, her mind was a sanctum closed to others... the only inviolate place in her existence. During months of counseling, her therapist, Julie Klein, had probed for access and been rewarded with no more than a shadow play on the therapeutic screen.

Amy had never permitted anyone to glimpse more than the reflection of her deepest thoughts. Yet, in ten hours, she would be expected to participate, as a group member, in the cathartic release of pent-up fears and emotions... expected to lay out the secret stuff of her life for the appraisal of strangers. The prospect filled her with palpable terror and seemed as inviting as submitting to the gang rape of her mind. For her, privacy was not optional, but an absolute necessity.

Through the years, she had become adept at providing a convincing appearance of genuine participation in the lives of others... so expert, in fact, that no one had ever challenged her pretense, until Riley Davis had done so recently. He was the only one to have guessed, that in many of her dealings with others, the real Amy Davis, like the wizard of Oz behind the screen, merely projected a persona to interact with them while she remained safely hidden. For her, dissimulation when under pressure, had become the mainstay of her strategy for emotional survival. The possibility of her façade being breached, however theoretically beneficial the process might be deemed to be from a therapeutic viewpoint, was absolutely unacceptable.

When Dr. Landry had mentioned the group session, her heart had been momentarily flash-frozen by a burst of fear, then leapt in bounding escape into her throat with such force that she had literally coughed several times from the sensation produced. Although Landry had said nothing about revealing private personal information, she suspected that such disclosure was the covert purpose of the exercise. And, while her intellect could appreciate the logic, her emotions could not accept it.

It was dawning upon her that she may have made a grave miscalculation in choosing the clinic. Her presumption had been that therapy at Renaissance would be solely individual and conform to the cognitive-behavioral model that she knew dominated the field of psychotherapy. In that paradigm, all the causes of turmoil buried in the patient's past are de-emphasized while present thought patterns, which have become automatic, become almost the exclusive focus of intervention. The here and now is the working terrain of cognitive therapy... never the past. Had she suspected that her past were to be examined, however ephemerally, she would never have come despite the excellent reputation of the clinic for producing remarkable cures.

She had achieved a measure of acceptance of the damage the past had inflicted upon her and she wasn't willing to risk losing that precarious equilibrium by challenging it unnecessarily, particularly after the sordid revelations of incest she'd discovered during her recent trip to Morganton.

Long ago, she had learned that the sexual abuse at her father's hands had been the genesis of the conflicts, not only of her childhood, but of her adult life as well. Hence, any honest revelation of her history must include that insight.But how could she risk speaking of it in front of others? She still struggled with being honest with herself about what had happened.

The abuse had all started so early in the primitive mists of childhood that it had not been purely abuse. Her mother, crippled by the trauma of her own tragic childhood, had been wholly inadequate at meeting her child's physical needs for affection. As a result, her father's attentions had been a welcome compensation, allowing her to fulfill instinctive needs by attaching physically to a parent.

Since no child has a frame of reference for adult behavior, the drunkenness, in which the beating of her mother and her closeness with her father occurred had not been experienced as unacceptable beyond the noise and violence which, at that stage, never involved her and was usually mercifully brief.

When she reached four or five years of age, however, the caressing advanced to invasive aggression that shocked, frightened, and confused her. Her protests were ignored. What she felt didn't matter at all to him and the initial pleasure of intimacy fled. She grew to fear his advances, to reverberate with the terror her mother displayed. She came to understand that something too awful to speak about aloud was happening.

It took years for the guilt, like a creeping cancer, to emerge from the crevasses of her memory and nest in her awareness.

Revulsion for her father and self-disgust had incubated malignantly within her, spreading toxic tendrils into every corner of her mind, contaminating her view of herself and grotesquely deforming her perception of the role of men in the lives of women.

The guilt had handicapped her so severely that by the time she had escaped from his power, she had become like a stunted pine rooted on a barren cliff blasted and warped by the sea winds into a cowering distortion of normal. This was the blighted image of herself which she would drag behind the protective screen of dissimulation when someone got too close. She could never risk complete disclosure lest others, seeing her without her disguise, should turn away in disgust.

Her ex-husband Riley Davis had been correct in at least one of his accusations. She had indeed hidden from him during their marriage. Their courtship had been like a game of immature make-believe for her. She had enthusiastically assumed the role of a sensual, even seductive woman. She had actually reveled in the overt sexuality which she used, first to attract, and then to hold the bright young lawyer. Some genuine excitement and even arousal had been generated by playing the part of a young woman connecting with a desirable man who pursued her beauty. But, in the end, the game and not reality had predominated and Riley never came to know the real Amy. He romanced and married a vibrant shadow, never glimpsing the reality of the wounded woman beyond it.

When he began to beat her during his bouts of alcohol and cocaine intoxication, the enchanting young woman fled into the wings and the frightened helpless child emerged on stage. The cycle of abuse she'd suffered as a child began again and wasn't broken until Amy was forced to attend counseling after charges were laid against her husband who had physically abused her in public.

Even if she did take her courage in both hands tomorrow morning and attend the session with the other patients, who did she dare let them see… the depressed nurse?… the abused child?… the seductive young woman?… the raging victim of abuse capable of murder? Surely, not the real persona behind the screen. All her options were framed in the fear of discovery and rejection.

In spite of the emotional disarray she was experiencing, Amy's thinking was still clear enough to realize that most of the things she feared as an adult, if they came to pass at all, never materialized with the severity she had anticipated. However, such rational thought could not erase the specter of tomorrow's emotional violation which continued to hover over her as dawn approached.

She began to indulge in some self-talk, a therapeutic self-help skill she had learned from Klein.

"I can't go to that session tomorrow morning."

"But you're expected, aren't you? They'll all be waiting, won't they?"

"They don't know who I am. I've only seen three people who even look like patients here. If I don't show, it won't matter. Besides, Dr. Landry said the session was meant to introduce us... Well, I don't choose to be introduced."

"What harm could there be in attending if you only make a formality of it?"

Her conversation was not covert. She spoke aloud, the two interlocutors representing the opposing sides of her ambivalence.

"I'm afraid. Not sure of what, but I know I don't want to meet those other people."

"They're just people like you… people with problems, people who are depressed. You probably have a lot in common with them."

"People like me! There are no other people like me... you know it and you know why. If my face were scarred into a horrifying mask, I'd be permitted to hide it. Just because my distortions don't show outwardly, I'm not going to risk exposing them."

"You're being extreme, Amy. You *are* like others. And, even if someone someday learned our secrets, they wouldn't necessarily reject you because of them."

"I'm not only afraid of rejection. I don't want to become some kind of freak to be studied or to serve as a bizarre curiosity. Don't forget what happened at the zoo with Carly's daughter."

Just a week before her departure for St. Lucia, a close friend had invited her to accompany her on an excursion to the zoo with her two children. In the llama enclosure, they saw a young animal with a stunted extra leg growing crookedly out of its shoulder. The sight had stimulated questions from the oldest girl.

"Mom, look at the llama calf... It's got five legs but one's twisted and ugly. It doesn't even touch the ground... How come?"

Trying to provide a learning experience, her friend had explained to the fourteen year old that the animal's inbreeding was the probable cause of the birth deformity.

"When animals or people choose mates, they shouldn't choose relatives... it reduces the gene pool and monsters are born."

"Monsters, mom?... What do you mean?"

"Monsters, dear, that's what the word means, real monsters, not like in fairy tales or science fiction. Monsters exist because of what is called inbreeding. Sometimes the defect shows, like the extra leg with the llama, but most times it's not as obvious, perhaps a mental disorder or some other affliction."

"Why does it happen, mom?" asked the young girl seemingly fascinated by the phenomenon.

Perhaps seeking closure, or having reached the limits of her expertise, her friend had summed it up.

"God did it, dear... sort of a curse for violating His laws... We can't stop it with animals, but we do stop it with people... There are laws against it. It's called incest."

"Wow... incest makes monsters?" her eyes were wide.

"Not always, but it can. That's why it's against the law."

Listening to her friend, Amy had been stricken by an irrational panic which seized her heart and lungs in a vice-like grip. She'd had to excuse herself on a pretext, and being unable to calm herself even when alone, she had run to the parking lot and taken a cab home without saying goodbye. Coming on the heels of the events in Morganton, it was more than she could bear.

In the days that followed, the smothering weight of her depression, like a pillow pinned over the face of her vitality, rendered every act of existence an agonizing effort. A permanent grimace seemed graven on her features. Her mind, like a laboring womb, struggled vainly to produce lucid thought and, only in the most superficial mode, was she capable of intellectual functioning.

Although the increase in the intensity of her depression had been steady and gradual, it had been the zoo incident and the painful regurgitation of the memories that it provoked which had pushed her to make the contact with Renaissance.

When her alter ego finally replied, emotion shook the voice.

"Yes, I remember. It almost pushed you over the edge. Maybe you're right."

"I am right. NO GROUP SESSIONS."

"I agree, no group sessions."

"Individual counseling, or we go home!"

"What about the twenty-five thousand you spent to be here...?"

"Stuff the money, if necessary... Individual sessions only, or we leave."

When Amy finished her exercise, although she felt much better, it was already five a.m. and she knew by then that sleep could only be commanded by its chemical masters. Common sense pushed her to her feet and she made her way to the bathroom cabinet where sleeping pills and a glass of water were to be found.

She soon tumbled into a medicated slumber that extended well past the ten o'clock morning group session which all the other patients attended.

CH012: DETROIT, MICHIGAN

The phone in a leather case hanging from the side of the wheelchair burbled irritatingly and Carmen Gallo nodded to the giant standing beside the door.

"Everyone out… now!" bellowed the giant and the three women who had been attending to the old don's toilet immediately set down their esthetician's tools and scurried toward the door. A pair of hair scissors slid from the tray where they'd been laid to clatter to the floor.

Gallo removed his left hand from the manicure soak bowl drying it on the silk of his robe while he studied the buffed nails on his right hand.

"Get the phone…" The old don's voice quavered from the effects of his Parkinson's disease but it retained its authoritative tone.

The giant strode over to the chair after closing the door behind the women. He answered the phone on the seventh ring.

"Who's calling?"

The voice on the other end said brusquely, "I need to speak to Carmen Gallo…. I was given this number."

The giant repeated, "Who's calling?" and then paused to hear the reply. "Just a minute," said the giant before placing a huge thumb over the receiver. He looked down at the old man in the chair who was still examining his nails. "Says he's *judge* Angus McLean."

The gray head lifted and repeated, "Angus McLean?"

"Yea, that's what he said, boss."

Nodding his head and pursing his lips, Gallo lifted a hand to the giant, "I'll take it alone. Get lost for ten minutes."

When the door closed behind the bodyguard the old don put the phone to his ear and spoke.

"Judge McLean... you're a voice from the dust... I thought we might never speak again… What's it been… fifteen years?"

"Not quite, Gallo. Closer to ten…"

"Ten… fifteen… who's counting? As old as I am numbers don't mean much anymore," the old man shrugged as he spoke. "Why are you calling after ten years?"

At the other end of the line there was a moment's pause before the judge replied. "You remember a promise you made to me when we talked about your son and the Dicaprio murder trial?"

"I remember that I said I owed you. I think I told you that you could count on me for a favor. I never forget my promises. Is that what this call is about?... You need a good turn from me?"

"Yes. We need to meet someplace discreet."

"You're too old to run for public office, judge, you can risk being seen with me now."

The old Italian was smiling, imagining the discomfort of the man on the other end of the line.

"No offense intended, Mr. Gallo, but we still move in different circles."

The voice seemed strained.

"Relax, judge… I don't move much anymore at all… traded my legs in for wheels about four years ago, now I never leave my house."

"Does this mean we won't meet?"

"*We* won't meet but I'll send Michael to talk to you wherever and whenever you choose. I'm a man of my word."

"I wouldn't have called if I didn't believe you were. This 'Michael' is he your…"

The old man cut him off. "Yea, my boy. He's the one you let go on my word… He's my right hand. Speak to him and you're speaking to me."

"This thing I need done… this favor… it's not urgent but I have to put my mind to rest on it. When can I meet with your son?"

"Like I said, judge, wherever... whenever... you choose."

"I'm at my summer home on Mackinac Island. Can he get here?... It's discreet and safe."

"You got there, he can get there," replied Gallo. "When do you want him there?"

"Is tomorrow afternoon too soon? And I prefer he'd come by float-plane and not on the ferry. No sense taking any risks..."

"He'll be there tomorrow around four o'clock. Fax me a map of the island."

"No need. My place is the big gray granite chateau on the easternmost tip of the island. My estate has four hundred acres separating it from my nearest neighbors. It sticks out from the air. The water's plenty deep and there's never much boat traffic during the week. The pilot should have no problem."

"Very well. Michael will see you tomorrow... and you'll see that you didn't make a mistake helping him avoid the frame-up. He's a fine man."

"I'm sure he is," answered the judge and then, almost as an afterthought he added, "If I hadn't believed your story that the boy was innocent, I never would have agreed to expose the Dicaprio conspiracy. I stayed on the right side of the fence. Justice was served."

“But I still owed you, judge.”

“I never thought I’d need your help, Gallo, but no one can tell what the future holds for them can they?” The judge spoke with a tone of sad resignation as he thought of the deaths of his son and daughter.

“No, I never believed the tea leaves either, judge, but if you cannot predict events you can always influence them rather than sitting passively by like some chump watching a parade.”

“That’s why I made this call. I’m not sitting still.”

“Very well. Michael will see you tomorrow, judge. I’ll be getting back to my manicure and haircut, now... Small pleasures are all I have left. Have a nice day.” And he snapped the phone shut and pushed the button on his chair to summon the giant.

CH013: MACKINAC ISLAND, MICHIGAN

Despite the bright sunlight and cloudless sky, a brisk breeze tumbling down from the Canadian north had kept the afternoon cool. Angus McLean wore a tweed jacket and a wool scarf was draped about his neck. On the table before him a silver coffee pot with a long elegant swan neck sparkled in the sunlight. Beside it, a half empty cup had attracted the attention of a yellow jacket wasp that minced along its brim, abdomen bobbing and antennae flaring over a drop of congealed liquid.

Below the terrace on which he sat, Mary and the children had coerced the butler into a game of croquet in which the three of them connived to thwart the poor fellow's efforts to play. Michael shrieked with delight as he smacked his ball against the butler's, driving it twenty feet to the edge of the lawn. Mary laughed, her long unbound hair flung about by the breeze, as she chided Michael in jest for his attack on the other player.

His dear wife Mary had come alive in the children's presence. Always much younger in appearance than her true age, she had magically rejuvenated to the point where she could have been cavorting with her own children.

Angus smiled. She had been so near total collapse and then, suddenly, the resurrection. It had been marvelous how two children had achieved such a profound transformation in several short weeks when a team of high-priced therapists and a whole convent of nuns had failed miserably during months of seclusion and therapy sessions. Even the old judge himself felt younger now that the halls of the chateau once more rang with childish laughter and the sound of running feet. If only he'd been wise enough to enjoy such tumult when his own children had been young.

The eternal regrets of fathers... missed opportunities.

It was almost four o'clock and his vigil for the plane had brought him to the patio thirty minutes ago. He was curious about the impending encounter with Michael Gallo. Ten years ago, the boy had been an arrogant aggressive youth imbued with the awareness of his family's power and blinded by the illusions of invulnerability that handicap the young.

He had been an easy victim for the Dicaprios.

The Dicaprio and Gallo crime families had dominated the Mafia activities in Detroit for three generations and turf wars and conflicts punctuated their mutual history.

As the suburbs grew in the seventies, a struggle for supremacy in the new territories surrounding Dearborn and Bloomfield Hills became inevitable between the longtime rivals.

Michael, at age twenty-three, had been given responsibility for setting up the extortion operations of the Gallo syndicate in the new malls springing up like mushrooms around the city's perimeter. As the two families attempted to consolidate their new interests, clashes between them had been infrequent but vicious. Following the bombing of a Dearborn bakery in which a Dicaprio lieutenant and family member had been killed, witnesses had come forward to finger the younger Gallo for the crime.

An ambitious district attorney with political aspirations took on the case like a personal crusade against organized crime and Michael Gallo had been indicted for murder.

Judge McLean had never doubted that the brash young mobster, even at twenty three, had already committed his share of crimes. Maybe even murder. But this belief, however well founded in probability, wasn't a legitimate consideration when the case landed in his court. McLean was a stern champion of law and order and the district attorney had steered the case his way hoping for quick expedient justice. And he almost got it.

The case had been a well-publicized affair and was drawing to a predictable close when McLean had been kidnapped for five hours.

Old man Gallo, apparently frustrated at the impotence of his lawyers in court, could see his son going down for the count, and with him, the Gallo's dreams for the future.

On his way back from dinner at the Canadian Consul's residence, McLean's limousine had been forced to the side of the road, commandeered and driven to Gallo's estate in Northfield. McLean had been frightened but also outraged. In front of the old don he'd fumed about ignorant 'wops' who couldn't tell the difference between Palermo and Detroit.

The old man had absorbed his tirade in silence and then asked politely for twenty minutes of his time. McLean had had no real choice but the old man's apologies and the circumstances convinced him to listen.

A Dicaprio defector, well-rewarded by the Gallos, had come into the room where they sat and spent a full hour detailing an elaborate conspiracy between the district attorney and the Dicaprio family to frame Michael Gallo for the murder of one of their own which they had engineered. Names, dates and information were provided and the don pled for consideration of the 'truth' by McLean.

It helped that McLean was a republican and the district attorney a democrat and that McLean would be able to virtually name his own candidate for the position of D.A. if he displaced the democrat. And, best of all, he could topple the incumbent in good conscience because all he would do was reveal the truth.

The outcome was predictable; exposure of the plot, the ruin of the district attorney and the serious maiming of the Dicaprio expansion into the suburbs.

Immediately after his acquittal, Michael Gallo had been whisked off to the ivory towers of Ivy League academe not returning until he was admitted as a member of the Michigan bar several years later.

The old don, much to the embarrassment and consternation of McLean had appeared one Sunday afternoon, shortly after the trial, at the judge's residence to pay his respects. At that abbreviated session he had made the offer of assistance that would result in Michael Gallo's visit to Angus McLean this afternoon over ten years later.

* * *

'Hawkeye' McLean had always lived by the adage that on time meant fifteen minutes early. Anyone who dared to appear in his court less than five minutes before the appointed hour was already guilty, in his eyes, of a substantial offense and none were pardoned. Accordingly, he did not seem the least surprised to hear the approaching hum of a plane at three fifty-five on his pocket watch.

Mary and the children paused to look up, shading their eyes against the sun, as they squinted to bring the silver silhouette in the sky into focus.

The plane wheeled in a large circle so that it was coming directly out of the east, high over the water but descending rapidly, the crescendo of its engine climbing as the craft itself dropped to a few hundred feet and then hurtled over the trees and shoreline to whine aggressively above the estate as if on an weaponless strafing run.

The yellow jacket wasp launched itself up and away from the coffee cup in a flick of terror.

The speed and noise of the plane's approach were so startling that Caroline gave a small cry and went to her knees bending to hide her face while clamping her hands over her ears. Her brother pivoted in place following the aircraft's trajectory until it cleared the chateau and momentarily winked out of sight in the forest beyond before reappearing in a lazy bank to the south.

"Grandpa! Grandpa!" the boy cried dropping his croquet mallet and dashing up the incline of the lawn to where his grandfather sat unperturbed.

Mary had gone to Caroline's side and the two of them were now standing and watching the plane again.

As Michael covered the last ten yards between himself and his grandfather, the plane squared itself off at right angles to the end of the island and came in skimming the waves, the engine noise falling to a harsh mechanical muttering as it slowed precipitously.

"Grandpa! He's coming in," shouted Michael excitedly and now almost at his grandfather's elbow. "Cool, isn't it?"

The boy's voice was full of animated admiration.

"Who is it, Grandpa?... Is it the police?... Is something wrong?"

The old man answered calmly.

"No, Michael, nothing's wrong… It's just a man I sent for, coming to pay me a visit."

"Ask him to take me up for a ride Grandpa. If he came to visit you in his plane he must think you're important and he'll do whatever you ask."

The old man laughed at the boy's effervescence... "Whoa now, laddie, I'm not so important that he should be ready to do whatever I ask of him."

"Sure you are Grandpa... You have guards with guns at the gate and every one still calls you 'your honor'. If you asked him I'm sure he'd want to please you... and I want to fly in a plane like that."

"But you've been flying often Michael. You flew here from Georgia."

"It's not the same grandpa… Those big planes are just like sitting in a movie theater... It's not exciting at all."

The boy had dropped to his knees beside his grandfather's chair and latched onto his right arm with both hands.

As he studied the child with his blue eyes pleading and his bronze hair falling across his brow, the old judge felt a lump rising in his throat. The lad's mother had been a tomboy who had begged for adventure just as her son was now doing. He knew he couldn't refuse.

"Very well, laddie. I'll promise nothing but I'll ask him. Now go down with Thomas and meet the plane. Maybe he'll let you help tie it up."

The boy was up and gone before the old Scot stopped speaking. His bare legs flashed below his shorts as he dashed down the hill to catch up with the gardener, Tom, who had come out of the shrubbery to head toward the dock and the plane, taxiing in from the lake beyond.

Angus McLean arose from his chair and with small shuffling steps gradually drew up to his full height. The cool air had a gelling effect upon his muscles and, to avoid pain, he moved in incremental degrees until he felt stable enough to mount the steps into the parlor.

He had decided that his visitor would find him ensconced behind his imposing walnut desk set upon a low dais in his study and surrounded by the trappings of his position... the law books lining the walls, the pictures posed with presidents and others who walked the corridors of power. But his plan to receive the young Gallo in such a manner was more than a simple attempt to impress, for the study was the only room in the building that was regularly swept for eavesdropping devices. As well, the doorframe to the room incorporated within it a metal detector like those used in courtrooms.

Finally, a loaded nine millimeter automatic velcroed to the side panel of the desk clung within easy reach of the judge's right hand when he sat at the desk. '*Overly cautious, perhaps*,' thought the old Scot, but since his kidnapping years ago he had determined never to be taken unawares again.

At the dock, the Cessna purred to a halt, the engine shutting down with a final acrid cough. Tom, a young man of twenty-five who, at six foot five, towered over most everyone, had the well-defined physique of a body builder. Doubling as both gardener and bodyguard, he was paid as the latter and only his love of nature and the need for distraction on the tiny island permitted him to putter around the grounds. Agile as a cat despite his size, he leapt lightly onto the plane's float and fastened a line to a strut. The pilot tossed him a second line through the cockpit window and the plane was well-tethered by the time the door opened.

The pilot paused with one foot on the step, removing a pair of sunglasses as he put on a smile to greet the two people on the dock.

"Well, that was very efficient... Looks like you may be used to having planes drop in."

His gray eyes moved easily over the dock, his greeters and the woods and lawns beyond. His hesitation, half out of his plane, seemed more of a pleasant welcome than the careful scrutiny of the environs that it was.

"Oh, no sir, we don't get planes here," volunteered Michael cheerfully, "but it's much like tying up a boat and we do that often." He was smiling broadly with the innocence and enthusiasm of childhood.

Beside him, Tom remained with his arms crossed over his chest displaying in a partial flex the bulk of his biceps and forearms. His face remained impassive as he studied the pilot before he spoke.

"So you're alone?" he asked.

"Yup, don't often get the opportunity to get behind the stick much anymore so when I do, I take advantage of it."

Obviously satisfied that there was no apparent danger, the younger Gallo committed his feet to the pontoon and then hopped to the dock extending a hand all in one smooth motion.

"Michael Gallo," he said.

Tom unfolded and stretched out a hand locking firmly with Gallo.

"Tom Perry... Welcome to Greystokes."

Turning his attention to the boy, Gallo tousled the child's thick hair and asked, "And who might you be young man... the master of Greystokes?"

"Oh, no," blushed the boy replying almost sheepishly, "That's· my grandfather, Judge McLean... I'm just Michael."

"Just Michael?..." the newcomer repeated with mock surprise in his voice, and then he squatted to a position in front of the boy and took his arms at the shoulders speaking earnestly… "Michael's my name too, son. Do you know what Michael means?"

The boy seemed a little taken aback by the question about which he'd truly never reflected and stammered... "No… no, I don't. I thought it was only a name."

"Much more than that, Michael. Michael means 'a man like God' and our namesake is the most powerful of all God's angels.... What do you think of that?"

"Wow!" said the child obviously awed and pleased by the explanation.

Gallo had stood up and placed his arm around the boy's shoulders and, without waiting for an invitation, turned to head up the walkway to the lawn. Tom followed closely behind the two who had become quickly engrossed in a conversation about flying.

At the edge of the terrace the butler was waiting to pickup the relay of guiding the guest. Tom, who knew that Gallo and McLean would need to confer privately called out to the child.

"Michael, I've got some plastic sheeting that I have to put over some seedlings. Could you give me a hand?"

Michael, his reluctance to part from his new friend clearly visible on his face, hesitated looking back at Tom. "Plastic's not heavy, Tom," he opined.

"I know, Mikey. But it is bulky and stretching it out is a bit like making a bed… It's much easier to do with a helper."

Gallo lifted his hand from Michael's shoulder and placed it encouragingly on his back with light pressure.

"Run along and help, Michael. I need to speak with your grandfather and then I promise I'll be back and" he paused for effect, "If you've worked well and Grandpa agrees, how about a little plane ride?"

"Wow, a plane ride!" the child echoed excitedly. "Sure, that would be cool!" and he ran to join Tom.

There were no introductions with the butler who simply said, "Please follow me, sir," before crossing the terrace and entering the chateau.

They passed through French doors to a large drawing room furnished with one long bare trestle table and several armchairs upholstered with well-worn leather. Superficial cracks spider webbed the leather of the back and seats of several chairs, testifying that, despite their Spartan appearance, someone had spent many hours sitting there. The chairs and table appeared to be antiques, now serving primarily decorative purposes.

Facing him as he entered the room was a medieval tapestry full fifteen feet high, suspended against the wall by a long wooden rod which ran through supporting loops at the upper edge of the artwork. A hunting scene was depicted with three tall thin anemic-looking men in period costumes standing around an equally unrealistic stag crumpled on the ground, its tongue lolling out of its mouth. Incongruously, a frail, ephemeral beauty stood off to the side of the men. She wore a formal gown, the stark lines of which matched the expressionless stare the artist had woven into her eternal features. Her right hand rested daintily on the head of an emaciated hound sitting rigidly at attention. Gallo wondered who would ever have paid good money to purchase such a dreary piece.

Behind the tapestry, a wall of gray granite rose to a vaulted roof where broad beams, eerily tattooed with soot from the huge open fireplace, seemed to have spectral faces within them as if some malevolent highland deity had imprisoned enemy spirits of the clan in the very substance of the wood.

The judge's private office was up three stairs at the far end of the room. The butler stopped at the stairs and wordlessly indicated, with a wave of his hand, that Gallo should enter.

The young lawyer, of course, knew the full story of his family's indebtedness to Angus McLean. Logically, there should be no reason to fear attack or betrayal but his instincts had been alerted by the brooding aura of this isolated chateau with its cold gray stones, stiff furniture and soulfully dismal beams. The whole place was like a movie set saturated with a sense of ominous foreboding. He paused to look around once more as the butler retraced his passage back through the room.

Cautiously, he went up the steps and stood on the threshold of a much warmer room chock full of bookshelves and chairs laden with stacks of law reviews and professional journals. He felt immediately more at ease... The odor of the law... old paper and moldering book bindings.

The wall behind McLean's desk was covered with black and white framed photos. In the largest one, Gallo recognized Dwight Eisenhower standing beside a young man whom he took to be the judge in his youth. Though the collection dated the époque of the old judge's influence, it testified to his ready access to power. Gallo smiled wryly thinking how the photos of his own ancestors had decorated post office walls.

As he stepped into the room, a small red light began blinking in the doorframe above his head. McLean pointed to it catching Gallo's attention before speaking.

"The door frame contains a metal detector... I don't allow firearms in my office." His tone was blunt and factual.

"I'm clean, your honor, the detector must have picked up on theses," replied the younger man fishing a bulky ring of keys from his pants pocket and plucking an impressively thick silver fountain pen from a shirt pocket.

He came forward and placed them on the edge of the desk before holding open his down-filled flyer's vest with both hands to show he had no shoulder holster.

He continued, "You saw me at my worst in my younger days when I believed in guns," then, picking up the pen, he spun it in his fingers. "Seven years of university and law school have taught me the power of the pen, so, I rarely arm myself nowadays."

The judge's face remained impassive but his eyes which had been riveted onto the young man before him, softened and he gestured to a chair facing the desk.

"Please sit down."

Gallo had classic Mediterranean good looks with an aquiline nose and an olive hue to his complexion. His hair was full and carried a natural wave. He sported a day's growth of jet black beard as was now quite fashionable among the young. McLean, however, could see that the disarming set of his face when he smiled disguised the ability to use his eyes as a tool of intimidation if the occasion called for it. At least, they had that skill in common.

The old Scot spoke when his listener had retrieved his keys and pen and settled himself in the chair. "I'll get right to the point Mr. Gallo. I have a problem with a man who threatens the integrity of my family. He is dangerous to us and must be dealt with."

Gallo nodded to indicate that he had assimilated the essence of the situation. The judge went on.

"Do you know the tragic story of my children?"

"No, I'm afraid I don't, your honor."

"Then you need to hear some of it. I have... rather I *had* two children, one boy, one girl. Remarkable spirits both of them, the light of their mother's life and..." he paused momentarily, his eyes dimming with sadness as if a rheostat in his brain had been twisted, "...my heirs."

His voice quavered and lost volume until he cleared his throat and resumed.

"The McLean clan evolved from simple shepherds to become the dominant power of the Glengarry highlands. For two centuries our clan, at least our particular branch, has affected the history of wherever we've lived. My children were poised to continue that tradition. It's a family imperative that I sense you may well understand."

Gallo did. He had long since discarded the idea of repudiating his origins. His own father's attitudes mirrored the depth of the judge's passion as he spoke of family, roots and traditions.

"Well," went on the old Scot, "it wasn't to be. Colin, my son was gunned down senselessly in a botched robbery attempt three years ago and, in May of this year, my daughter, was killed in a single vehicle accident in Georgia where she lived."

His shoulders shuddered and the hunch they carried became noticeably pronounced. Silence reigned for several moments while the judge struggled with his emotions and Gallo attempted to take in the staggering impact of a family, anchored in tradition, being snuffed out in one generation.

"Our lives, my wife's and mine, came crashing down like a house of cards in a whirlwind. She very nearly lost her mind and I mourned not only my children but also the future extinction of the McLean family. Killing us, if fate truly needed McLeans as victims, would have been easier than losing our children."

He paused again, overcome with grief, sliding his head into his hands and staring at the desk.

Gallo felt he needed to share the burden of the conversation but he didn't share the judge's obvious belief of the role of fate in the affairs of men. His experience had led him to search for less mystical explanations when disaster struck, particularly if circumstances seemed to defy simple coincidence.

The apparent naivety of Mclean's beliefs that his family and its members were the mere playthings of destiny shocked the pragmatic young lawyer. The old man's superstitions could blind him to any serious consideration of foul play in the decimation of his family while the probability of just such a cause for the tragedy seemed glaringly evident to Gallo.

He hesitated for a moment, fearing that McLean might react badly to any challenge to his convictions, then decided to risk it. "Are you absolutely convinced that the deaths of your children were accidental?"

The judge seemed galvanized by the impudence of the question. He raised his eyes quickly, skewering the young lawyer with his infamous gaze.

"What do you mean?" he demanded, his voice hard and flinty. "You'd better have a damn good reason for what you're suggesting."

Gallo wasn't intimidated, sensing the apprehension behind the old man's ire. Besides, the matter had to be discussed openly or his visit here would be no more than a farce if McLean's request for a favor had anything to do with his children, and Gallo was certain now that it did.

He replied calmly, "Just that my experience in such matters... matters of deaths... I mean, has made me a supreme skeptic about the elements of chance and accident. It's common practice to make any murder appear accidental... After all, that's how we lawyers earn our livings isn't it? On one side or the other, we either support or attack the notion of an accident."

"I don't believe in accidents either," snapped the judge testily interrupting Gallo, "but if you discount fate, which I permit myself to point out has absolutely nothing to do with accident, you're still without a plausible explanation."

"Of course, I'm just playing the devil's advocate, Judge," rejoined the younger man, "but if you had an enemy, a blood enemy who sought to punish you and prolong your suffering, he might attack you through your children."

"And who in hell would fit the bill of such an enemy… because I can't think of a single one?"

Gallo leaned forward in the chair and settled his elbows on the edge of the desk before answering.

"Consider this, Judge, if you will. When you exonerated me of murder, four Dicaprios went to prison along with that slimy DA. Two of the family members bought it in the joint and the other two are still there. If that isn't enough, just think back to the fratricidal war that broke out within the family when the truth got out that Vinny Dicaprio got roasted in the bakery by his own uncle. A lot of people were snuffed and when it comes to forgetting, Sicilians make elephants look absent-minded. It doesn't take much imagination to make a case for your face being on someone's dartboard … Perhaps 'a child for a child' …?"

The judge sat up, his brow furrowed, and for a long minute he seemed to be studying the ceiling, replaying the notion Gallo had introduced over and over again in his mind. *'Attack me through my children'*. The logic of it all became overwhelming. He sighed deeply, a prolonged sibilant whisper of air pushed out through partially pursed lips.

When he finally spoke, his tone was ponderous and somber. "I pray to heaven that you are mistaken in your suggested scenario, counselor."

Gallo was perplexed by the comment. For him, any adverse event could be more easily accepted if it made sense... however ghastly that sense might be. A smoker dying of lung cancer made sense, a child killed by an automobile when running out between parked cars still left the world with a semblance of predictability and consequence. Tragedy existed but rarely as the random unpredictable act of fate. *How could McLean not welcome a more plausible explanation?*

"Why would it be more tragic if I were right, Judge?" he asked, his eyebrows raised.

McLean seemed to be looking past Gallo, somehow peering into the future when he replied." Because, counselor, if you are right, then I am still vulnerable and my grandchildren could be in danger. Anyone wishing to mortally wound me would now take aim at my wife and those children. The implication of your spin on things is horrifying."

Gallo understood. Love made us vulnerable. As long as a man loved he could be hurt and, if he loved deeply enough, he could be destroyed by the loss of his loved ones. His point had been made and the old man had accepted it.

"Just a theory, Judge… but where does this 'man' you mentioned earlier come into the picture? How is he a threat to you or your family?"

The judge had collected himself somewhat and continued his story.

"My daughter eloped with a young doctor from Georgia... almost broke my wife's heart. She'd planned twenty-two years for a wedding she never saw. On the other hand, I wasn't surprised. Annette always had a rebellious streak in her and she had shocked us before, although not on such a scale… Well, they settled in Georgia and eventually had two children."

Smiling, he added, "I think you've already met young Michael and seen his sister Caroline with my wife, Mary."

"I saw them both," confirmed Gallo, nodding.

"We saw the children infrequently but Annette and the kids spend several weeks each summer here with us at Greystokes. When Colin was killed, my wife invested all of her affection for him into Michael and the bond between them became intense, almost essential to her existence. They talked for hours on the phone and Mary showered the children with gifts which seemed to offend the father, Dr. Jason Turner. Their father is the man who threatens my family."

The flinty edge to the judge's voice returned with the mention of Jason's name." He doesn't realize that we can care for the children better than he can. He wants them back when he returns from the nut farm he's in right now."

"Is he insane?"

"Not insane… weak… flawed emotionally. His mother was an eccentric musician and his father ran off, then died falling down a flight of stairs, if memory serves me well. He grew up lop-sided and the only balance he ever knew in his forlorn life was when my daughter was alive. He's had a nervous breakdown… a woman's affliction… and he's holed up somewhere in the Caribbean trying to get all of his beans back into the bag."

"Is that why the children are here?" asked Gallo.

"Yes… and that's why my dear wife is still alive and sane. We need the children and the children need us. No McLean will ever be raised without both a father and a mother. We can offer the children that and he cannot. I can't put it more simply."

Gallo asked, "Have you talked about this with him?"

"Would you arm your enemy before the battle, Mr. Gallo?"

"So, he doesn't know what you intend?"

"He may suspect, but he knows nothing."

"And where do we come in?" queried Gallo sensing that he would now hear the heart of the matter.

Angus McLean drew himself up until his bent back touched the leather of his chair. "Formally, I am retaining your services as a lawyer to act in the matter of the custody dispute of the children."

"And informally?" Gallo's voice lowered, instinctively preparing for the secret.

“Informally, his opposition must be overcome, his objections nullified... How you proceed is none of my business and I never want to hear about details. Just make it so that my grandchildren are raised by my wife and I.”

“Why us, judge? Why call in our marker on what is essentially a family problem?” Gallo was looking for explicit instructions but none were forthcoming.

“Mr. Gallo,” said the judge, the tone of his voice condescending, “do you really expect me to answer that question?”

“I understand, your honor.”

“Then take this as a retainer,” and the old man flipped open a long checkbook on his blotter and began to write.

Gallo protested, “No need for money, judge. This is a favor.”

McLean ripped out the check and thrust it across the desk ignoring Gallo. “Fifty thousand dollars for expenses and retainer.”

Gallo’s eyes widened. “You really do want this badly,” he said.

“I want you to solve my problems like I might have done once if I were still your age. I also want you to arrange for the inauspicious guarding of my grandchildren until we know whether your theory about my children’s deaths is correct or not. Tom is to be briefed on all security measures. He has my full confidence and he can become your man in matters relating to the children’s safety.”

Gallo sat for a moment fingering the check and considering the implications of accepting the judge’s bargain. An image flashed on his mind’s eye of him explaining to his father why he had refused to assist the man who had kept him out of prison. He looked up and locked eyes with McLean. “It’ll be done the way you want it.”

“And I’m assured of discretion... that I’ll never hear of the details of how you proceed?”

"We'll make sure you find out if I'm correct about the deaths of your children and if there is any continuing danger to your grandchildren, but nothing more."

Gallo rose from his chair and extended his hand.

The old man leaned over the desk and took it. The lawyer was surprised at the force of the judge's grip.

"And one more thing, please, Mr. Gallo... Michael wishes to have a ride in your airplane, if possible."

Gallo grinned. "Already arranged."

CH014: ST. LUCIA

His session that afternoon with Dr. Landry had left Jason pondering his 'dependency'. It had also left him irritated.

Landry had the benefit of two weeks of intensive self-revelation by Jason, and yet the therapist had been sparse in his commentary about what he'd learned about his patient until to-day. This individual session had been like a mini-symposium on dependency and how Landry saw it as the dominant theme in Jason's life. He'd gone so far as offering the interpretation that Jason's own identity had become confused with those of the dominant women in his life, particularly Annette.

Landry was working on his third wife and Jason suspected that the good doctor was harboring an unconscious bias. When marriages were durable attachments of many years duration, the shrinking of the partners' individual identities as the couple expanded might be perceived as 'unhealthy' by someone who had never experienced such integration or had fallen into the habit of seeing everything through the prism of the self and its wellbeing. Jason needed to believe that his therapist had committed just such an error and arrived at a faulty conclusion, as a result. The alternative was to believe that he, himself, harbored an unpalatable emotional flaw.

Dependency.

The word, like a metal shard twisting in his brain begged to be expelled in the interest of peace and sanity. He had to get it out, purge himself of the morbid introspection that ruminating on the morning's session was spawning. It was already night and he was at the beach where he had retreated to find a measure of peace and relaxation. He looked around him.

With the sound of crinkling cellophane, a miniature wave rippled and fell upon the beach. A wavering foamy fluorescent line of lace flashed momentarily against the black sand before sinking into obscurity.

The metronomic rhythm of the water seemed to cueing the scrabbling choreography of a palm-sized blue land crab that scuttled forward in the wake of the receding water to pick at invisible bits of sustenance before scuttling back as the next wave rolled in. From his perch atop the black basalt boulder coughed out from a volcano's fiery throat eons ago, Jason watched the crab. Its repetitious action seemed evidence that at least a measure of humdrum routine at all levels of existence was inescapable.

The night air was fresh and laden with the musky scent of tropical blooms. The moon's reflection rocked like a lily bloom on the gentle swells of the inlet and stars salted the vault above. Behind him, the raucous chorus of tree frogs chirping in the vegetation provided a blanket of sound that muffled all evidence of civilization. As the minutes passed in quiet contemplation, he felt alone but not isolated. Solitary, yet integrated into nature, the peace of his surroundings coaxing him out of his concerns over therapy into a kinder mind set.

Meditation as a conscious exercise had never worked reliably for him, but Jason recognized the need for its revitalizing power. Each evening for the past week he had retired to this isolated spot. He had come to bandage his bludgeoned emotions with a poultice of silence, to gently shake out the tangled fibers of his mind and restore function to his intellect, to harmonize his internal processes with the eternal vibrations of nature. In short, he sought the restoration of his losses... healing. He had applied himself assiduously during these nocturnal retreats to practicing the process of meditation, the results becoming more rewarding with each effort.

Tonight, he allowed himself to drift easily into a muted awareness of external concerns much like the exhaustion of the day flows silently into restorative sleep. The tension he had felt humming in every cell while thrashing through the content of today's psychotherapy, seemed to leach out of his body and into the boulder as if the basalt were a sponge.

His breathing became regular and abdominal. He slid his legs into the lotus position and, rather than producing a sensation of abnormal constraint, it felt entirely appropriate. He could feel the relaxation of the musculature of his face and a pleasant heaviness began infusing his limbs as he surrendered his body to the usurpation of the trance. He emptied his mind and allowed the sounds, sights and rhythms of the night to seep into his soul like a spiritual balm.

How long he had sat wrapped in the shroud of meditation he didn't know. But life intruded in a flash of dark fur streaking across the beach. A mongoose had snatched the blue crab in the midst of its promethean routine with a crunching bite that the mute crustacean could only protest with helpless swings of its single outsized claw. Hunched over its impotent victim the hunter crushed out the life of the crab in rapid-fire bites. Tossing its head back the mongoose swallowed a morsel and then grabbed its prey's mutilated body and raced back to the leafy darkness from which it had emerged with such deadly agility and purpose.

The whole minuscule drama, brief and violent though it had been, penetrated Jason's awareness as if through an emotional filter of detachment and acceptance. He didn't stir. His observation had been unconnected to the content of the event. The experience of something that could have, would normally have, been startling and, at least mildly disquieting for him, was devoid of emotional content. The fact that internal peace could be so pervasive provoked a hushed amazement in him. The happy implication for his battle against depression was profound.

Had his night ended at that moment, the knowledge it had brought him would have been worth the travail of the day. But it didn't.

Still silent and detached, almost a piece of the boulder itself, Jason became aware of movement far down the beach. Someone was approaching tracing a meandering course through the gentle effervescence of the lapping waves. The person's progress along the strand seemed incidental, not purposeful.

The figure, still a distillation of shadow only barely distinguishable from the surrounding night, wandered at times high onto the beach and at others into the waves, bending occasionally as if to examine something in the water or on the sand.

As she approached, Jason could make out the figure and long hair of a woman. Inexplicably, her appearance on the beach seemed entirely synchronous with the rhythm of the night and produced no sense of intrusion. He watched her as he had earlier watched the moon on the water, the crab on the beach.

About twenty yards from where he sat atop the boulder, the woman knelt in the sand and began tracing with a twig some message upon the wave-polished ebony surface. Her memo was obviously long because she raised up until her body formed a right angle in the darkness and kept writing as she moved along the sand.

Suddenly, a wave several times more forceful than its fellows splashed around her ankles and ran up her calves in bubbly enthusiasm as if taunting her by scrubbing away her efforts. She stood upright, momentarily surveying the result of the wave's effects upon her script, then she pivoted, hands on hips, and, in playful defiance, flung the twig out upon the water before shaking her finger after it.

She stood for a few more moments as if absorbed in contemplation. And then, in a graceful folding motion, sank down upon the sand and hugged her knees while staring at the moon.

Ordinarily, Jason would have reflected upon his presence as an unseen witness to the scene. He would probably have felt the need to either slink away unobserved or do or say something to let her know he was there. However, tonight's experience was anything but ordinary and no such thought or impulse crossed his mind. It was as if he were observing her from another dimension separated by the breadth of a galaxy from the reality of her world.

They sat in twin solitudes each enveloped in the sounds of the night. He turned his gaze as well to the moon inhaling the ghostly features of the moonscape to experience any beneficial sensation the exercise might arouse within him.

When he next looked back at the beach, she was gone from the sand but in a moment he saw her head emerge from the sea several yards from shore. Her ivory shoulders, reflected in the moonlight, rose rhythmically as she breast-stroked toward the moon oscillating on the sable surface of the cove.

She advanced through the water with calmness and grace, her long tresses alternately swirling then trailing out into the tiny wake her efforts created behind her with each purposeful thrust of her body. Her feet never broke the surface and she seemed to glide forward as if carried on the back of some benevolent sea wraith. He wondered if she intended to swim to the edge of the world but felt no apprehension as she moved so far out to sea that she was barely visible. She had swum through the moon and well beyond when she finally paused, turned and retraced her passage with the same powerful silent strokes.

As her feet found purchase on the sand a dozen yards from the shore she ceased stroking and her body slowly emerged from the womb of the water as naked as a newborn entering the world. Jason noticed her milky nakedness with the same detachment he had observed the whole night's panorama. In fact, her lack of raiment seemed less incongruous than if she had emerged from the waves clad in a swimsuit.

She had the body of a young woman with soft curves and pert breasts that neither swayed nor jostled with her movements. Strands of dark hair forked around her nipples in a vain attempt at modesty. Her face remained swathed in shadow.

As she reached the water's edge he could see she was headed toward the components of a bikini that lay upon the sand where she had left them. After smoothing the water from her skin with sweeping caresses, she hefted her mane of hair and twisted it in her hands to squeeze out the water. That task finished, she shook her head to loosen the tresses and then flung it back to allow a yard of hair to fall in disarray upon her back. During the motion, the moonlight behind her had sprayed rusty highlights through the fan of hair and momentarily illuminated high arched brows, raised cheekbones and a straight narrow nose.

She bent to pick up the bikini and shook the sand from it. After rinsing it, she stepped into the panties and deftly holstered her breasts in the top. She stood for a minute facing the sea, her paleness almost apparitional in the subdued light of the night.

She retraced her steps down the beach and when halfway back to the path by which she must have entered, she broke into a steady lope running with the practiced ease of an athlete accustomed to regular exertion.

Jason remained cocooned in the tranquility that permeated both his body and mind. While part of him sensed that a return to his room and sleep was expected of him he was loath to disturb the peace he had discovered. Almost unconsciously, he unlaced his legs and flexed his muscles. Gathering up the towel he had folded to sit upon, he carefully sought the hand and footholds down the side of the boulder to the sand. However, with each physical movement he seemed to be moving further from the rapture he had experienced in the trance. He sensed that if he allowed his conscious mind to resume control of his activity, he might never find the pathway back to that state again.

Jason recognized that, through the experience, he had only partially fulfilled his enormous need to find a safe haven within his own mind. The thought that he might lose the ability to return to such peacefulness was so disconcerting that he acted quickly to abort the process of reviving.

Curling up in the sand at the base of the boulder, he could feel the sun's warmth stored in the deeper layers. He pulled the towel over his torso, scooped a pillow in the sand and let himself tumble back down the rabbit hole to the refuge he'd at last discovered. Solitary peace was a unique and vastly reassuring experience for him. Alone but still whole.

The next morning, he was awakened by the slanting rays of the rising sun. Jason Turner had begun his healing. He felt it. He knew it but was afraid to question precisely how or why, lest the process cease.

CH015: ST. LUCIA

Jason settled back on his towel on the sand, his arms crossed under his head. High above, towering cumulus clouds, like the laundry of the Gods tumbling from a celestial hamper upon the floor of the sky, played hide and seek with the sun. For brief interludes the shadows of drifting cloud would blotch the bay, beach and bluffs, providing welcome respite from the searing heat. In his imagination, the cloud shadows crawling across the water and transforming the turquoise depths to more somber blue as they passed, became monstrous manta rays patrolling beneath the surface.

He looked forward to his free time on the beach each day and used it to read or to reflect upon the content of his therapy sessions which he had requested be changed to the mornings from the afternoon.

"Well, Jason, you've acquired quite a tan since your arrival."

Jason who'd been lost in contemplation of the seascape shaded his eyes and looked up into the bearded face of Brigham Landry draped in the shadow of a broad-brimmed straw hat.

"I hesitate to comment," smiled Jason, "you might detect some unconscious death wish being acted out on this breeding ground for melanomas."

The therapist laughed heartily.

Dr. Brigham Landry was a wealthy man who dressed like a thrift store refugee. All his nondescript clothing hung on his tall, bony frame like cast-offs on a scarecrow. A craggy angular face with Lincolnesque nose and brows gave the impression of a roughed-in clay sculpture that had been fired into permanence before the final touches had been applied. His robust gray beard framed a generous mouth too large for a normal man but which complemented his face quite nicely. However, it was his eyes that people noted first and never forgot. They were an electric blue with flecks of hazel scattered like traces of mica in a quartz crystal. When he looked you in the face, his gaze, piercing but benevolent, conveyed the impression that he was examining your soul. Jason imagined that God's eyes might look like Landry's.

"I've never seen you as being self destructive, Jason. You've a finely honed penchant for morbid introspection, but nothing lethal... Mind if I join you?"

He'd already begun settling his considerable bulk as he spoke. Part way down, his feet slipped in the loose sand and he lost the struggle with gravity falling the last three feet to the beach in an awkward flop onto his buttocks and back, that evoked the image of the 'Jack and the Beanstalk' giant flopping to the earth.

Landry's face registered surprise but no embarrassment as he recovered his balance and shifted into a tripod stance, his arms out behind his body on the sand.

"Ground's further down than I remembered it being..." he grunted.

Jason smiled at the picture the world-renowned therapist presented in his cut-off Levis, Harvard sweatshirt, and bone white legs that accounted for fully half of his six foot eight inch stature.

Pointing at Landry's legs, he said, "I gather you're not a sun worshipper."

"On the contrary, I'd like to spend more time out here. There's no substitute for the benefit derived from absorbing the peacefulness of nature. Taking more time to enjoy it is on my list of good intentions, but for the moment, I remain holed up in that therapy room like some prisoner doing a life sentence who gets a new visitor every ninety minutes... Wouldn't be here even now, except that Bishop Lansdowne is laid up with dysentery... I was coming to ask you if you would look in on him. He doesn't trust our local physician."

"Be glad to… I haven't any medicine but I assume there is a pharmacy in Castries."

"Well, we get most of our medicine from our local clinic dispensary just up the road since it's more convenient. They have quite an impressive supply. You should find what you need without a problem."

There was a minute's pause, as both men sensed they had come to the closure of their small talk, of which the Bishop's bowel problems had been the centerpiece.

Jason spoke first.

"I sense you don't do much without specific purpose, Dr. Landry… Is this visit business or just pleasure?"

His eyes were on the therapist as he spoke, but the big man was looking at the sea and didn't return his gaze.

"Business,… but off the record, Jason. I've noticed that our last two sessions haven't been that fruitful and I thought I'd take the opportunity to talk with you on your own turf, so to speak, here on the beach."

He had turned to meet Jason's eyes and a disarming smile was beginning to crinkle his features.

"I'm not certain if your decreased participation in our sessions is a sign of progress or of resistance to the process?... It could be interpreted as either one."

Jason looked away.

Beyond the two men, standing chest-deep in the water, a lone fisherman whirled the glistening fan of his cast net into the air, the lead weights which hemmed its periphery landing with an audible sizzle on the surface of the sea.

Jason seemed to be studying the fisherman and didn't answer immediately. The question wasn't unexpected but he needed to prepare his answer. He was hesitating, reluctant to share with the therapist his own reflections on Landry's interpretation of the cause of his depression. He decided to buy some time for more reflection.

Turning back to Landry, smiling, he countered.

"You mean to say that you get ninety minutes of free time and you use it to engineer an open air therapy session with a patient you just saw this morning?"

The tall man shrugged his shoulders and a hint of embarrassment could be seen on his face.

"What can I say Jason, I may have left the rat race of Philadelphia but I've discovered that I carry the seeds of my workaholism inside me… The disapproval of one's own mother… it'll turn you into an overachiever, every time..."

"If you don't become a misogynist first..."

"Few men really turn on women, Jason. True misogynists are rare. Most of us just mix a bitter brew composed of equal parts of need and resentment and use it to fuel our interactions with the women in our lives."

"Firm in our ambiguity..." Jason cracked wryly.

"I guess you could say that ...Ambiguity about captures the essence of how we struggle with our conundrum."

"Can't live with them, can't live without them... that what you mean?"

“Not certain that it’s quite so simple. God, or whomever, has decreed that man enters the world from the womb and immediately grasps instinctively for a breast to survive. A good argument can be made that perhaps our whole existence as males is just one long pilgrimage to return again to the breast and the womb.”

“And that’s not simple?” asked Jason cocking his head to look into the face of his therapist who had looked away to the sea again.

“No, not simple at all, but perhaps that’s how God intended it. Man’s eternal task may be to re-forge that union with a woman, to become a part of her again… And, the equivalent task for a woman, seems to be to love her husband more than her child… Twin impossibilities for most ordinary folks.”

“I’ve never heard it put it quite that way before.”

“Never realized it myself until just now… the wisdom of the moment so to speak… profound today, puerile tomorrow.”

“You could be right about the search for unity… but I think most of us men stop short of the goal and settle for a nice breast and just the entrance to the womb…”

“You don’t really believe that, do you, Jason? At least, it isn’t true for you, is it?”

“Maybe I just wish it were. I still remember your lecture on my dependency,” and he smiled to soften the implicit criticism of Landry. “A lot of men seem satisfied with that kind of superficiality in their relationships with women, and, frankly speaking, I think it would be a relief if I could feel the way they do about it.”

Jason had drawn up his knees and was hugging them as he made himself small enough to fit into his therapist’s angular shadow.

“Not much chance of that with the mother you had… “began the doctor, but before Landry could complete his thought, Jason interrupted.

"Lay off my mother, doc. You know how I react every time she comes up in our discussions." There was irritation in his voice and he'd averted his eyes as if examining a blemish on his kneecap.

"That's what I'm trying to get at Jason. You resist exploring how your childhood, during which you were the sole intimate of such an extraordinary woman, imprinted you. In my opinion, it set a pattern that your intense relationship with your wife just continued."

"Wasn't that your point about male-female interaction?... I can't imagine a struggle to 'return to the womb' as anything but intense. Shouldn't it be the same for all of us men?"

"All of us didn't have a famous concert pianist for a mother who gave up a career on the stages of the world to teach piano lessons in Albany, Georgia so she could raise her son as a single parent."

"I didn't ask her to do that."

"You were her child, Jason. That fact alone became an imperative for a woman like her."

"Obviously, my father didn't share her commitment."

"Few fathers do..."

"And that's part of my problem too..."

Jason smiled wryly and looked back at the therapist who answered in a calm voice, knowing that Jason was beating himself up for having left his children.

"We can talk about your kids in a few minutes, Jason. You're too hard on yourself when it comes to them."

"Well, my mother is a tough act to follow... In fact, so is my wife..."

"Exactly. I've noticed how you seem offended when I raise the issue of your dependency, even indirectly."

"It's just that I'd prefer talking about my hemorrhoids... at least we could both agree that I really do *have* hemorrhoids."

"It has a lot to do with your depression, Jason."

"My hemorrhoid condition?" he smirked.

"No, your dependency."

"We may be getting into value judgments here, Brigham. You know I don't share your views on how close people should get in a relationship."

"Well, to avoid a futile disagreement, would you agree that both your mother and your wife were extraordinary women?"

Even the mention of the two women in the same sentence brought a rush of emotion to Jason's throat. He silently nodded his acquiescence.

"And that you feel as if part of you died with each of them, leaving you immeasurably diminished?" continued the therapist.

Jason nodded again.

"If I remember your history correctly, you were torn between medicine and a career as a concert pianist yourself, weren't you?"

Jason nodded a third time.

"And yet, you haven't played a note since your mother died?"

"My music was a part of her… I think I played so she could see herself… a small part of herself that she had invested in me."

He paused and rubbed his chin with a forefinger. When he spoke again his voice was flat and matter of fact, squeezed dry of all emotion, and at odds with the expression on his face.

"When she was gone, so was my motivation to play. I guess, when I think of it, I've never played unless I've been inspired by a woman I've loved."

"A bit extreme as a reaction to the loss of your loved ones, don't you think, Jason? How many parts of yourself do you have left to bury with the women you love before you give up something essential to your own continued existence?" asked the therapist.

Jason shifted his hand from his chin to his forehead. He was obviously troubled.

After a long empty moment, he asked, "And what part of me did I bury with Annette, Dr. Landry?" His voice had become almost tremulous and his eyes were downcast.

"Well, only you can answer that, Jason… what's left now that she's gone?"

There was another longer pause.

When Jason spoke his voice was still husky with emotion.

"Until several nights ago, I could have said 'not much' but now, I'm more hopeful… I'm discovering, while I'm here, that there may be more to me than I thought."

"If that's true, maybe what I've sensed in our sessions is healing and not resistance." Landry sounded genuinely relieved.

Jason managed a half-smile.

"A spark of hope, Brigham ?... Small beginnings?"

"I don't know what happened to you Jason but the change I've seen in you in therapy recently couldn't be the result of anything small."

"I had what you might term a private spiritual experience that had a very beneficial effect on my moods. I do feel better but I'm not out of the woods yet. The fact that I can get irritated with you for labeling me 'dependent' is progress, in my mind."

"I never meant to label you, Jason." Landry's tone was almost apologetic.

"Well, then I guess I've labeled myself… My expectations of what a relationship should be have always been so lofty… but the results of my best efforts have been dashed to bits… not once, but twice… I'm almost afraid to try again."

"Is that how you feel, Jason, like a failure…?" Landry sat up straight and placed a reassuring hand on his patient's knee.

"Essentially, yes. At least, emotionally. Like I said, I'd prefer not to care so profoundly for the women I love, to be more adequate on my own, but then something pretty profound and visceral in me rebels at the proposition that we should remain distant enough to be safe from the kind of devastation that I'm wading through now."

He reached down with one hand and began sifting sand through his fingers, working them deep into the cool moisture below the surface then rising with the damp blackness to lay it out for attack by the sun, the photons leveling the rough edges of the minuscule mounds one grain at a time.

"With Annette, I thought I had found the path, the grail, the goal… whatever you want to call it. I invested every atom of my being in our relationship and the return on my risk was more than I could ever have hoped for and then… BAM! The cosmic fist smashes down and she's gone… and most of me is gone with her. It's more than enough to make me question whether I'm flawed in some elemental way. There's not much resolve left to start again, you know… not much more than a hope for a new beginning."

"And the children?"

The older man's voice was soft, encouraging.

"What do they mean to you?"

"The children…" and Jason's voice trailed off for a moment… "Well, you know, Brigham, I love them… Hell, I'd die for them but I am so inept around them."

He shrugged his shoulders and let fall another handful of sand.

"It was like I needed Annette to translate for me, to make me acceptable and important to them. I see them now with her not around and it's like she was the link coupling us. We're like railcars edging slowly apart. They know it and so do I but we don't say anything because there just aren't words enough to mend the problem. We were a unit with her and now we're just components drifting along without even the mechanisms to dock with one another. I can't even think about them without a band of guilt being snapped around my heart like a slap on an open wound."

He had found the freedom to talk of his pain with Dr. Landry during his therapy and a measure of relief had followed. But relief wasn't answers.

"What'll I do, Brigham? I know I'll survive now. I can even feel the weight of the depression lifting, but how do I get back into my life?... Pick up the pieces?... Connect with my children?"

The outgoing tide was rolling a bent palm trunk slowly away from the shore. Three black children were laughing and splashing, crawling aboard the trunk only to be thrust off by the momentum of its spin.

"Children don't need as much as we do to survive in good health, Jason. Look at those kids out there," and he pointed to the boys on the log.

"What adult could find joy and companionship just crawling on a log with a friend? You could be reading more into the expectations of your children than there really is. You may not be everything they need but you could be enough... Ever dare think of it that way?"

Landry had lifted his hat to scratch his head.

"Maybe I have been thinking too much about my own losses," admitted Jason, "but I know the fear I've seen in their eyes... it's real. Unless I'm totally projecting my own doubts that we could make it on our own, they are in danger, too. When I think of myself as a father I feel pretty inadequate most of the time lately."

"I imagine your mother may have said something like that long ago."

A half smile curled Jason's lips as he seemed to be imagining his mother in the past.

"You didn't know my mother, Brigham. She may have played out that sentiment as a recurring theme during one of the many times I heard her get up in the middle of the night and improvise at the piano for hours... but she never would have said it. She was a woman of profound emotions but few words."

"And you've become a man of profound emotions and few notes..."

"No notes, Brigham. I don't play at all anymore."

"What would she say about that decision, Jason?... What did Annette have to say about it?"

"That was the joy about Annette, Brigham." said Jason tossing a handful of sand in the air then watching it fall before continuing, "She never wanted me to be anything but what I was..."

The sarcasm in his voice was muted but unmistakable.

"Well, maybe this is as good a line as any on which to end this conversation," said Landry. "I've found the answer to my question and I'm satisfied."

He grunted as he stirred himself in preparation for departure.

"I'm glad you stopped by, Brigham... I appreciate your concern."

Jason didn't want to feel responsible for having ended the impromptu session.

Landry guessed the source of his malaise and reassured him. "I truly am satisfied with our visit, Jason. You're making quite remarkable progress. It was just that you seemed to change almost overnight and I felt I needed to check things out between us."

As he finished speaking he hefted himself up to his full height and looked up and down the beach.

"You've got the place pretty much to yourself Jason... You seem to thrive out here. Maybe that's the secret of the change. Nature has a way of piecing together the scattered bits of our lives if we'll just allow her to heal us..."

The sun was behind Landry and Jason had shaded his eyes to keep from squinting. "Who could argue with that?" was all he said.

Trudging away with the sand wedging up under his sandals Dr. Brigham Landry spoke half over his shoulder. "Remember, Jason, trains gets re-arranged all the time... few cars end their journeys hooked to the same companions they started out with… life can be a little like that too," and he gave a blind wave of his hand as he headed back to the villa.

Jason sat immersed in thought hugging his knees and staring at the whitecaps etching the horizon.

* * *

Beyond the boundaries of the bay and the protection of the basalt promontory frothily shrugging off the surges of the Atlantic, a vigilante wind was assaulting the sea decapitating, in gushes of white vitality, any wave that raised its head. The distant commotion gave birth to large dark swells that rolled obliquely across the mouth of the cove to spend themselves in sibilant charges against the black sand of the far shore.

The net effect of the sea's dynamics was to produce a clockwise current that curled around the cove and herded blossoms and other bits of wind-harvested flotsam imperceptibly toward the churning open water just beyond the cliffs.

Almost distractedly, while he reflected upon his therapist's comments, Jason had followed the seaward progress of the coconut tree trunk, the plaything of the three young boys, as it was wafted farther into the swells. At first, the increased heaving of the heavy log seemed to heighten the challenge of remaining astride it. Animated shouts of glee bounced against the craggy cliff face and rebounded across to him. The children's poverty and deprivation hadn't dampened their enthusiasm for simple joys.

Abruptly, one end of the deformed trunk, warped during its life by years of prevailing winds, reared three feet out of the water on the crest of a swell and, like an angry serpent tired of being taunted, it spun and lashed the surface where a child paddled beneath it. A guttural cry of terror from the scene catapulted Jason to his feet. He could see only two heads bobbing where three children had been a moment earlier. One boy had begun thrashing toward the beach as if pursued by the demons of hell. The second child was attempting to cling to the offending log and cried out again in panic...

"Help.... Help!"

Jason was already sprinting along the sand to the east end of the cove where the drama was being played out. The trunk was almost 150 yards off the beach. His heart pounded with exertion and horror at the prospect of the death of a child.

As he raced into the water just before plunging headlong, he caught a flash of red hurtling into the void from the cliff's edge as a woman's body knifed into the water.

When he broke back to the surface his arms pistoning him toward the log, he could see another swimmer, far closer than he was, moving with smooth powerful strokes that ate up the distance separating her from the child and the log. He took a bearing and gasped to fill his lungs for a mad dash to join them.

Upon reaching the log he saw a young boy of perhaps eleven, eyes wide and face contorted by fear.

He sobbed.

"Daniel gone, he gone... oh, Daniel."

The woman was nowhere in sight.

Sucking in air as deeply as he was able, Jason plunged beneath the water. He expected crystal depths but when the water clapped its palms over his ears, instantaneously blotting out the turmoil on the surface, he blinked repeatedly but could see only a multitude of miniscule bubbles and gray depths. The turbulence of the previous night's storm had conspired to hide the boy.

He thrust himself down with heroic kicks equalizing the pressure against his eardrums as he dove. Darker shapes in the gray began to mushroom into vague perspective. He knew them to be the coral heads he'd snorkeled over a few days before when the water had been clearer. Luckily, the cove was relatively shallow in the area. With no mask to provide clear vision, a body in these waters would be no more than a blur. He searched turning his head from side to side during his descent. The child, even with his lungs full of water, shouldn't have sunk to the bottom yet. He reached toward a blotch vaguely resembling a stand of staghorn coral and pulled on a branch to propel himself over the edge of the coral head and into the gloom below.

His lungs began to slam at his glottis with painful rhythmic contractions demanding oxygen. He obeyed the imperative and thrust toward the light above him porposing his whole body to maximize the speed of ascent. His head and shoulders shattered the surface four feet from the tree trunk that was swiveling dangerously once again on the crest of a swell. Still no one in sight except the child who had barnacled himself to the monster that had struck his playmate.

He filled his lungs again and plunged back into the depths pushing himself through the opaque gray zone before the coral shadows loomed once more. Curling around another coral head he startled a school of large fish that detonated away from him in small silvery explosions.

He pulled himself through the water to a second coral head and, as he rounded it, he saw a flicker of red beside a darker object a few yards away. Approaching, he could make out a woman struggling to free a child's body from entangling sea fans. The child's limbs wavered lifelessly animated only by her tugs on his hair and jockey shorts.

Jason reached for the boy's head and wound his fingers into the wiry locks then, planting his feet firmly against the coral, he thrust upward with his legs and the child rose with him. The woman climbed past him toward the surface, literally snatching at the water, her desperate movements betraying her imprudence in overextending herself. His own lungs were screaming again but the child seemed to weigh hundreds of pounds and the surface seemed to recede even as he pedaled desperately toward it.

A gush of air. A flash of sky. Resistance gone. Sucking in air. Then the tug of the boy's weight reminding him.

"Go to the rocks… the rocks!" she shouted over the ringing in his ears.

The woman had already turned the child onto his back, lifting him under one armpit and obviously expecting Jason to mirror her efforts on the other side.

He heard her voice again, sharp and commanding but without panic, speak to the second child.

"You, there, boy. Let go of the tree and follow us… Now! Dammit… Now!"

He could see the other boy, eyes still screaming wide, relax his death-grip on the trunk and begin a hesitant crawl after them.

"Get to the ledge, straight ahead… He's bradycardic but he still has a pulse."

Her arm beneath the child's arm was positioned so that her fingers could overlay the carotid artery as well as keep his chin out of the water. It was all Jason could do to keep pace with her as they almost surged toward a low shelf of basalt carved by a millennium of erosive waves breaking upon it.

"Take his whole weight, I'll get up first and pull him up," she ordered.

Assuming that he'd comply with her instructions, she turned, grasped the edge of the ledge and, timing her efforts to coincide with the rise of a swell, hoisted herself lithely onto the slippery basalt.

"Pass him up to me… one arm is good enough…."

She spoke through a curtain of copper hair as she bent forward toward Jason and his burden.

He raised the boy's arm and was surprised by the strength with which she gripped it and lifted. The child was more than half out of the water.

Jason sidled between the boy's legs and heaved upward with his hands under the thighs but the force of his effort simply drove him below the surface. While still submerged, he searched for a foothold on the cliff wall, located an outcropping with his right foot and pushed again. This time he rose and the child's body disappeared over the lip of the ledge.

A moment later, when he pulled himself up beside them, she was already rescue breathing. The small black face was ashen gray. The eyes stared blankly from beneath half-closed lids. Behind and below them, the second child had seen the water frothing at the ledge and chosen to strike out for the beach swimming for all he was worth.

Jason knew that if the victim's stomach were distended with water, as it surely was, the pressure would increase the difficulty of forcing air into sodden lungs. Timing his thrusts with the rescue breathing he pressed twice firmly and rapidly into the epigastrium just below the ribs. Water fairly shot from the child's mouth and Jason thought he felt the diaphragm jerk in spasm against his fingers.

"He's working at breathing… keep going… you're doing great…," he puffed.

He surprised himself with the calm undertone of his voice until he realized that he was functioning just as he'd been trained to do. An adrenaline assist. Reflexes honed to razor sharpness by years of learning and ER practice coming into play. He checked the pulse.

"Weak but up to over 70… wish I had my stethoscope…"

She smiled wryly at him through ribbons of hair, her head bent prepared to deliver another breath.

"Use your ear, doctor… We didn't always have stethoscopes…"

"Yes, of course…." and he bent and placed his ear to the child's chest first on the right then on the left.

"Adequate air exchange bilaterally… The water's being driven into the bloodstream and his lungs are clearing" he reported.

Just then the boy's arms shot into rigidity beside his body and he buckled at the waist in a wordless spasm. Another gush of water exploded from his lips. He coughed several times and then began to whimper. His eyelids fluttered and light re-appeared in the pupils… confusion and fear… but alive. His chest rose slowly several times, air coursing through his swollen trachea with a vibrant high-pitched whistle and then he cried again, lustily and full force, arms and legs flexing instinctively as his spirit re-infused the body from which it had been driven by the sea.

Jason listened again at his chest… a few scattered wheezes but the air was reaching the bases of both lungs virtually unimpeded. It was better than he had expected.

He glanced across at the woman. Her eyes were closed and the fingers of her hands were tented against her temples. Her head was tilted back and he thought he saw her lips quivering in what might have been a whispered prayer… or simply exhausted relief. She was beautiful and, when he noted how her long bronze tresses fell across her breasts, with a flush of excitement that tightened his throat, he recognized her as the woman he'd seen on the beach several nights before.

She finished her moment's pause and checked the pulse once again.

"Can you hear me Daniel?... Tell me if you can hear me, son…" she asked.

The child's large eyes rolled up to fix on her face above his head... a tortured voice scrabbled up the ravaged slopes of his throat. Something unintelligible... then he coughed and said weakly… "I hear you, missus…"

"You are going to be fine Daniel. You have a nasty bump on your head," and she smiled as she let her fingers outline a large contusion swelling up above the child's right eye.

"Headache?"

"Yes, missus… big headache..." he replied more strongly, grimacing as he spoke.

"Can you see my fingers, Daniel?"

She waved her hand to draw his gaze and then held up two fingers.

"How many fingers do you see, Daniel?"

"Two, missus, I see two."

"Good boy," and she bent and kissed him on the forehead.

He smiled wanly and she lifted his head to cradle it on her knees where her legs were folded under her. The sun was blazing down mercilessly and she positioned a hand to shield the child's eyes.

"Just lie still, Daniel. Don't try to move, son," she whispered as she caressed his shoulder reassuringly with her free hand.

A large swell struck the cliff face below with a 'whump' and foam and water hissed around their knees covering the ledge. Surprise and fear flashed back into the boy's face and, this time, Jason spoke to reassure him.

"We're safe here, Daniel. We're both with you. You don't need to be afraid of the waves."

As he spoke, he lifted the child's legs and lay them on his own. The more flesh and the less water the boy felt, the calmer he would be.

From above them on the cliff a voice called.

"Are you alright, Mr. Jason Turner, sir?" There was sincere concern in the query.

Jason recognized the distinctive East Indian accent.

"Yes, Mohammed, I'm fine but we need to get this boy off the ledge and to St. Jude's hospital immediately."

"We are three strong men up here, sir, and we have plenty of rope... Shall I drop it down to you, sir?"

Jason peered upward and saw Mohammed and the fisherman who had been casting his throw nets. The man must have run for help as soon as Jason started to the scene. He held up his arm.

"Yes, let the rope down carefully."

The rope bounced in its descent, the wind swinging it momentarily to the right. Luckily, it was the pliable braided half-inch soft nylon used to moor yachts and wouldn't bite into the skin.

He took it and allowed his muscle memory to fashion a fireman's sling around the boy's thighs and under his arms. Ten years of boy scouts a century ago and this one occasion made all the ritualistic knot tying that he had done for merit badges worthwhile.

The boy was whimpering again and had clutched the woman's arm tightly in terrified hands.

"Oh, missus, Daniel afraid..."

Calmly, her voice soothing and reassuring, she held his gaze while she signaled with her hand for the rope to be hoisted.

"Daniel, you are safe but you need to stay quiet in this rope chair... I'll be with you as soon as I can," she soothed.

Despite her efforts, he began wailing mournfully but permitted her to transfer his grip to the rope that was now lifting him.

Jason stood up on his toes guiding the child's ascent as long as possible.

"Mohammed, watch his head. Don't let it swing into the rocks."

The East Indian, lying on his belly, reached out over the cliff top and, with all his force, held the rope away from the rock his rapidly moving hands functioning almost as a pulley. The ascent was without incident and three pairs of hands plucked the child from sight.

Mohammed's face returned.

"Do you wish now to come up, Mr. Jason Turner?'

Jason surveyed the forty rugged feet to the top then glanced at the sea washing foamy at his feet.

"I'll swim back, Mohammed, but perhaps the lady…"

His offer was cut short as the woman dove lightly into the water and surfaced heading toward the beach.

Jason looked back up at the East Indian.

"Mohammed, take the boy directly to St. Jude's casualty room and tell them what happened. I'm sure he'll be alright but he needs to be watched."

"I will, sir… you may count on me, Mr. Jason Turner," and he was gone.

CH016

Jason's years of regular swimming had taught him to love the water. During thousands of laps in the pool three days a week he had learned to think while his limbs moved smoothly without specific attention.

Now, as he stroked easily toward the beach, he thought about the woman who had just saved the child. She had called him 'doctor' and yet he had never met her. He knew he wouldn't have forgotten if they had been introduced. He was virtually certain that their encounter on the beach that night earlier in the week had been one-sided, so, how did she know who he was?

As he imagined her in his mind's eye, he felt a soft tremor begin inside him like the quivering of a silken web strand laden with a dewdrop or a violin string under the caress of the bow. Some subtle emotion was struggling to be recognized, acknowledged.

He didn't know her; had never spoken to her before to day, but together, they had saved a child's life and the intensity of the experience seemed to wash away the need for formality between them.

As he swam, the awareness of his attraction to her began to drift as softly as snowflakes into his consciousness and he found the sensation both soothing and disconcerting. Lately, he had been attempting to re-engineer his values so that solitude without a partner could become a peaceful fulfilled state. But stirring, probing, deep in his unconsciousness, like a seed in rich soil deprived of light, was an elemental need to be joined to a woman.

His toes flittered across the sandy bottom and he drifted with the remnant of his momentum for a few more feet before drawing his legs under him to stand. She sat on the sand arms wrapped around drawn up knees... The same posture she had assumed the night he first saw her. Her face was turned his way and her eyes followed him with such attention that he felt embarrassment, as if she had been reading his thoughts and had found herself standing naked in them.

He ran his hand through his hair squeezing water onto his shoulders, more for something to do than with purposeful intent. Stretching his arms wide, he bounced them backwards against the limits of their range of motion and felt the stretching of his pectoral muscles as he did so.

"Well, that was some adventure... more than I signed up for when I came here but it seems to have ended well..." he said flashing a self-conscious smile at her that invited some comment.

He was close enough to her now to see a twinkle of amusement in her eyes which were hazel and had bright yellow flecks glistening in the pupils like gold dust. He was struck by the similarity to Brigham Landry's eyes.

"Yes, it turned out to be an adventure but it could have been a tragedy if you hadn't happened along," she said.

"You're quite a swimmer."

He was standing above her and she shaded her face from the sun with her hand as she looked up at him. He flushed at the directness of her gaze and her compliment.

"Thank goodness you arrived before I did, or I wouldn't have found him. Where were you, anyway?" he asked.

"The sun and I have an adversarial relationship," she replied. "If I allow myself to become too familiar, he punishes me by blotching my face with freckles, so I often sit and read under the large Banyan tree up on the point," and she gestured to the lone giant perched precariously at the eroding edges of the cliff.

"I was there, just musing on the vicissitudes of life, when I heard the cries."

"So you leapt from the cliff top?" He asked incredulously, knowing all the while where she'd come from.

"Didn't leap, dove… but yes, I came from the top."

He grinned, "Quite a daredevil…"

"Not really. Instinct took over, I think, what with a child being in danger and all…" She let her words drift into nothingness, lowered her eyes and shrugged in a gesture of self-deprecation. The admiration she saw in his eyes made her distinctly ill at ease. Her view of self couldn't accommodate the sentiment it aroused.

As if by common consent, she had arisen from her crouch and, as she brushed the sand from her buttocks, they started off down the beach in the direction of the Renaissance buildings walking side by side.

"I'm curious," he said, "you called me 'doctor' on the ledge. Do you know me from somewhere?"

She didn't look at him, her eyes seems focused on some thought floating a few inches in front of her that she was examining before deciding whether to put it into words or not. Instead, she responded with her own question.

"Do you recall ever seeing me?"

He hoped he didn't blush as the night scene of her standing naked in the moonlight flashed across the screen of his mind.

"No... um, we've never been introduced…," he replied weaseling neatly out of the unexpected pinch her question had created.

She laughed, a lilting twinkle that ran half way up the scale then back down, before stooping to snatch up a handful of sand that she studied for a moment as if it contained some omen to be read and heeded. He was certain he had blushed when her laugh had startled him but he didn't know exactly why.

"Well," she said suddenly stopping, and tendering her empty right hand to shake, "I'm Amy Davis and I'm a patient at the Renaissance Center."

"Sounds a bit like an introduction at a closed AA meeting," he said with an attempt at humor, extending his own hand and taking hers.

"I'm Jason Turner and I'm a patient at the Renaissance center too."

He was surprised at the firmness of her grip and remembered how she had hoisted the child so easily up to the ledge.

"I know that much, I must admit… I asked Mohammed who you were after I saw you once in the middle of the night just sitting quietly at the grand piano in the foyer… Were you meditating?"

"No, just remembering… I used to play…"

"Used to play?"

Her question was probing and it made him uneasy. He decided to utilize her stratagem and answer with a question of his own.

"What were you doing up in the middle of the night watching me at the piano? I thought I was alone… just me and my memories."

"Nothing menacing, I promise you. It was quite incidental. I was returning from a walk and a swim. I find it relaxing to be the only one awake and about… It sort of lets me be myself without the need for pretense, or for that matter, etiquette. Alone, I can do whatever I want. I guess that's something I'm learning to do more often but I still find it easier at night than in the light of day with others observing me."

She was stirring the sand in her left palm with her right forefinger and studying it.

He was glad she seemed absorbed. It freed him to appraise her without appearing impolite. She was a head shorter than he was but still tall and she had long legs with trim thighs. Her body, which had seemed petite to him on the night of his voyeuristic encounter, was more medium build with her arms and shoulders showing an unusual amount of muscular definition for a woman. Her neck was long but not overly slender and, when he looked carefully at her face in profile and imagined her hair bouffant and full, he realized that she was also the woman from the plane. Could she have been the woman from the taxi too? He found his reflections startling and unsettling.

She looked up and caught his eyes on her.

"You look like you've seen a ghost... I realize I'm not at my best, what with my hair all stringy and full of the sea, but I didn't think I looked frightful." She pursed her lips in mock disapproval. Unlike the admiration of her character that he had expressed earlier, a man studying her physical beauty was something Amy was accustomed to and found unthreatening.

He struggled to control his emotions and master a normal tone when he spoke. He hoped that the knot of muscle that began working in his jaw at times of stress wouldn't be noticed and betray his internal disarray. Annette had called it his 'stress spasm' and teased him that he could never lie to her because of it.

"You remind me of someone...," despite himself, he stammered... "Someone that I used to know..." and his voice trailed off lamely.

She responded brightly, "I know... red hair and freckles... Little Orphan Annie... I've been told that before."

He turned to look at her in surprise and it was his turn to chuckle in amusement. With her humor, she'd freed him from his growing discomfort.

"Nope, you have pupils."

"Well, thanks... Little Orphan Annie with pupils," she retorted.

He laughed again and she joined him easily.

"You and Little Orphan Annie have absolutely nothing in common."

"Be careful, Dr. Turner, you don't know me yet… and remember, I'm a mental patient."

Her eyes twinkled mischievously. She was beginning to enjoy her role… the beautiful woman toying sexually with an interested male. She hadn't played the role overtly in years, since before her marriage.

"I don't think of myself as a mental patient," he protested. "I'm just, well, depressed…"

"Twenty-five thousand dollars worth of depression, unless Dr. Landry passes on professional discounts to fellow physicians, is probably more than '*just*' depressed."

"Well it was pretty bad. I really couldn't function acceptably but I've improved a great deal since I've been here."

His tone had suddenly grown grave.

"And you?" he asked.

"Oh, a mixed bag of problems, I guess. I've been trying to get a handle on my emotional life for years now and never been able to truly do it. I heard of Dr. Landry from a friend and I had twenty-five thousand dollars just gathering dust under my mattress… so, here I am in this tropical paradise where virtually nothing reminds me of my problems…"

She affected nonchalance as she spoke by picking up tresses of her damp hair and combing it with spread fingers, having let the sand she'd been examining drop from her hand.

"I think I've concluded that my own steps toward recovery have been attributable more to the peace and tranquility of this place and the sun, the sea, the sand…," he gestured with an arm, "than the therapy. But, if I get well, it doesn't matter how it happened, it's worth the price."

"I feel that way too. But, my best moments are when I'm volunteering at the little charity clinic and see how much better off I am than the truly needy people here in St. Lucia..."

"Clinic?"

"Yes, there's a little place just down the road. It belongs to some small Canadian non-governmental organization. They set it up years ago and it's staffed by rotating medical volunteers but Canadians only get two months of decent weather a year, so no one wants to junket in the Caribbean during the summer. They have no nurse or physician right now and, since I'm a registered nurse, I fill in three afternoons a week. I find the work fulfilling. It helps me to value myself a little more highly… I've had a problem with self-esteem. At least, according to Dr. Landry, it's a major area I need to work on."

She blushed and suddenly realized that the admission was taking her too much out of character. Too much honesty. Too soon.

"According to the great Dr. Landry…" he repeated with obvious sarcasm. "I guess it's because I'm getting better, but I've found myself disagreeing with him more often on interpretations of behavior. He might be wrong, you know."

"His omniscience can get on my nerves too, and at first, I had some serious misgivings about being here, but now, I'm grateful to him and the clinic. If I hadn't come, I'm sure I'd have simply sunk deeper into the mire of my psychopathology..."

"Mire of your psychopathology... You really have a way with words," he said, raising his eyebrows in mock surprise.

"Hadn't noticed. Like I mentioned, I have a problem with self-esteem… everywhere except at the clinic that is. There, I feel almost important, or at least needed, I guess. I'm not sure how to put it into words… so perhaps I'm not as good with them as you think."

"Do you always try to slide out from under a compliment like that?" he asked. She blushed and made a pretense of examining a cuticle.

"You've had too much psychotherapy, doctor… you've begun practicing it," she replied, brushing the last vestiges of sand from her hands with crisp efficient movements.

They were approaching the Renaissance beach and the cook, a ship of a woman weighing over 300 pounds called Mama Jo, was waddling toward them as fast as her stumpy legs could carry her.

The woman's body was as broad from front to back as she was tall. Her saturated metabolism had stored fat cell upon fat cell until her upper arms approached the thickness of most people's thighs and jutted out from her body at angles like the wings of a wounded goose. Her face was knurled and seamed with fleshy crevasses that provoked the memory, in Jason's mind, of the manatee woman at the customs bench in the Castries airport. They were surely close relatives.

She puffed prodigiously from the effort of walking in sand and, when she spoke, it was in little emphysemic clutches of words wheezed out to the rhythm of rapid respirations.

"Miz Amy, child... is you alright?... me prayed... to dee… Lord God… Oh, me prayed… when me hear… you try… tuh save… poor drown… Daniel… He be mine… me grandchild…"

"Mama Jo, he will be fine. We got to him soon enough. He was talking and smiling and, after one night at the American hospital he will be home."

"Oh, tanks be tuh God…" cried the cook and sank to the sand with her hands clasped and head bowed. Her flower print dress tented out around her bulk on the sand giving the impression that she her body weight was causing her to sink into the beach.

Amy dropped to one knee and put her hand on the woman's arm while the cook wheezed out expressions of gratitude to the heavens.

Jason felt awkward. He sensed he should be doing something besides standing there but his instincts abandoned him in situations of effusive female emotion. Sidling uneasily closer to Amy, he placed a hand tentatively on her right shoulder thereby connecting him indirectly to the woman's upheaval. Amy glanced up at him approvingly.

Mamma Jo finished her ablations and raised her eyes to Amy.

"My heart… me gives… it to you... Miss Amy ."

Then, suddenly the woman's eyes, set like liquid brown marbles deep in the hollows of her face, widened in alarm.

"Heavens child!… you be hurt… see dee blood… all dee blood…" And a pudgy finger stabbed the air aiming at Amy's left side.

Amy didn't turn to look but Jason twisted to follow the finger and saw a darker hue of red pasting the crimson tissue of her one piece swimsuit to Amy's body from breast to hip.

"It's only a scratch, Mamma Joe. It doesn't hurt and I'll clean it up when I get to my cabin... Don't forget, I'm a nurse…!"

"But him…," and she gestured to Jason, "… be a doctor… Miss Amy… an blood… like dat… needs sewed… for sure."

But, even as she spoke, it was apparent from the calming of the animated furrows of flesh on her face that Amy's words had reassured her.

As Amy stood up, the woman's arms came up in a silent plea for assistance in rising. Amy took one arm and Jason the other but even their combined efforts required several repositioning of their stances before the woman was finally standing.

"Dee sand an' me... ain't no friends... him suck me down... an hol' me tight... every time," huffed the woman.

All three were puffing with exertion as they herded her towards the slope of the steps leading to the kitchen. When she was safely supported by the two railings and inching upwards with the creak of the tortured stairs groaning an accompaniment, Jason spoke.

"She's right, you know... that's not an inconsequential laceration judging from the blood flow. How did it happen?"

She grinned sheepishly and re-arranged her long bronze tresses so they camouflaged her injury more effectively. She didn't look down at the wound.

"My breasts have never been a point of pride in my life", she lied, " but they've never been a hindrance either like they are to many women. Today, is really the first time I can remember one of them getting seriously in the way. I scraped myself on the ledge when I hauled out.. It stings a bit, nothing more."

"I suspect that you're minimizing again. If it were someone else's laceration, mine for example, I sense you'd show more concern."

There was no tone of lecture in his voice... just a simple statement.

"Aren't we all like that... medical personnel I mean?"

"In fact, in my experience, we're not... I have a good friend, a general surgeon, who almost calls a code if he gets a boo-boo of any significance."

She laughed lightly.

They were already on the walkway leading to their cabins and the shadows of palm fronds tossing in the wind above them flashed across the yellow brick in kaleidoscopic patterns of light and dark. She seemed to have quickened her pace and kept to his left to hide the wound from him and avoid more expressions of concern.

"Believe me, Jason... may I call you that?'

"Please do..."

"Well, believe me Jason when I tell you that I've coped silently with worse boo-boos than this scratch."

"In the jungles of Vietnam sludging through the undergrowth during your stint with the special forces, I assume."

The sarcasm in his voice was soft and teasing.

"You're amusing Jason. I wouldn't have expected it of you... humor from a depressed doctor and all."

"You've forgotten that I am a mental patient here. My soul is damaged and I seek escape from my misery in multiple personalities of which you've only seen one", and he hummed the theme from the 'Twilight Zone' and let at least three caricatures of his normal facial expression play sequentially across his features.

She laughed and put her hands on her cheeks while shaking her head in a gesture of disbelief. The action fanned out her hair, which glistened in the sunlight. Her shoulders were as smooth as polished stone and mottled attractively with what she had alluded to as the sun's curse.

He felt an almost overwhelming desire to touch her skin.

A parrot bulleted across the path in front of them with snapping wings, a blaze of red and green. As different from its caged cousins in the north as individuals of the same species could be, it reminded Jason of how far from his world they truly were.

"Well, here I am, home away from home," she said stopping in front of the path to her cabin.

"Promise me you'll call me if the wound needs suturing… after all, what are neighbors for…?"

He was loath to see her leave.

"I promise... thank-you for your concern."

She held out her hand and he took it lightly in his own. It wasn't a simple handshake and they both knew it.

"Till next we meet then? Perhaps I'll attend one of your nocturnal recitals."

She'd intended the remark to be nothing but pleasant banter, however, his eyes suddenly clouded over and he looked at the ground and began tracing the line between two tiles with his toe.

"I don't play anymore… but, perhaps we could go for a swim together. I still do that."

"When my enemy the sun has run from the night I'd be happy to join you," she said.

They had still been holding hands and she tugged gently to signal that she was leaving.

"Then it's a date?"

She'd already turned toward her cottage and the sunlight slating through the overhanging palms teased flashes of amber from her hair.

Over her shoulder she called, "Yes, doctor, it's a date," and she tossed a little wave of her right hand in a parting gesture.

"Jason," he called out, "just Jason."

He watched till she disappeared inside then stood for several minutes looking at the potted orchids hanging on either side of the doorway and imagining her still there.

CH017: JECKYL ISLAND, GEORGIA

The shadows were lengthening and stretching the silhouette of the palm leaf palapas, under which Mark West sat, into a narrow caricature of itself. Fifty yards away, the pounding surf generated a pungent aerosol of salt and sea scent to drift imperceptibly over the patio's restaurant leaving a residue invisible everywhere but on the lenses of his glasses.

A capricious breeze riffled through the desiccated palm fronds of the palapas producing an intermittent electric buzz, as if some huge winged insect had been caught among them and was struggling to escape. Despite the onshore breeze, the air was still heavy with the fading heat of the day. He touched the condensation-beaded side of his second scotch and ice to his temple.

Beside him on the table, lay the accusing tatter of his manuscript on Healthcare Management. No physician with aspirations of bestriding the medical world at the head of a large HMO could ignore the imperative to publish. It had gotten to the point where a physician-executive, without his name prominently in print, wasn't worth the price of a used stethoscope. So, Mark West was never far from his incomplete manuscript. In fact, it was the excuse he had used to be here in Jeckyl Island. Like a nagging sciatica, from which it seemed there would be no lasting relief, the unfinished tome dogged him wherever he went.

However this afternoon, as he waited the arrival of Randal Smith, the private detective Milton Kleinberg was sending to brief him on the background checks of TurnerWest's physicians, the manuscript and its quiet curse would have been a dangerous distraction. He needed his wits about him since the vice-president of Cumberland had told him he had several potential courses of action to destabilize Turner's position on the merger that needed West's collaboration.

That he had asked West to discuss them with Smith seemed to indicate that the detective enjoyed Kleinberg's full confidence although Smith hadn't been identified to him as the liaison person Kleinburg had mentioned earlier that he would send. He picked up the manuscript and stuffed it under the table onto an empty chair... out of sight, out of mind.

The anticipation of the actual information on TurnerWest's physicians, that Kleinberg had described as 'promising' in their cryptic telephone conversation, had kept West off his golf game that morning to the point where he'd paid the caddy off at the fifteenth hole and asked to be dropped at his car. He was anxious to move into action as quickly as possible since Jason Turner's absence was scheduled to be two months at the most, not much time to effectively undermine his partner's support among the other physicians in the group.

Smith was already a half-hour late and whatever West's vices may have been, he was obsessive about punctuality. His emotions had been growling in discontent since the ice from his first scotch had melted to a hazy gloom in the bottom of the tumbler. He was to the point of cursing Kleinberg's choice of messenger when, between the booms of the surf, he heard the scuff of feet on the stone of the walkway leading from the indoor portion of the restaurant. He turned to look.

A man of medium height and corpulent build was slouching over the stones in his general direction. He wore a white Panama hat, the brim of which wavered as he walked. A vividly patterned short sleeved shirt revealed muscular forearms and massive fists disproportionately large for his stature. Beige knee-length shorts with multiple pockets, which would have seemed out of place with anything but a pith helmet and knee socks, completed his attire. In one hand he casually carried a thick orange file folder.

If he was Smith, West wondered, '*What the hell is the point of a clandestine meeting at the tip of Jeckyl Island when he dresses like a clown trying to be the center of attention?*'

Although there were only a handful of customers enjoying a sunset cocktail, every head swiveled to study the newcomer.

'Damn, this is starting out well,' West mumbled sarcastically as the man continued toward the table at the edge of the patio where West had sequestered himself. He began talking loudly as he approached.

"Dr. West?"

The voice had a gravelly quality to it that made the words sound heavy.

"I'm Randall Smith... sorry I'm late. I hate bridges and that damn causeway was so long it reminded me of a nauseating trip I made to Key West once. Gotta say, I'm not impressed with these streaks of sand that get everybody's vacation juices flowing. My room here is a pit with puke-yellow carpeting that smells like they shampoo it with cat piss. I've seen better decorating taste in YMCA locker rooms."

Arriving at the table, he tendered his huge right hand.

West tried to hide his instant disgust and took the ham-sized paw but his irritation was audible in his voice.

"Good thing I was Dr. West. You almost gave me your whole report before you knew who I was, Mr. Smith."

The fat man, whose belly bulged over the top of his shorts like bread dough rising over the edge of a mixing bowl, didn't react. He pulled up a chair and sighing deeply lowered himself into it, then dropped the orange folder on the table.

"What are you drinking doc?" he said picking up West's empty glass and sniffing it. "Can learn a lot 'bout a man by what he drinks."

West screwed up the edge of his mouth skeptically.

"And what do my drinking habits say about me, Mr. Smith?"

Smith grinned slyly, "I'll save that till later doc. I'll just say that there was about as much chance of me not picking you out in this group as there was of me offering a bone to the wrong end of my Rottweiller."

West's face reddened.

"Whichever end of your dog you prefer to attend to hasn't much to do with our business, Smith. Shall we get on with it?"

The detective smirked as if he were enjoying West's pique.

"Hey, why not?" and raising an arm he snapped his blunt fingers loudly.

"The spic waiter over there has got the same problem that killed the cat. He's been standing behind that bar watching me since I stepped through the door… Think I'll give him a chance to study me up close… Maybe pose for him in my new outfit. Whattaya think of my duds, doc? I can see you've got an eye for style… Think I might get lucky to-night with one of those school marms?" and he waved to a group of four young women sitting at a table on the far end of the patio.

To West's amazement one of them actually waved back.

The sooner West could finish with this character the better. His eyes said as much.

The Chicano waiter, despite having been out of sight behind Smith's back when he snapped his fingers, appeared as predicted.

"Yes, sir, may I help you?"

Smith winked at West who shook his head dismissively.

"Sure can, Pedro. Get me four bottles of Corona and stick them in one of those champagne buckets with some ice."

The waiter acknowledged the order and left.

"My duds, doc?" Smith repeated sarcastically.

"Still no opinion... C'mon now, we need a little small talk to fool anyone spying on us. Maybe there's a techno-snoop listening to us from that grove of bamboo over there with one of those parabolic mikes they use to pick up the players' profanity at football games," and he laughed aloud at the obvious growing contempt on West's face.

West turned away wordlessly as if to study the surf. Smith continued on without pause.

"Do you know, I swear I heard Dan Marino fart once over one of those mikes... a real nose reamer. The players were huddling see, and suddenly they all jump back except Marino, and then the guy with the parabolic mike and headset on the sidelines starts dancing around busting a gut laughing. Damn near dropped the thing... Amazing what technology can do, ain't it doc?" and he grinned at the side of West's face.

"Look doc, we don't have to like each other. I'll bet you were expecting some hard-eyed Ivy leaguer in a Brooks brothers' suit who gets his hair cut at a stylist. Someone who knows which fork to use for his dessert at a formal banquet and which finger works best to gouge out an eyeball."

Smith paused as if expecting some comment from West but when none was forthcoming, he continued.

"Sorry to disappoint, but Kleinberg chose me. You didn't. I've been in a dozen of these operations before and he knows what I can do. You may think I'm uncouth and a social embarrassment from the basement of society but that isn't going to be reflected on my check, and believe me, it won't even put me off my breakfast... Now, Maybe you better get used to me being an important part of all this and start dealing with reality 'cause if you don't

I'm going to heat things up by ordering a chaw of Redman tobacco and a Styrofoam spit cup!"

West swiveled slowly to face the detective. He was no longer putting any effort into disguising his sentiments. His eyes roamed over the other man's pale pasta face which was now lit with an orange tinge by the rays of the sinking sun. The fellow's expression was flat giving nothing back, but his washed-out brown eyes had an electric intensity to them that echoed the challenge he'd just slapped on West.

"Well, Mr. Smith, it won't be the first time that I've worked with someone I otherwise wouldn't waste words on, so let's finish with the homey 'plain folks' shuck and just give me the information you've collected on my colleagues." West had dropped all pretense of civility.

"I can live with that, doc," said Smith as he shook out of the file folder five small sheaves of paper each stapled and bearing the name of one of TurnerWest's doctors.

"I'll give you a brief resume of each one. You can study their files overnight but I'll need them all back in the morning."

His eyes narrowed and hardened as if to add meaning to his words.

"They are not to be copied, in fact, they're on paper that can't be copied. I never risk having the sewage I dredge up on folks get out of my control... don't ever want the smell traced back to me. Making a stupid mistake like losing control of information would be too much like owing money everywhere and still leaving your phone number listed, if you get my drift. I ain't into masochism, so I make keeping control of my data, rule number one."

West didn't waste any words on the veiled threat.

The detective picked up the first report with 'Thomas Calvin Mellows' printed like the title of a book on the cover sheet.

"This one's my favorite. He'll be a pushover. A practicing Baptist with a history of groping his female patients when he was working in Portland. There's a good chance he was poking his nurse as well when his first wife gave him the heave ho and held their kids for ransom. To top it off, he's also a gun nut with a pistol range in his basement. Had a weapons charge out west too. Seems he fancied himself an unofficial SPCA sniper. Wiped out one of his neighbor's dogs from two hundred yards away when it was howling one night."

West couldn't hold back. His dislike for Mellows surpassed even the instant aversion he'd formed for Smith.

He chuckled despite himself, "Well, Cal, you old letch... this will be a distinct pleasure."

Then, to the detective, " Is there a record of this we can access?"

"Nothing official. If there were, you'd have found it when you credentialed him. His panty probing came to light when one of the victims went to his wife... motivated by female solidarity for sure. Anyway, no money changed hands. The wife blew him in to his partners who had nightmares of the executive director of NOW accompanied by a black female district attorney and a feature writer from Women's Week paying a surprise visit to the practice. They hastily arranged a private little midnight confrontation in somebody's basement at which Mellows denied everything. Seems he was pretty convincing but, his lying nurse was ambitious, and her accusations of dirty deeds in the X-ray suite added to the patient's complaint, brought the poor beggar's life down like a teetering tower of turds."

"How'd he get out of it?" asked West who was leaning forward over the table fairly licking his lips at his good fortune.

"He left town with his prayer book and a backpack. Partners bought him out at fire sale prices and the wife took that bundle of cash and everything else. All he got was a promise not to blackmail him and the right to continue to practice medicine."

West was fascinated. "So, where'd he go?"

"He ran to a Baptist sponsored clinic in Nicaragua for two years. He did everything from burr holes to bunions for nothing but his room and board and free diarrhea pills."

Smith leaned back in his chair and sucked audibly at a morsel of food wedged between his teeth before continuing.

"Came out of that toilet covered in roses, however. Some pious young thing, whose daddy owned half of Omaha, went to 'find herself in the service of her less fortunate fellows' in the third world."

"Yes, his wife's from Omaha," added West.

Smith went on.

"She was not only beautiful but rich and smart. Guess he charmed the pants off her, too, 'cause they married and he came home like a conquering hero; God having rewarded the repentant... Georgia is about as far from Oregon as you can get so he starts calling himself Calvin instead of Thomas and sets up practice here."

West was shaking his head in disbelief and satisfaction.

"The hairless hypocrite… and we heard nothing about it."

"The whole mess was buried under a lot of money and a promotion for his lying nurse as nursing director at the biggest hospital in Portland. Not surprising that nothing was admitted on his resume."

He paused again to dig at his teeth with his thumbnail.

"His kids never contact him. Devil only knows what his ex-wife told them about their wayward father… The woman scorned bit and all that… Just one of the fifty good reasons I never married. Anyway, Miss Omaha Chamber of Commerce, 1988 knows nothing about it at all. You can bet on that."

"Do we have any proof?"

Smith flipped to the last two pages of the document.

"No proof that he actually did the groping but proof that he dealt his way out of a tough spot. Here's a copy of a notarized agreement between him and his partners. A simple copy of it stuffed under his door should be more than enough to have him change his name back to Thomas and make a beeline for the nearest U-Haul. Dumb fart should have taken a lesson from me and kept only the original, no copies."

West saw an opportunity for a shot at Smith and took it.

"Bet you didn't start out your business with that tidbit of wisdom. A man doesn't usually learn to look down 'till he's already slipped in manure at least once."

"Touché, doc," said Smith and marked a point with his finger on an imaginary scoreboard hanging in the air.

"Listen," said West, "I'm going to go over this file carefully because, after Turner, Mellows is the worst enemy we have. Somehow, I don't think it would take much in today's climate of paranoia about sexual harassment to have history repeat itself."

The waiter had brought Smith's Coronas hidden under a linen towel in a champagne bucket. One bottle was already open and Smith chugged it directly from the bottle. He wiped his lips with the back of his hand.

"Beer, doc. You'd be advised to drink nothing but beer in public. It's the most anonymous booze money can buy. Everybody 'cept Mormons and reformed alcoholics drinks some beer. Doesn't say a thing about you!"

"Oh, I'm not so sure about that. In your case it says you like Mexicans…" quipped West.

"Says I *might* like Mexicans. Truth is I think they're all a bunch of garlic-tainted greasers. Had to shoot one once when he tried to convince me I could breathe easier through two holes carved in my chest than through my nostrils. Didn't even lose a night's sleep over him which is more than I can say for the first Gook I popped in Vietnam. Still see that guy's face every time I get blitzed."

He took another swig of the Corona, wiped his mouth again and continued.

"I did the greaser a lifetime ago when I was on the force in San Antonio. Nobody likes wetbacks down there except the politicians, so I was in good company. I could tell you I left there to get away from the beaners, but that wouldn't be the truth and I got scruples..."

"What is true," and he held up his Corona, "is that I prefer their beer to our domestic swill. Hey, every culture has at least one good point. Take the French for example, arrogant, cantankerous weirdos. Fight at the drop of a hat but haven't won a war since Napoleon. They take in any scumbag dictator who gets turfed, turning their country into the toilet bowl of Europe… but… where would we be without Champagne?"

"And where would the world be without amateur philosophers?" interjected West snidely.

If Smith noticed the sarcasm, he gave no sign of it.

"Interested in your dermatologist, Dr. Nguyen Trang? He's got a story that could be published as well."

"Wouldn't doubt it about that weasel. When he's skulking around, his little slit eyes seem to follow you everywhere and just when you try to look in and see what he's thinking, they go blank. Shutting down your eyes like that, it's an acquired skill. You don't learn it without having a head full of worms you don't ever want seen. Tell me his story."

He settled back in his chair and crossed his arms expectantly, almost relaxing for the first time since Smith's arrival.

"Well," began Smith after taking another swig from a Corona while he leafed through Trang's dossier, "Dr. Guy… I think I'll call him Guy. Anyway our friend Guy did his medical studies in France right out of gook high school. No weeding out process over there in Nam with undergraduate degrees to eliminate the idiots. In Guy's student days you could have been the brightest kid in Vietnam, but if your old man wasn't a colonel in the ARVN, you might as well slip on the flip-flops and head for the rice fields 'cause you weren't going nowhere."

"Look," interrupted West, "I'm impressed all to hell with your savvy social insights but I can do without the cultural commentary. I was in Nam, too, so save it for the schoolteachers later. I'm sure you'll get some ooo's and ahhh's and maybe even more, but don't waste the war stories on me."

His voice snapped like a quirt on horseflesh.

"Sayyyy... you aren't married, are you, doc?" asked Smith in a brilliant non-sequitur.

West's face clouded in perplexity for a moment while he processed the question before he answered derisively.

"Do me a favor and take the bottle caps off your Coronas before you drink them, Smith, the aluminum's affecting your brain… No, I'm not married, but what's that got to do with Trang's story?"

West had obviously slipped off the short end of his patience and fallen back into a focus of intense dislike for the Texan.

"Well," drawled the Texan, "It explains why you don't hear every night what a jerk you are. That's not to suggest that everybody who knows you thinks that, but it's something you might hear more often if you was married… I mean, if it was me, I'd want to know. I might even thank the guy for the insight…"

He paused, a broad smile of condescension on his face.

"I got only a few rules but one of them is 'tell it like it is'… and that's how it ties in, doc."

He paused again for effect then continued.

"Now where was I?"

West wanted to flatten the guy's nose but he needed the information in the files, hence, violence wasn't a reasonable option at the moment. Resignation seemed the best choice left open to him so he sat silently fuming while the fat man droned on.

"Yea, I remember... Guy gets into slice and dice school in France and comes out with honors… Dr. Trang he is and, even if he's only a dermatologist and not a real surgeon, he absolutely, I mean passionately likes to cut on folks. So, when he gets back home to Nam the black pajamas guys are still hiding in tunnels in the south. The North Vietnamese regulars aren't around yet…"

He paused again and looked directly at West who had averted his eyes momentarily.

"I hope you're still following me, doc… Well, Guy gets tired, real quick, of rashes and dispensing steroid creams. So, he applies for the job of head torturer for the second brigade of the ARVN, the unit his dad used to command… Did I tell you his dad got killed in a latrine by the Viet Cong?... If I didn't tell you, I need to, 'cause it helps explain Guy's irritation with the VC… helps to explain why all the lamp shades in his house had VC tattoos on them and why he used to give out change purses to all his friends at Christmas made out of high quality tanned VC scrotums, drawstrings and all. The guy is good with skin, you gotta give him that… Anyway, seems his daddy was on an inspection tour to the Mekong one day when he gets the squirts and has to use a field latrine."

At this point, Smith pauses to laugh out loud at the mental picture his story conjures up.

" Well, unbenonced to the colonel, a fourteen year old VC kid is hiding in the crap up to his eyeballs. Been there all night just marinating since he dug into the place from the back. The kid's got a rusted old French .45 caliber revolver with one bullet in it, sitting on a rag on top of his head to keep it dry. Don't ask me how he recognizes from the view he has that it's a colonel on the can, but he shoots him right up the butt. Hits his heart or something 'cause they find him with a funny surprised look on his face. Dead as a doornail and still sitting on the seat. They caught the kid and were holding him for Guy when he escaped. I think ol' Guy was still looking for him 'till he had to leave Nam suddenly at the end of the war... Am I boring you, doc?" said Smith in a bemused tone.

"You know what I think without me saying it, Smith"

"You're right, doc, I do. It's in your eyes. You need to take a lesson from Trang. Learn to pull the shutters across 'em."

West refused to be drawn into the detective's game. "So what do we have on him? Skinning a few VC alive twenty years ago isn't punishable by anything here in the US. For all I know the locals might make him an honorary member of the KKK, if the story got out."

"Not done with the story yet, doc..." grinned the Texan.

"Here's the best part. See, Guy's married to ex-president Thieu's niece. Ol' Thieu, old as a stone, is still alive in France somewhere directing the Vietnamese mafia. Her whole family is up to their slanty eyes in the Vietnamese equivalent of the Chinese Triads... You know about the Triads don't you? Extortion, drugs, etc... Well, the Vietnamese gangs are all over the West coast cities and Vegas and are moving east. They're spreading faster than herpes and even have the distinction of ordering the first drive-by shooting ever done in Salt Lake City. To make a long story short, there's some pretty nasty fruit hanging on the branches of Mrs. Trang's family tree."

"So? What's your point?" asked West impatiently.

"My point is that Dr. Guy married Mrs. Trang for political reasons. If you've ever seen her or her picture, you'd understand... face flat as a skillet... looks like some five year old drew on her eyes and mouth with a broken crayon. She'd have been a throw away if Guy hadn't needed a leg up the political ladder after daddy got shot. Well, Guy knew how to make the best of a bad thing. Found him a real cute piece of fluff about thirty years younger than him. He keeps her in Malaysia but he'd like her closer. Only gets to check on his Malaysian investments, so to speak, twice a year now. It's a real love match."

"So where's our leverage?" asked West impatiently.

"Hang on, doc and listen to the story… Guy had two children by her and none by Mrs. Trang. Apparently Madam's ovaries aren't any more impressive than her face. Or may be he just could never bring himself to jump her bones. I don't know, but the only kids he has and the woman he loves are in Malaysia and he can't get them into the US. He's tried twice, but no go. He can't tell Mrs. Trang bye-bye either like other docs do when they tire of their old wives 'cause her family would make what happened to Guy's daddy look like a good way to go out."

"Can we get his family into the US?" asked West, looking hopeful.

"You and me and all the king's men couldn't, but Kleinberg can fix it in the twinkle of an eye. He's slept in the Lincoln bedroom more than Mrs. Lincoln ever did."

"Great! So, Trang's in the bag."

"Yep, that's about right."

"And what about the others?"

"Let's see," Smith said distractedly, shuffling the files into some priority.

"Got the rest of them here, I think… Goldman, Chen and Singh. If I put Trang back into this group it sounds like some UN committee set up to investigate the feasibility of doing brain transplants in Singapore for refugees who need more education to get into Canada… How'd you choose these guys for me to investigate, doc? Are you trying to 'racially purify' the TurnerWest group?"

West skewered him with a glare, then the corners of his mouth began to crimp up into a grin. "You're not married either, are you, Smith?"

"Ok, ok, doc, I get your drift. You've probably guessed by now that I like to push your buttons."

"Your 'pushes' are about as subtle as a thumb in the eye and you need a rewrite on your humor, too," snapped West.

"Thanks for the tips… as I said 'tell it like it is' but you didn't answer my question and I need to know what criteria you've used in selecting these five men for investigation?"

The sun had dipped below the horizon and the sky suddenly glowed orange and red as if a torch had been pitched off the edge of the world to ignite the oily conflagration of hell. The school teachers who had been watching the sunset silently, suddenly broke into rapturous applause, standing up, as if Mother Nature might notice the ovation and somehow devise an encore.

West's face was flaccid in thought but Smith guffawed loudly and one of the teachers looked his way, then visibly slowed down her clapping.

"Doc, it's amazing what some people will do on vacation… Stuff you couldn't pay 'em enough to attempt at home. Those gals have obviously spent time in Key West going cross-eyed watching for the 'green flash'. It's really something to see. A knot of sunset freaks gathers each evening, on this pitifully dirty little beach, and when the sun pulls the plug and sinks, somebody yells… 'I see it… the flash!' and soon, everybody's yelling about the flash. Collective hallucination, but about the closest you're gonna get to a spiritual experience with a group of fags."

West's attention had drifted back to the table and he spoke quietly.

"*I* saw the flash in Key West."

"Yep, an' you ain't married either. I'd keep those little confessions under my hat if I was you, doc. You might get misunderstood and lose all your male patients."

West winced at the man's crassness. He'd been thinking about how much he should reveal to someone for whom he felt such profound antipathy. He needed to deal with Smith as Kleinberg's agent but he'd decided to hold back and discuss only the most basic elements of his thinking. At best, the guy was a goof… at worst, he was dangerous.

"The list was made up of partners I know to be in Turner's camp. Mellows is the only real danger and I feet the others are lightweights we might pull to our side of the line... that's the logic."

"Impressed by anything you've learned?" grinned Smith.

"Yes, I must admit, the background on these two suggests exactly how we can get to them."

"I didn't find anything quite as tantalizing on the last three but we've got good points of leverage there as well."

He was drumming his fingers on the other files in front of him on the table.

"What do you have on Sol Goldman?" queried West.

"Him, we can get at through his two sons. Seems Dr. Sol Goldman has a younger brother whose rise to fame has eclipsed our lowly internist's accomplishments. When the Goldman generations get together all the conversation centers around his brother Alvin Goldman and his exploits in the OR. The guy's a pediatric neurosurgeon at St. Judes. High profiler ever since he got into Harvard medical school years before."

Smith looked up at West, then back at the dossier.

"Poor old Sol barely got into the program at Eastern Tennessee University's med school…. I mean think about it…. Eastern Tennessee!"

And he raised his eyebrows and wrinkled his nose like sulfur dioxide was rising off the page from the very name.

"But the saga of two Goldman brothers continues on through the generations. Sol has one bright son, his youngest, and one turnip... but both want to go to medical school. Sol and Gelda, his wife, have put a small fortune aside to guarantee their progeny's success if... mind you... if they can get them into Harvard or Yale... But most definitely not someplace like Eastern Tennessee. There are already two elements of déjà vu in the second generation of the family with the bright and the dumb duo, rolling out of the genes in the same order as the internist and the neurosurgeon."

West could see by the detective's animation that he loved to tell his stories. His pasty pock-marked face fairly beamed with enthusiasm. Grudgingly, he had to admit that the gumshoe did it well.

Smith was so wrapped up in his tale that he didn't notice a mosquito tanking up on his forehead. The little mutt was sucking for all he was worth and turning his abdomen into a regular blood blister. He'd stuck his proboscis deep into a transverse ravine in the terrain of the corrugated skin and he rode the waves of expression that washed over Smith's face like the turbulence of a midair refueling.

West was smiling watching the insect and the detective smiled back figuring his work was finally getting the recognition it deserved from the physician.... Ignorance truly was bliss.

The story unfolded.

"Now back in Memphis, Alvin, the neurosurgeon just can't get the reproductive thing right... it's like he has defective sperm with twisted tails or something... You know how the Jews feel about a male heir... Well, no such luck! He goes to the well three times and comes back without a single foreskin to show for it... three girls! Count'em one, two, three... and it don't matter that one has a mustache and arm hair like a mechanic... he still missed."

"Now the race is on again, two boys against three girls. Sol and Gelda take heart... they may get to be dinnertime conversation at family gatherings on

Rosh HaShannah in a big way if they can pull it off. They've already got the only Bar Mitzvahs and their little burr-headed boys get a real beanie full of gifts from the adoring grandparents each birthday."

And he paused to take a drag on a corona before continuing.

"Meanwhile, one of Alvin's daughters manages to eliminate herself from the Goldman stakes. She gets knocked up by a teaching assistant in her first year of pre-med. Marries him, a goy no less, and she's out of the running."

Smith held up two fingers as a visual aid for the next part of the story.

"Sister number two is a good looking chick who's always been a rebel... you know the belly button ring.... Anyway, she's bucking for an activist's seat on the board of directors of NOW... She's studying sociology, escorting poor pregnant black girls through the gauntlets at abortion palaces, gay rights marches... The whole nine yards. Mom and pop are gaga in disgust but she's going to do her own thing. Exit number two contender carrying a protest placard."

He drew a deep breath before continuing.

"Now we get to daughter number three, the beauty queen, who, for twenty thousand dollars of electrolysis, has exchanged the mustache for a million little holes in her upper lip... Looks like one of them inborn errors of metabolism that the Ashkenazi Jews have cornered the market on... But... the good news is, she's a genius. Started winning science fairs in kindergarten and was handing daddy instruments in the OR before she was tall enough to see into the holes he drilled in kids' skulls."

Smith drew another deep breath.

"Alvin figures she's a shoe-in for Harvard... and he's right. No threat from someone wanting to marry her so the career path is clear. ...Meanwhile down in Albany, the Sol Goldman duo plods along. The oldest kid who's got muscles on his muscles but no brains, has had more tutors than Madonna has had lovers. However, he's scraped through high school on the strength of his ability to run with the football and Daddy's donations of time and money to the team. But Harvard?... Gimme a break!... The younger boy shows promise ... No science fair wins but he wants to be a doc and he's got the smarts to do it."

"So can we get the dunce into Harvard?" asked West.

"Unless Senator McCain becomes president, the kid will be in with a football scholarship… full ride."

"The Lincoln bedroom again?" cracked West.

"You got it, doc. It's a pricey little motel, but the bed vibrates and breakfast is included."

"So that's Goldman," said West pursing his lips in satisfaction. "And Chen? What about him?"

Smith shook his head in derision... held up two sheets and said, "Nothing to twist him with. He's as clean as a new set of Jockey's. Hasn't done anything but study since he was five years old. All his kids are swift and will make it on their own and his wife never sticks her nose outside the home."

"What about the immigration angle? Anything there?" West asked, hopefully.

"Nope. The guy's been a regular conveyor belt to the States and everybody's here already."

"Well, where's the angle, I have a feeling you've got an idea. You look like you're going to come out with some corny crack and then lay it out for me, so, get on with it."

"Doc, you take all the fun out of this," and Smith feigned disappointment with arched brows and a pout.

"Come on, Smith, I haven't got all night and you want to bed your teacher, right?... The sun's down and they're off to the piano lounge of the

Holiday Inn for a rowdy evening… Spill it!"

"Simple, doc. Dirty tricks… You say he's Turner's boy right?"

"Right. Thick as thieves, Turner recruited him from L.A."

"Rumors, Doctor's lounge scuttlebutt. Spread it around through the nurses, they love doctor gossip anyway. He reads mammograms, right? So, let it out that Turner's been spreading rumors about how many bad reads of booby portraits Dr. Chen, radiologist extraordinaire, has been making. By inference, it will make him responsible for the deaths of all the women in Albany who would have died from breast cancer no matter what was on the film."

He smiled malevolently, then added.

" You can leave this little task to me; that's how I earn my money. I'll get the rumor mill grinding."

He paused and dabbed at his forehead with a napkin. The mosquito tried to escape but had taken on too much blood and buzzed downward in a murderous trajectory like a drunk crop-duster right into the side of the flower vase in the middle of the table. Smith reached out a huge thumb and squashed it.

"Hate the ones with no whine…" he muttered.

Then, "Let's finish with Singh and call it a night."

"Carry on," said West.

"Singh's simple. He looks black, but he ain't negro. However, he's been turned down as a member of the yacht club at the lake. It's important to him. He'd be grateful if you pry open the lily white door for him. This is something I'm counting on you doing for the cause, doc."

West nodded his head.

"I think I could swing that, but so could Turner."

"Turner's at the funny farm for two months… Do it while he's gone. If we need more to reel Singh in, we'll play the immigration card…. He's probably related to half of Bombay."

"Ok, now, I've still got to have one or two more votes even if we get everyone we've discussed. How long will it take to have you work up, say, three more names?"

"Any of them foreigners?"

"One, a family doc from Canada."

"Canada's easy. I mean offshore foreign."

"No."

"Should be able to be done ten days after I get the names."

"Good."

West's face tightened and he leaned across the table and lowered his voice.

"Mellows is a loose cannon who fires even when Jason Turner is gone. He's got an evangelical hate on for me and he's seeking converts to their cause everyday. I need him shut down immediately, if not sooner."

"Still worried about the parabolic mikes, doc? No need to whisper. That's only in the movies."

Smith grinned and when he got no reaction, shrugged.

"Mellows won't be easy. I need authorization for the funds involved but I figure we can shut him down in two weeks… three at most."

"No sooner?" queried West.

The detective's face flashed irritation.

"Even God took a week to finish the earth… be reasonable, doc. I need to undermine him first and subvert a couple of his people. Three weeks is minimal time… No one else could do it in less than three months."

"Ok, then. Three weeks, but I can't be seen to be involved."

"Hey, you're the bossman of TurnerWest in Turner's absence. You'll have to be involved putting pressure on scalpel man Mellows once the plan is underway, but I'll keep your hands clean if that's what you mean."

"Yes, I can't be involved directly in any dirty work or it risks alienating the votes we need to override Turner."

"Then rest easy."

"Are we finished?"

"Unless you want to get all weepy and thank me for all the good work I've done, I guess we are."

Smith had his stupid grin back as he spoke.

West was pushing away from the table.

"Fat chance of that!" he chirped.

"Do I get the files for tonight?"

"Take them... but don't even try to copy them."

"Listen, Smith. We need to get something straight between us... You don't ever threaten me! Nobody threatens me with impunity."

West was standing and had taken an expensive looking silver pen from his inside pocket that he was fingering with nervous energy, twisting its top open then snapping it shut. His eyes were riveted on the detective's face.

The air thickened between them.

"Well, doc," the Texan drawled as he got to his feet slowly never averting his own glowering gaze.

"In my opinion, I ain't even threatened you, yet... What's more if I ever do, you won't have any doubts about what's happening."

The two men remained bolted together at the eyes, neither blinking.

"Be forewarned," growled West in a voice gone menacingly soft.

The sarcasm was lard thick in the detective's reply.

"Doc, I'm shaking in my boots and about to pee myself… So, if you'll excuse me… Oh, and don't forget your files."

His huge hand pushed the sheets across the table aggressively then he turned and strolled away without another word or a backward glance.

West picked up the files. He knew that someplace down the road he'd have it out with the fat Texan but there was time enough for that much later. For now, he needed him.

West had decided to walk to his room down the outside of the hotel on the beach. The sky bordering the sea had dimmed to a leaden plumb purple and darkness crouched behind the blunt dunes to the north preparing a stealthy advance across the scrub and sand.

A wavering line of pelicans skimmed the water returning to their roost, shadows vibrating against shadows. The leaves of the miniature palms squatting alongside the walkway clattered dryly in the wind like the fleshless fingers of the dead. A bat swooped and chittered, then wheeled away.

Mark West's pride had been bruised by the disrespectful arrogance of Smith but overall the information had been worth the aggravation. Removing Mellows from the game before Turner's return was more than he had expected. If the surgeon could be made to suffer before he was broken, that would simply enhance the coup. West lolled the possibility around in his mind to amplify the pleasure, like savoring a particularly tasty morsel by holding it in his mouth before swallowing it.

CH018: ALBANY, GEORGIA.

Gloria Mellows sat propped upon a profusion of pillows in the magnificent four poster bed she'd had fashioned from tropical hardwood. She'd clicked off the A&E classic movie and turned to her scripture study, seeking solace from her worries. Cal hadn't been himself for almost a week and she knew something was seriously wrong. She was attempting to immerse herself in the Gospel of St. John, her preferred passages, when the phone rang.

"Hello, this is Gloria."

"Hi, sweetheart... it's just me." Cal's voice was thick and the cadence of his speech was unnaturally stilted.

"Cal, have you been drinking?" her voice was taut with apprehension.

"A bit... Nothing to worry about... Anyway, I'm almost home."

"Oh, Cal, you know how it upsets me when you do this. You promised..."

"I know, I know… it wasn't planned… I'm sort of drunk by accident… Do you want me to stay in the coach house tonight?"

She sensed that he wanted her to become angry and consign him to the apartment above the garage which had been his occasional refuge when he drank. She was an abstainer and they inevitably fought when he indulged excessively.

"No Cal, something's wrong and I want to talk about it tonight… How much have you had to drink?"

"Too much… not sure we could talk, honey. Maybe tomorrow."

He was almost pleading.

"Where are you now?"

"Actually, I'm parked downstairs..."

"Downstairs? I didn't hear you drive in…"

"I've been here for about two hours… treating myself to some one-on-one therapy with Dr. Jim Bean, here in his mobile office"

"You're down in the car drinking whiskey alone?"

Her voice was pulled between irritation and alarm.

"You got it… Just me and my lousy memories getting pissed together…"

Gloria had swung out of bed and gone to the window. The garage door gaped blackness. The moon was up announcing the night and the yard was sprayed with a patina of pale light. Her mind was rebelling at the implications of the fact that her husband was sitting, drinking alone, in his car. He never drank alone. She spoke into the portable phone.

"Step on your brakes, Cal."

"What?" his voice oozed perplexity.

"Step on your brake pedal," she repeated firmly.

A crimson glow suffused the cavern of the garage and twin gleaming spots, the eyes of a monster glaring out from its lair, flared red against the darkness.

"Ok," she said wearily, the sadness welling up in her voice, "I see where you are."

"Didn't you believe me…?"

"I hoped you were somehow joking, Cal… I didn't want it to be true."

Gloria had slumped back onto the bed, her shoulders bent as if the weight of what was happening were about to crush her physically.

The ravishingly beautiful Gloria Mellows was an optimistic idealist. She had, over the years, acquired the enviable skill of rendering the unpleasantness of life bearable by renaming it 'trials' or 'adversity' and declaring it to be 'the fertilizer of spiritual growth'. At the same time, she selectively enhanced events that demonstrated the advantages of living Christian principles in a world virtually devoid of principles.

Her recollection of Nicaragua for example, had been effectively purged of the squalor, the meanness and degradation of grinding poverty. She was amnesic for the appalling brutality of a fratricidal political conflict where human lives were no more than points on an ideological scoreboard and murder had become commonplace. What she remembered were the smiles of the peasants, their naïve charm and their elemental devotion to God… to the God she adored and trusted to preserve her from the horrors of reality.

And so, when reality crashed through her defenses despite prayers and pious protestations, she felt defenseless and vulnerable.

"Cal, I need you to be here, now… We have to talk."

There was a long pause before he answered.

"Gloria, I can't face you right now and I'm sure that as soon as you see me and smell my breath your instincts will take over and we'll be saying things out of anger that we won't be able to take back… I'll talk but let's do it over the phone."

She wanted to reassure him that she could contain herself no matter what she saw but she wasn't sure she could.

"Alright, but something is lost when you can't see the person you're talking to…"

"Something is gained as well, darling… I might not have the courage to tell you what you have the right to know if I could see your reaction."

There was an awkward silence.

"You do want me to tell you what it is that has me by the throat, don't you?" he asked.

"Yes… yes, I guess I do. But put down the bottle… Promise me you'll leave it alone for right now."

"Promise…"

"Cal, what's happened… You've been acting strange for over a week now… the kids are even noticing it."

"Yea, I've been drinking…. Seems to be the only way to stifle the screaming inside. You remember how it was with me in Nicaragua?"

"Yes, but you changed then and that's been ten years ago… What's happened now? Is it something I've done?"

"Oh no, sweetheart, nothing you've done has ever been anything but a blessing in my life... I love you more than I love God…"

"Don't blaspheme, Cal…"

"It's true, Glor, I love you more than I could ever tell you."

"Then, if that's true talk to me, share with me!"

"Are you lying down?" he asked.

"Yes. "Her blanched knuckles gripped the phone as she lay stiffly on the pillows.

"Ten years ago in Portland, I was accused of sexually assaulting a patient… The patient went to my wife with the story."

"What did she accuse you of doing...?"

"Fondling her in the office on two occasions when she came in for breast exams... She had a breast lump."

"Did you do it?" her voice hummed with tension.

"No!" he said emphatically, "I didn't, but I didn't take the precautions of having the nurse in the room as a witness. Although, after the way the nurse lied later, it probably wouldn't have made any difference if she had been there…"

"What did the nurse lie about?"

"That's just it. It would have been difficult as hell but I think I could have beaten the false accusation of the patient, but the nurse… right out of nowhere… I still don't understand why… She told my partners that she and I were having an affair on the side. It blew me away… I never even came close to her!"

"And didn't your wife believe you?"

There was a bitter hollow laugh distorted even more by the confines of the car and its transmission through the phone.

"My wife was sleeping with one of my partners. I know it now but I didn't suspect it then. I was too wrapped up in building the practice to see what must have been obvious to everyone else. She turned on me like your mother does on Jehovah's Witnesses."

"That's uncalled for, Cal!"

"Sorry, honey, but it was savage. They came at me one evening, my four partners and my dear wife in a meeting in our rec room. I'd been drinking and I couldn't help but think of the kids asleep upstairs. They tore me apart. Threats. Accusations. Ultimatums. Like a pack of coyotes savaging a rabbit…. It was four hours of pure hell… Just pure hell… Even now, my gut wrenches when I think of it. I can still see all their goddam faces boring in on me!"

"Oh, Cal," she was crying… "please stop the profanity… I'm having a hard enough time with all of this without that."

"Hell, Gloria," he sputtered, "listen to what I'm saying, woman… They're doing it to me again!"

"What do you mean?"

"I mean it's like a damn recurring nightmare… Mark West, who's a prick to begin with, barged into my office last Friday and slammed down an affidavit on my desk signed by some Crosby woman swearing that I fondled her breast during an examination."

"Did you, Cal?" her voice quavered.

"Hell, no! No more this time than I did the last time, but it's the same damn thing… My nurse won't back me up."

"Wasn't she there?"

"To my recollection, she was. I always have her there, but I didn't document it in the chart and, this time, both she and the patient say she was called out of the room."

"Well, we'll tell the truth, Cal. We'll fight it. You have rights don't you. God knows who's telling the truth."

He laughed again more softly and without the edge in his voice. "My dear sweet Gloria. You live in another world, darling. I'm not criticizing you, believe me… but you're naïve."

"How, Cal?... Why can't we prove they're lying?"

"There is no proof, darling… There never is any proof in accusations like these. It's always a question of credibility and reputation."

"Does anyone know what they did to you in Portland?"

"That's the point. I didn't fight it there. I saw the hatred in my wife's eyes and my partners gnashing their teeth at my jugular... I sold out... gave up. Basically, I said to hell with the truth. I signed a paper and got out. That's how I ended up in Quintera at the mission clinic."

"You didn't defend yourself?"

"I was convinced it wouldn't do any good… my wife, my lying nurse, my partners who hated my guts. I didn't stand a chance."

"But it's not the same now."

"No," he said, "ironically, it's much worse."

"How, Cal?"

"Because somebody is behind all this pushing it. Hell, maybe even creating it. Whoever it is wants me gone real badly. Once they dig up the Portland garbage, I'll look like a recidivist molester grabbing at the breasts of all my cancer patients... There are several female lawyers, even in this little town, who would love to have a doctor's gonads hanging on their trophy wall... You really don't know how bad it will be, Gloria..."

Suddenly his voice broke and he sobbed. "You don't know what they'll do to you and the kids. They won't stop at anything... I can't put you through it..."

"Call Jason, Cal... He knows you. He's credible. You're not alone in this."

"He's out of touch, Gloria. I've tried since last Wednesday to get to him. They only take messages from direct family members and refuse to confirm that he is even there."

"Then, fly down to see him. You have no choice."

"Maybe.... I'm not sure what he could do, but I know this isn't just a coincidence. He might be able to help me get to whoever is behind it before it all blows up."

"Honey, come up now, please," she pleaded. She could hear him blow his nose.

"No... Let me sleep in the coach house ... I'm bad company, tonight, believe me. I love you Gloria," and the line went dead.

She sat stunned for a moment or two still holding the phone to her ear and calling "Cal?... Cal?..." Then she lowered her hand slowly to the bed. Quietly, the tears streaking her cheeks, Gloria Mellows slipped off the bed and knelt against it.

"Dear Heavenly Father...."

* * *

The next morning Gloria awoke asleep on the floor beside her bed. She rose to her knees expectantly hoping to see her husband lying in his accustomed place as she had prayed he would be. The bed was undisturbed but where he would have lain there was a sheet of paper folded in half. She quickly snatched it up and read.

Dear Gloria,

You and the children are the reason for my existence. I've lain awake all night trying to figure a way out of this nightmare that would spare you all but I haven't succeeded. No matter what happens, know that I will always love you. I'm going away. Please don't search for me. I know you won't understand but you must believe me that I've examined all the options and this is the only avenue left open for me.

Love forever,

Cal.

Gloria Mellows collapsed on her bed pouring out her anguish in soul-rending sobs.

CH019: ST.LUCIA

Jason was showering when the knock came at the door. He didn't hear it. The hot water was provided by a hissing white enameled contraption on the wall that ran water-filled copper coils through a blue gas flame.

Higher up the wall, a pale lizard the same shade as the paint and three inches long, glared at him cocking its head from side to side occasionally as if one lidless eye were tiring of staring at the intruder. The water heater was its home. The first time it had scampered out, Jason had almost stumbled backwards and fallen through the circular curtain that formed a shower stall in the middle of the marble Jacuzzi. The showering arrangement was a poor marriage of luxury and practicality.

When he finally shut off the water and the flame extinguished with an audible pop, he heard her voice.

"May I come in, Dr. Turner?"

He felt a quiver of excitement tingle through him and began to towel his hair furiously, which added a coarse vibrato to his response. "Of course. I'll be right out. Just have a seat please."

She sat on the flowered couch sinking back onto the cushions and letting a little sigh escape her lips. After all, he wasn't present to hear it.

On the end table beside her, under a lamp, a thumbed paperback copy of Albert Camus' '*L'Etranger*' lay splayed open, spine up. It was written in French judging from the cover and she picked it up. Flipping through the pages, she saw notations in a clear crisp hand in the margins on virtually every page. Whole paragraphs had been underlined. The comments were also in French, and with her limited knowledge of the language (she'd taken night school courses before she and her husband had embarked on a two week wine tasting tour through France, several years earlier), she could make sense of only a few phrases. The notes seemed to be comments on literary devices.

He had padded out noiselessly on bare feet and she startled when he spoke. "Hi," he smiled, "has the sun already gone down?"

"Uh, no, this is a professional visit."

Her hair had been dried and was fountaining luxuriously over her shoulders. She wore a short lavender dress with narrow string straps that left her shoulders bare. Pulling the left strap down, she bared the upper edge of her breast enough to reveal a gauze pad held in place with paper tape.

"It does need stitching, unfortunately... so, here I am," her voice was almost apologetic. "I didn't intend to interrupt..."

"What, my shower?... No big deal, the lizard wanted his nest back anyway..." "The lizard?" a quizzical expression played across her features.

"Are you using one of those *other* personalities you warned me about, Dr. Turner?" and she wrinkled her nose slightly and raised her brows to emphasize her perplexity.

"Not at all, you are quite safe... It's just that I share my shower with a pale little lizard who lives in the water-heater. Our relationship is a symbiotic arrangement. I expose myself in the bathroom to attract the mosquitoes from the rest of the cottage and he eliminates them before they pass on their little packets of malarial parasites to me."

He was grinning as he spoke.

"Oh, yes, I have one of those too," she said with enthusiasm. "I've got this ghastly piece of art hanging over my bed, which I'm certain must have been painted by a blind man. My lizard lives behind it. He's quite the little warrior. The other night he tackled a palmetto beetle..."

She paused to squirm visibly.

"I think that's what they're called down here, but to me, they are just flying roaches. Anyway, he jumped the roach on the wall and they both fell six feet to the floor in a fluttering tangle. They struggled for a good five minutes before he killed it and dragged it under my end table. Next morning I found it chewed up a bit, but he seemed to have only pulled the legs off. Drumstick special I guess, eight for $1.50."

She squirmed again.

Jason had positioned himself on the arm of the sofa at the end furthest from her. He wore only a towel wrapped around his waist. His torso glistened with moisture and his toweled hair was a shade darker than when dry. He gave no sign of discomfort with his state of undress and she warmed to his obvious informality.

"Please, don't call me Dr. Turner... It feels awkward, if I am to call you Amy, and I'd like to do that..."

"A slip, Jason, I was entering a strange man's room while he was showering. I felt a little formality would be good for my reputation."

"You *have* a reputation?" he queried

"I actually probably have several... Like I said before, I'm a mental patient here, remember?"

"We're almost wearing that one out I'm afraid...," laughed Jason.

"Well, your reputation with me is impeccably intact and calling me Jason won't alter that."

He saw the mischievous twinkle creep back into her lovely hazel eyes as she paused before she said more softly, almost suggestively, "I wonder what I'd have to do to alter my reputation with you…?"

She was playing with him and enjoying every nuance of the game.

Although *she*'d spoken the words, *he* blushed at the thoughts they provoked in him.

She laughed musically, obviously amused at seeing him nonplussed.

"There you go again with your words," he chided. "Let's get down to the business of healing. How deep is the laceration?'

"Full thickness, I'm afraid, and a bit of a tear with ragged edges. About three inches long, it catches the edge of the areola."

"I'll dress and be right with you. I have no instruments or suture material here. Do you have access to this clinic you mentioned earlier?"

He was speaking through the open doorway of the bedroom, as he searched through his closet with a tinkle of hangers, hunting something appropriate for clinical work.

"I have a key and, in fact, I had promised to be there an hour ago. It's my afternoon to work but events have taken over my timetable."

He didn't comment, but in two minutes, he appeared at the door wearing jeans and a green surgical scrub top. He held out his arms to display the shirt and then pointed to the 'Albany General Hospital' logo on the pocket and said, "*Voila, le medecin*!"

"Then we shall rush away to your surgery, *monsieur, le docteur*," she gushed with a passably correct accent.

* * *

The clinic was a plain two-story concrete block affair painted white. There were no other buildings around and it sat indecorously on the roadside like a single tooth jutting from a vagrant's jaw

"Full of country charm," quipped Jason, as they pulled up in the Renaissance van that Dr. Landry kindly lent Amy for her charity work.

"Not much from the outside ... Actually, not much from the inside either, but it's adequate and acceptably well equipped. As you can see, the locals value it highly."

A dozen people were huddled under the umbrella of a lone mango tree that shaded the left side of the building. They rose hesitantly at first, then recognizing Amy as she stepped from the vehicle, they ran as one, forming a jostling line across the front of the building.

A woman nursing a child and an elderly man and woman crippled with obvious arthritis, remained under the mango but were struggling to get up and to the clinic doors.

Amy was fumbling with a worn brass key trying to fit it into a scarred lock which had obviously been the target of thieves who had damaged both the lock and the metal-covered door with pry bars. Jason doubted the robbers had been successful in gaining entry, judging from the effort Amy had to make to force it open when the key finally did turn.

She flipped several switches and a series of fluorescent lights stuttered to life. A noisy air conditioner thrummed into activity beside the door where it protruded from the building's façade like a leprous lump. The odor of baked antiseptic floated unpleasantly out the door.

Noticing Jason's reaction to the stench, Amy explained, "That's the autoclave. They sterilize the instruments when they close each afternoon and, without ventilation, the fumes permeate the whole place by morning. You should see the machine. It's worth more at home as an antique than three newer models would cost, but it's all they have, and it's functional."

She led the way through a short corridor where a battered desk, besieged by a profusion of papers, had been driven back in retreat against one wall. Just past the desk, two doorways, one on either side of the hall, opened onto two examining rooms with jury-rigged homemade exam tables. Both tables had been covered with shiny oilcloth that was cracked at the corners and lacked a pattern in the center, where a thousand sweaty bodies must have lain over the years. The table legs were fashioned from bare two by fours.

In each room, a plastic-lined bucket sat under a utilitarian sink with a brown paper towel roll standing on end upon it. Water had seeped into one of the rolls blossoming the lower few inches into a bloated, dark brown, ruffle. There were no shelves but two bent metal instrument trays, listing to one side like amputees without prostheses, leaned against each table. One room had a battered goose neck lamp and a stubby stool. It must have been the gynecological suite.

At the end of the hallway, a metal stairway led off to the right, up into the darkness of the upper floor.

A single large room on the ground level occupied the back of the building. This room had open shelves covering every available inch of wall. A single barred window, too high to see in or out of, was set above a large stainless steel sink that looked like a utility fixture more appropriate for a restaurant than a clinic.

The offending autoclave, with a door clamp that looked like a hatch cover from the '*Nautilus*', sat on a counter next to the sink. Beside it, an antique glass Bunsen burner with a tray for slides, kept company with a microscope that seemed as old as the rocks in the yard.

The shelves of the room were crammed with bottles and containers of all descriptions.

"This is like a trip back into the twenties," Jason exclaimed, as his eyes, roving over the room and its contents, paused at a toilet stuck in an alcove the size of a telephone booth.

"Pre-Oslerian, in my opinion," added Amy, "but like I said, it's this or the herb peddler. The people at St. Jude's do their best and provide excellent care, but only for children. The local hospital does a decent job on routine surgery and acute care of the very ill, but the walking wounded from the rural areas really have no place to come but here."

He was still inspecting the premises when she interrupted him. "Well, Doctor, shall we get started?"

"Sure, let's get someplace where I can examine that wound."

"Not with *me*, Jason," a thread of supplication was stitched through her words, "I meant, let's get started with *them*. I've still got four more hours before it's too late to close my laceration. These people..." and she pointed to the expectant face of a curious child peeking in through the front door, "have been here since early morning, probably. They deserve our attention, first."

"But I can't practice here... I'm not licensed." His voice had an incredulous tone.

"I thought I was coming to tend to you."

"Believe me, you will. But in the meantime, there is an incredible experience waiting for you right here, and it has nothing to do with me..."

She could read the hesitation on his face.

"Trust me Jason, please, and relax... No one here is going to sue you. Things are simpler than at home... We're still needed by the people here, and there are no lawyers at all... Some vultures on the lamp posts along the Castries highway are as close to the malpractice environment of home that you'll ever get down here."

When he didn't respond to her attempt at humor, she moved closer to him and took his bare forearm gently in both hands. She was looking into his eyes, almost pleading.

"Please Jason… *help me to help them.*"

Her touch awakened something in him and, when he looked down at her face, he was transfixed by what he thought he saw in her eyes. Captured in a loop of memory that wound round his heart and tightened, pulling him away from reality, it was as if he were suddenly drifting in a fever. Her image began to slowly blur and, in its place, Annette's face appeared but the eyes never changed… the two women shared the same eyes.

"Jason, please… trust me."

Her voice, too, had become Annette's. He felt suddenly light headed, disoriented, and it must have shown in his face.

"Jason, are you alright… Do you need to sit down?"

Despite his temporary malaise, he sensed the dangerous impression of debility she must have detected in him. The last thing he wanted to portray to her was emotional instability. He'd just told her today, that he was almost well. Besides, he, too, was alarmed at the flush of emotion, and confused by the blending of his memories of Annette with the reality of this young woman he'd barely met. He needed to reassert control over his body and mind. And he needed to do it quickly.

He held up a hand to signal that he was in no serious distress. Then, to be certain that his throat had had time to release enough for him to speak, he gained a few more moments by massaging his forehead slowly with his fingers.

"I'm fine, really… I'm okay," he reassured her, as she had been attempting to lead him by the arm to a chair in the corner.

"I sometimes get head rushes like this, but I've had it checked out and it's benign," he lied.

"Maybe we shouldn't see any patients today," she ventured and the previous tone of supplication in her voice had been replaced by one of genuine concern.

"No, you're right. Let's get started."

He moved to the sink and began to lather his hands with a large cube of yellow soap, effectively silencing her protests.

Two cases of severe conjunctivitis in young children (one little girl's cornea had already been scarred by the gnawing erosion of the bacteria) caused him to shake his head in disbelief. Near blindness, for lack of a dollar's worth of garamycin drops. It was as if he had traveled from another planet to a truly primitive society where nature's cruelty remained unchallenged by medical science.

A third child, older than the others, hobbled in without an accompanying adult. An angry looking '*hurtin me leg*' had been '*paining*' him for several weeks. Jason palpated the tissues around a large, red, swollen lump on the boy's thigh, in order to delineate the extent of the infection. The skin over the highest point of the mound was taut and shiny with the pressure of the poison dammed up below it. The boy cringed when he pushed on the apex of the abscess to locate the point of greatest fluctuation.

"Abscess, but luckily, not too deep… I'm going to scrub again. Do we have xylocaine with epinephrine?"

"Two percent?" she asked.

"That will be fine. Four cc's please and can you prep him with betadine and get some sterile draping? I'll also need a number eleven scalpel and lots of sponges. That thing will be a little Vesuvius once we get in, if I'm not mistaken... Oh, yes, we'll need some sterile saline for irrigation," he added as an afterthought.

"Reality check, Jason... Best I can do is boiled water kept as sterile as possible."

"It'll have to do, won't it?"

Five minutes later, the boy's leg had been cleansed and a sterile field established with drapes clipped together with hemostats.

Jason had gloved but gowning was out of the question. He stepped to the boy's head where he smiled as reassuringly as possible.

"It will be alright, son. You'll feel a needle stick... no worse than the bite of an ant. But you must lie still while I'm working. Ok?"

The child was trying to put on a brave front, but his lower lip quivered and beads of sweat had appeared on his forehead in such profusion that they were coalescing like mercury droplets and tracing glistening tear tracks in the direction of his ears. He nodded his agreement.

Jason took up the syringe of anesthetic and advanced on the abscess. Along an invisible line that bisected the swelling, he injected the pain-numbing solution. The child's thigh muscles flexed at the needlestick, bringing the abscess into sharp relief but, after the initial discomfort, he lay still.

"We'll give it a minute to take effect...," he said. Then to the patient, "How you feeling, partner?"

The boy nodded in reply, but said nothing.

"He looks fine, Jason. Scared, but otherwise okay."

"I'm ready for the scalpel," he said to Amy and held out his gloved hand.

"Sorry, reality check again. We have no sterile gloves my size, so you'll have to be your own surgical assistant."

She smiled apologetically.

Picking up the scalpel handle he deftly fastened the pointed blade to it. Using the pinpoints of blood from the anesthetic injections as orientation points, he stabbed, then slowly drew the blade along the skin laying open a two inch track. A thin line of blood, followed by a surge of pus the color of guacamole, welled up after the scalpel. Like lava, the infection first sprang forth under pressure, then settled down into a steadily advancing stream overwhelming individual leg hairs on its gravity-drawn course toward the sterile drapes.

"Like I predicted, Vesuvius. I'm going to waste a lot of sponges on this... Do we have packing gauze?"

"'Fraid not, Jason. You'll have to improvise."

"That's okay. I can pack adequately with sponges."

Quickly and efficiently, his fingers flew through the tasks of evacuating the effluent, rinsing and finally packing the wound. Amy could easily imagine his dexterity at the keyboard. Before finishing, he put in two interrupted sutures at each end of the wound to prevent undue spreading of the incision and, finally, he wicked up the gauze in the center of the cut so the osmotic pressure that would drain the continued secretions would carry over to the gauze of the pressure dressing.

"Well, partner, it's all done... You've got a brand new leg but I have to see you tomorrow."

As he spoke the words, he realized that he had committed himself to return to the clinic. He felt no regrets.

Amy's face beamed with pleasure and admiration.

After snapping off the gloves, he helped the boy up and off the table. The child's first step was hesitant but, when he felt no pain (the anesthetic was still working), he walked tentatively around the table. Then, unexpectedly, he jumped up and down twice, his eyes sparkling with amazement.

"Whoa! Take it easy... No jumping or running... Walk carefully until it's all healed," and Jason placed a calming hand on the child's shoulder.

The boy still didn't speak, but his grin literally split his face from ear to ear. He negotiated the corridor with a jaunty spring to his step that had both Amy and Jason laughing.

The next patient was an old man with gnarled limbs twisted like diseased grapevines. He was malnourished, and so painfully thin, that the cord like tendons in his arms were traced in stark relief under skin as insubstantial as black silk. It was as if his swollen bulbous joints had sucked all the vitality from the rest of his body. When he attempted to speak, a dozen ligaments in his neck flexed tightly, as though an inept puppeteer hidden inside his chest was vainly pulling strings to control his clumsy speech.

Jason had difficulty understanding what the old man said and assumed he wasn't close enough to the patient. However, when he leaned nearer to the lined and shriveled papier-mâché face, he could see that the man's jaw was scarcely moving. In response to Jason's request to open his mouth, the old fellow strained mightily but could scarcely move the jaw which seemed as effectively tethered as if it had been wired in place.

A quick exam revealed a firm oblong mass extending under the mandible from chin to throat. Probing the inside of the man's mouth with a gloved finger, after literally prying his toothless jaws open a crack, Jason could feel the slick upper surface of the tumor crowding almost to the roof of the mouth. When he attempted to have him take in a spoonful of water and swallow, the patient began to cough uncontrollably and seemed likely to expire from the effort. The cancer had closed off his esophagus and he was aspirating the fluid into his lungs.

The secret of his malnutrition had little to do with the arthritis that had twisted his joints into functionless deformities. He was starving to death because a rock-hard cancer had clamped his jaws shut with the grip of a pit-bull. While forbidding its victim nourishment, the malignancy, like a voracious wasp larva, would feed on the little vitality left in his body until he withered to a dehydrated husk.

The old woman, who was apparently his wife, stood dutifully just inside the door of the examining room. Even at a distance, Jason could detect the frosty walleye opacity of one of her corneas. Her other eye, cataract-free, read the message on his face and gazed at him with a dispirited resignation that he knew he had no power to dispel.

Amy had been dispensing birth control pills to a young woman and came into the room just as Jason and the old woman exchanged wordless messages. Their despair quivered in the air. She glanced furtively at the old man, and then back at Jason with a question in her eyes.

The physician said nothing. He was searching for the words to use with his patients, reworking the doleful message he had communicated so often before in the sterile confines of his clinic. But here, today, given the exalted expectations the St. Lucians had of foreign doctors, it was somehow different, more difficult. He was struggling.

Silently, the old woman broke gaze, leaned on her cane and toddled toward him. When she was close enough, she raised a frail quavering hand, with no more weight to it than a butterfly wing, and set it gently on his arm. Weariness flattened her voice.

"Thank you, doctor... It wer' needful for us to know."

Shuffling to the examining table, she lay her cane against it and, with her own and Jason's assistance, her husband slid from the table exhausting himself in the effort. He, too, patted the hand that had helped him up.

He managed to whisper "Cank..kew" through a mouthful of disease. There was a serenity in his eyes that freed Jason from the obligation to say anything.

As the old couple left, Jason asked, "I don't suppose we have any morphine?"

Amy didn't answer. She was staring at the retreating couple. She had no words... There were none that would be appropriate.

The rest of the afternoon passed within an envelope of sadness, although no further tragedy was encountered, in serving the few patients who remained to be seen.

Amy had barely closed the door behind the last patient when a frenzied knocking vibrated down the hall. Re-opening the door, they found the young boy with the abscess. He still wore a grin so broad that it forced his eyes into a squint.

In one hand, he held a piece of well-worn string tied around the legs of a small rooster hanging quietly upside down with its wings spread. The bird's legs had been plucked clean of feathers.

"For you, doctor," he said simply, extending his hand.

Jason eyed the cock and was about to politely refuse when Amy whispered.

"It's worth several dollars, Jason, and he wants to pay. The girls who look after the clinic will know what to do with it tomorrow."

"Well, thank you. It's a beautiful bird."

Jason was striving to portray genuine appreciation for the gesture. The lad released the string to Jason and the cock, as if it sensed that some weighty and perilous transaction was occurring, frantically flapped its wings raising dust, before giving up to swing like a pendulum on its leash.

"He fight real good... You be happy with him, doctor. I come tomorrow."

And he was off... almost running.

"Hey, walking only, remember?" Jason called after him.

"What's he mean '*fight real good*'?"

"It's a fighting cock, Jason. They raise them here. They are highly prized and valuable."

He looked down at the naked drumsticks.

"Wonder what they taste like?" he joked

"Gamey," she replied and they both laughed in much needed relief.

* * *

As she cleaned up the examining room, Jason washed his hands.

"It's been close to twelve hours since your accident, Amy. If we're going to close the laceration, we need to do it now."

"I've already drawn up the xylocaine and there's a suture tray in the next room. I'll be there '*ready to be repaired*' when you've finished washing up."

Getting enough dry paper towel from the sodden roll was a messy affair but, at last, his hands were dry. He crossed the hall and entered the next room, then stopped short at the sight that met his eyes.

Amy was sitting on the table, bare from the waist up. Her hair was pulled over her shoulders and the top of her dress lay crumpled in her lap.

"Come on Jason, you know we have no gowns and, besides, you're a physician aren't you?"

Her eyes sparkled with mischief.

"Y...Yes", he stammered, "but I haven't gotten used to you as a patient, just yet. It makes all the difference in the world, you know."

"Oh, does it really?"

She was playing with him, again.

He was trying to peel the true meaning out of her words. Was she being coy, or did he detect just a whiff of sarcasm?

"Well, of course it does. You should know that as a nurse."

He fumbled awkwardly with his hands searching for pockets to hide them, but his jeans were tight, and he would have had to thrust unnaturally about to find them. As if ashamed of his fumbling, he let his arms slide lamely to his sides, his fingers nervously picking at the fabric of his pants.

"Are you embarrassed, Jason? You're blushing," she laughed.

He relaxed a little and attempted a smile. '*No sarcasm, at least*', he thought.

"I'm trying not to blush. In fact, I'm trying to look only at your face. Inside my head, I'm shouting 'Come on, she's only a patient'…"

"And what were you saying, inside your head, the other night?..." There was a twinkle in her eyes again and she was enjoying herself, thoroughly.

"*The other night*?... I don't know what you mean."

He felt his face glowing, probably cherry-red. His ears started to ring.

"Your nose is growing, Pinocchio," she teased. "I mean, what were you thinking when I walked out of the water naked?... You weren't honest earlier when I asked you if you'd seen me before… Remember?"

He smiled foolishly, found the jeans' pockets, thrust his hands in and started rocking up onto his heels and back down, a nervous habit he'd had since childhood.

"I was meditating..." he muttered.

"With your eyes open?"

"Well, you disturbed me when you arrived."

"Then why didn't you tell me you were there *before I took off my bikini?*"

She was taunting him, enjoying his discomfort in a benign exercise of power she relished, but wasn't exactly sure why. He was going to explain himself. She wouldn't let up until he did. Her sexuality had precipitously stirred to life and her adrenalin was pumping. She reveled in the effect her partial nudity had upon him.

His mind was a maelstrom of half-formed thoughts and he was still struggling to keep from looking at her breasts. He didn't feel exactly threatened by her questions, but he was pinioned. She had the upper hand and, while he felt embarrassment at being evasive earlier, there was a *playful* undercurrent to what was happening.

If she hadn't been naked to the waist, he would have felt a little like a child being scolded by his mother. When the Freudian implications of that thought registered, he squirmed visibly.

She saw it.

"Well, Jason, why didn't you signal your presence to me *before* I stripped myself naked under your very gaze? You still haven't answered me."

She'd placed both hands on her hips in mock indignation and the gesture did things to the contour of her breasts that made it even more difficult for Jason to organize a coherent reply.

He stumbled over his words. "You were staring at the moon… So was I… I mean, I wasn't watching you. I started meditating again and then, I guess you got undressed, and I didn't notice it."

"*I undressed in front of you and you didn't notice it, Jason*? You're getting yourself in deeper all the time. That's insulting... *If it's true.*"

"It *is* true, I swear it…" he blurted out, his voice intense and higher than normal, almost infantile. Little boyish. This process was beginning to feel a lot like a punitive parent-child thing, and he was on the receiving end.

She burst into fragrant laughter. "You should see yourself, Jason. You look like a twelve year old caught by his mother peeking at a Playboy magazine under the bedcovers with a flashlight."

"I was thirteen and you, Miss Amy, or should I say '*Miss February*', are posed almost like one of the models I was peeking at when she caught me."

She blushed suddenly and crossed her arms.

Now *he* was on the offensive. "How could you see me on the boulder? I was in the shadows?"

"See you on the boulder? Your face struck out like a pie tin reflecting the moon's light… I could hardly have missed you."

"And, just at what point, did you see me?... *Before* you peeled off your bathing suit and pranced about naked as a sea nymph?"

His voice grew bolder as he spoke.

The tables in the tussle were definitely turning in his favor and the fact was obvious to them both. Her indignation was becoming increasingly genuine and her face glowed in open rivalry to the color of her hair.

"Now that's not fair, Jason... You *know* I wouldn't do that!" she exclaimed.

The twinkle was now in his eye.

"Oh, do I? Remember, I don't know about your '*reputation*', but I do know that most women harbor a secret exhibitionist *streak*... no pun intended... Besides, I don't remember you covering up much when you strutted out of the surf, right at me..."

"*Strutted*.... When I *strutted* out of the surf!" she blustered, as she sprang down off the table and covered the ground between them in an instant.

She was shaking her finger, literally in his face.

"I didn't *strut*. I wouldn't *strut* for you or for any other letch... I didn't see you until I was getting dressed and, when I did, I wanted to snatch up a rock and brain you for being an insensitive peeping Tom! Would have, too," she fumed, "except it occurred to me that you might want to add rape to your repertoire of sexual perversions!"

Her face was pinched with emotion, and she was actually biting her lower lip. The game was becoming dangerous as her role risked genuinely overtaking her.

Her hands were clenched into fists at her sides and he wouldn't have been surprised if she had started beating on his chest in frustration.

She felt like doing precisely that, then realized how impulsive such a reaction would have been, and spun on her heel turning away from him. As she fought back tears and pulled clumsily at the straps of her dress, wriggling to pull it up, she was filled with alarm at the intensity of the emotions she was feeling while in role. It wasn't supposed to be like this.

She sensed his hands hovering hesitantly above her shoulders like a butterfly above a bloom before she felt them settling gently upon her hair where it lay on her shoulders.

It was several moments before he spoke, and when he did, his voice was husky with emotion.

"Here is the truth and only the truth. When I saw you that night, I *was* in a trance and well beyond the power of speech. I wanted to tell you I was there, but the experience seemed almost like a dream. You weren't some flesh and blood woman for me. I never saw your face and, in my state of mind that night, I was naïve enough to believe that you might have been a vision sent as a signal… that your appearance was an omen of sorts."

He swallowed audibly and paused. She heard him sigh, a shuddering, almost whispered vibration.

"That night was a time of profound transition for me, the beginning of my return to health and sanity… I had begun to crawl out of the pit of depression where I'd been shut up for what seemed like an eternity. The miracle of that evening was cathartic, transforming... You couldn't have known it, but your appearance coincided with a profound reawakening within me. Since then, even though I didn't see you again until today, whenever I think of you, I feel the stirrings of elemental longings I thought I'd lost forever."

He continued. "Do you know what it's like to experience resurrected hope, the promise of renewed vitality… a return to life?"

He paused once more and neither of them stirred. He could hear her breathing, feel his own heart pounding. He was astonished at the risk he was taking, speaking so openly to a literal stranger, but he was compelled to continue even if she didn't respond.

"Whatever happens, I will be eternally grateful to you and, if we hadn't spoken here of the events of last night, I would never have whispered a word of it to another living soul… It was private, internal, almost a spiritual experience, for me. I would have treasured the memory.... never devalued it. Please forgive me for having done just that today... I'm so sorry."

The last words of apology caught like burrs in his throat, which was closing under the weight of intense emotion. He lowered his hands slowly from her shoulders, allowing his fingers to caress her back as he did.

She turned slowly to face him. Her eyes soulfully searching his face and he could see her tears glistening. The flecks of gold in her pupils held him, until he could literally see his own reflection in her eyes. He could tell she was desperately struggling to assess the impact of his words.

She was frightened by the implications of his confession. For a moment, they both remained locked in hesitation then, she slowly lowered her eyes and spoke.

"I'm so sorry, Jason. I was teasing you... It was a foolish and cruel game. I don't know what to say... I never suspected you felt about me like you do."

His heart sank. He could feel her slipping away. In desperation, he took her by the shoulders. "Amy, please tell me what you're thinking... *really* thinking... I was almost certain you were sending me a message... What's happening?"

She continued to hang her head, her shoulders slack. "I can't, Jason... I just can't."

"Can't what, Amy?"

"I can't explain... You'd never be able to understand..."

He could feel her shoulders shake, as sobs began to punctuate her words.

"Please, just let me... Just let me go..."

He pulled her to him, but she remained still, arms hanging limply, unresponsive.

They stood together with his arms around her for several minutes. Her cheek lay warm and moist against his chest, but it was the only response she made to the invitation of his arms. When they separated, he spoke first, bravely attempting a smile.

"That laceration needs stitching and I need to scrub again. Please, lie down on the table, and I'll be back in a minute."

On the table, she stared up at the ceiling which quivered and then dissolved into a blur of white as the tears welled up in her eyes. She had to hide to withdraw back into herself, her instincts left her no other choice but for the first time in her life she truly didn't want to.

* * *

The next morning after his therapy session, Jason was waiting for her at the van. Despite her resolve to remain calm, her heart leapt when she saw him. She'd lain awake all night tormented by regrets, cursing her inability to escape her protective role playing. She'd convinced herself that he would try to avoid her. Several other times in her life, she had come to the edge of potential happiness only to dart back into the burrow of her fear when the glare of discovery threatened.

For some reason, this time, despite the fact that she'd fled from him, she'd been spared and he had come back.

"Jason, I'm so very glad you're here." She stepped up to him boldly and kissed his cheek.

"Hey, the kid with the abscess will be back and I promised him I'd be there," he said.

"Truly, a man of your word."

He blushed vividly, " *Too many* words last night... I apologize."

She reached and took his hands in hers reassuringly and simply repeated her greeting... "I'm so pleased you're here."

"Me too," he replied sheepishly.

* * *

The next two weeks fell into an idyllic routine, more rewarding than either Jason or Amy would have believed possible.

Each morning, they attended individual therapy with Dr. Landry, although the therapist readily admitted that his services now seemed unnecessary for either of them. Each afternoon, rather than simply three days a week, they volunteered as a team at the charity clinic. In doing so, a profound spiritual renewal was taking place as they rediscovered the avocation and dedication both had almost lost as caregivers in a system that invited the alienation of practitioners from the ideals of medicine.

Then, after the sun sank below the horizon and the enchantment of the tropical night fell over all of nature, they would walk and swim together. By unspoken agreement, they avoided overt sexual behavior although they held hands and hugged at each encounter. Both of them remembered clearly the embarrassment of the incident at the clinic.

They were falling in love but neither of them dared risk enough to speak of it explicitly and both were aware of the perils of infatuation. Each, therefore, imposed strict restraint upon their instincts, knowing that the greatest threat to their relationship would be to plunge ahead impulsively into what they needed so desperately... to belong to someone... to escape loneliness.

What lay ahead for them was never a topic of discussion but, incrementally, and with great discretion and hesitation, they disclosed the trauma in their lives that had brought them to St. Lucia. She learned about his children, Annette's death, the struggle with his in-laws and the turmoil at TurnerWest.

Neither volunteered much about their childhood, but she unburdened herself on the subject of her abusive ex-husband and the ongoing struggle of coming to grips and dealing with herself as a battered woman.

And so, in lieu of becoming lovers, they became the best of friends. And, in the process, were returned to health.

CH020: CARRABELLE, FLORIDA.

It was six p.m. when the captain of the 'Critter Gitter' stowed the last of the trolling rods and pitched the three remaining baitfish high into the air to reward the patience of the lone gull which had cruised in avid anticipation over their wake while they trolled. Although no competitors were near, it screeched like a strangled cat, and plunged with undignified haste to skewer one of the Ballyhoo before it hit the water. A bobbing of the bird's head in full flight and the bait was swallowed in time for the scavenger to wheel and snatch a second fish just before it sank beyond reach.

The sun was sliding toward the horizon but the day had been torrid and its slanting rays still distorted the boundary between water and sky so that a boat, which was approaching from the direction of the coast, seemed to be suspended on a silver foil shimmering above the surface of the sea.

"That idiot's heading the wrong way for this time of day," grunted the captain as he shaded his eyes by extending his hat brim with the flat of his hand and squinting at the puff of white as it approached.

"May be he's going to overnight thirty miles out, beyond the K towers," volunteered a second taller and thinner man who had emerged from the cabin to join him on the deck. "Here's a cold one," he added thrusting a silver Budweiser can toward the Captain.

"Thanks! Well, we better be on our way back to port. Is everything secure below?"

"All secure. Think I'll stretch out while we run in. Call me if you need to be spelled," and, with that, the tall man unlimbered with a sigh on the padded bench across the boat from the captain's chair.

The twin Mercruisers coughed once and then began a grumbling duet while the captain checked gauges. He pushed the throttle handles forward and the engines, purring throatily, crescendoed into action thrashing the water to instant foam as the Mako surged up and forward like a skier rising off a mogul.

A compass heading of 300 degrees would take them laser straight to the gulf coast between St. George and Dog Island and with the swells slick and flat as an oil spill, it would be less than an hour's run at full throttle.

Almost instantly, the Mako was skimming the surface in an easy lope, regular puffs of low white spray like dust spurts beneath antelope hooves, marked her bounding course toward the invisible shore.

To starboard, the distant boat had settled from the mirage shimmer and was now riding clearly on the blue of the water. Her course paralleled the Mako in the opposite direction.

"Moving at trolling speed," muttered the captain to himself and with the innate curiosity of the fisherman, he altered his course slightly to pass close enough to the vessel for identification.

He'd fished these waters for ten years and knew most every boat. Unless this was one of the growing number of newcomers who'd discovered the beaches of Dog Island, they'd be well enough acquainted to wave or perhaps banter the day's news on the radio.

He turned his thoughts to the half dozen fish sloshing in the ice of the Igloo cooler and imagined himself before a plate of succulent Mahi Mahi after a cool shower and a change of clothes. Sucking at the beer in his hand, he felt good and would return to his office tomorrow morning without feeling cheated by life. The confident dual tones of the engines as they obediently surged off each swell was almost entrancing.

When he next focused on the approaching craft, he saw it suddenly wallow like a drunk stumbling on a dance floor. Its bow pitched awkwardly into a swell then rose once more and fell back. The boat's creamy wake suddenly disappeared like a chalk-line hitting the edge of a blackboard.

The boat was now close enough that he could see the outriggers had been deployed. However, there was no activity on the deck as he would have expected if the occupants had tied into a billfish and slowed or stopped to play it.

The captain kept watching as the distance between the two boats narrowed. He inched his helm slightly closer to the other craft and called his sleeping partner.

"Bill, take a look at this, will you?"

The tall man raised himself on an elbow, peered across at the other boat now rolling silently in the swells.

"It's a Bayliner. What are they fighting?" he grunted, forcing himself up to a sitting position, reflexively blinking, splinters of sunlight jabbing at his unadjusted pupils.

"That's just it. I don't see anything happening. She just stopped. Can you see anyone on deck?... Check it out with the glasses," and he gestured to a set of binoculars hanging on the wall in a mesh sack.

Bill fumbled the glasses out and trained them on the Bayliner while the captain throttled back to steady the Mako.

For a moment he said nothing.

"It's the 'Old Fart'. That's the doc from Georgia's boat isn't it?"

"You mean the guy with the knock-out wife?"

"I don't know about his wife, but he's bald and short. He told me once that his kids had named the boat after him, I remember that."

"Well, the old fart must have traded in his first wife for one of those twenty year olds. Haven't ever talked to her but I've seen her and she's a beauty... a hell of a lot younger than him. Can you see her on board?" asked the captain.

"Can't see anyone. Hail them on the open channel. Maybe they've got trouble below deck and are just out of sight."

The captain picked up the radio and called. "This is 'Critter Gitter' to 'Old Fart' come in please. Come in..."

His appeals went unanswered. The Mako had passed the Bayliner which was now about 200 yards astern and Bill could see the aft section of the boat clearly.

"Not a soul in sight but all the lines are out... Something's wrong!"

"I'm going in to make contact," said the captain as he heeled the Mako to starboard and curved toward the Bayliner.

In a couple of minutes they were alongside the craft which had two poles on the outriggers and two more in stern rod holders. All four lines drooped limply in the water.

"Hey! Anyone aboard?" called Bill as he dropped out one of the Mako's bumpers and reached with a boathook to pull the vessels together.

"Man, this is spooky... Hope no one's dead in there," said Bill.

"Tie us off and I'll check her out."

The captain had cut his engines and was moving to join his companion. When the gunwales were close enough together, with the easy balance borne of experience, he hopped deftly onto the side of the Bayliner and then dropped lightly to its deck.

"Anyone on board?... Are you ok?"

No answer.

He scanned the deck. The sun glinted off the open lid of a live bait well where the bubbles from an aerator stirred the surface in an easy effervescence. The buckle from a fighting chair cast a lazy swinging shadow below the seat to which it was attached. Beside the chair a gaff rocked on the deck. The business end had fresh blood on it. Several more blotches of blood had begun to bake into black stains on the heat of the sun-sizzled deck.

He glanced into the cockpit: throttle in the forward position, key on and the fish finder's green glow marking 80 empty feet below the vessel. A short bungee cord tethered the helm to a clasp fastened to the sidewall of the cabin with two brass bolts. It was an arrangement commonly used by single fishermen who watched their lines while trolling in open water.

"What do you see?" asked Bill.

The captain didn't speak but waved his hand and shook his head in reply. He was standing at the head of the stairs to the cabin. The door was made in two halves that swung together for latching and folded back into the interior when open. One half was swaying open, then shut, with the rocking of the boat. The other had been clipped open he stepped down into the shadows of the entrance and poked his head in.

"Anyone on board?"

Before him he could see two empty upholstered benches with a table between them. A large tackle box lay flipped impotently sideways in the center of the table, its contents scattered on the table and the deck below. A life jacket had been flung like a dead thing against the end of one bench. The narrow door to the head was swinging open and shut permitting glimpses of a porcelain commode and wash basin.

Only the small aft half cabin behind him remained hidden from view. He stepped into the fore cabin taking care to avoid the hooks of the scattered lures. He felt an impulse to stop and heeded it, calling out almost haltingly. "Anyone here?"

No surprise answer.

He forced himself to turn toward the odor of mildew and moist cloth baked in the claustrophobic confines of the aft cabin. Darker than the rest of the below deck space, its threat heightened by the absence of anyone elsewhere, the aft cabin nonetheless proved to be empty of anything significant. Bedclothes, many weeks, perhaps months past changing were heaped indecorously in the middle of a velveteen-covered mattress. Two fishing rods had been tossed in haphazardly.

The captain sighed in relief.

"Nothing down here. It's empty as a tomb."

"That's not funny, Mitch..." the tall man called down.

"Where the hell is the doc?"

"Damned if I know. Can you see anyone adrift?" he asked as he climbed back to the deck.

"Not even a bird. If he is overboard and he must be, he's not close... Poor bugger, he could be miles back there at the speed the boat was traveling."

The captain was checking the gauges.

"Tanks are dead empty," he said tapping the gauge with his finger... "If he came out from Carabelle, he didn't start out full, which doesn't make much sense either."

"You going to call the coast guard or you want me to?"

"Let's check the engine compartment first. It wouldn't be the first time someone keeled over from fumes and got trapped..."

As they pulled up the engine trap, a wave of even hotter air laced with fumes of oil and old gasoline rolled out but the compartment contained machinery only.

"If he'd fallen overboard on a Saturday or Sunday chances are someone would have pulled him in but not today. There isn't one boat per ten square miles out here today," the tall man's tired eyes swept the empty horizon.

"He could drift forever and never be found even if he'd been wearing a life jacket, which I doubt he was."

He spoke in the subdued tones of a man contemplating a fate he'd risked many times pursuing solitary pleasures on a boat where a simple misstep could spell tragedy.

"I'll try to raise Panama City... Look for his registration in that document pouch," said the captain pointing to a plastic pouch pressure-snapped to the side of a seat.

"Panama City coast guard, this is the 'Old Fart'... Come in please..."

The crackle of static punctuated an immediate reply.

"This is the US coast guard at Panama City, 'Old Fart'.... Over"

"This is Mitch Steiner, captain of the 'Critter Gitter'. I'm on the vessel the 'Old Fart'. We have an incident to report. We have found a 30 foot boat with no one aboard. We have reason to believe someone may be lost at sea...Over"

"Go to channel 24 Mr. Steiner please and stand by to give details..."

The tall man had found the boat's registration among the papers in the pouch and proffered it to the captain.

"This is Panama City coast guard station calling the 'Old Fart'... Come in please"

"Old Fart here..."

"What is your current position, please."

The captain glanced at the GPS digits and read into the mike.

"North 4592663 West 725941, over."

"And the name of the registered owner of the vessel, please. Over..."

"Dr. Calvin Mellows..."

CH021: ST.LUCIA

Amy was waiting for Jason at the van for the short trip to the clinic. It was another paradisiacal day.

Last evening as they swam, a surgeon wind had slit open the bellies of the clouds and a vertical river had poured out of the sky. They had been forced to dive under the surface repeatedly to escape the stinging volleys of rain that raked their skin like liquid birdshot.

Finally, driven from the water by the torrents, they had huddled together laughing ecstatically in the lee of the boulder where Jason regularly meditated . Their laughter had been drowned by the tattoo of the rain upon sand, rock, and vegetation... the strength of the storm's assault literally bending the leaves of a nearby banana plant to the ground. After ten minutes of snuggling to make themselves too small to be worthy targets for nature's playful vengeance against man, they realized they would have to make a run for the villa.

Towels knotted about their necks like children playing Superman, they had raced down the beach literally shrieking with excitement. Amy's trained legs easily outdistanced Jason's best efforts and he didn't catch her till she slowed her pace on the slick stones of the lower patio.

Breathless, they slipped quickly inside and then stood, chests heaving to repay their oxygen debts, while they watched the downpour of the rainy season's mighty baptism of the tropics.

Later, they had hugged, shivering with cold and exhaustion, before running off to their cabins to recuperate.

After a warm shower, Amy lay on her bed feeling no need for sleep as the rhythm of the rain on the cottage thatch provided a backdrop for her journal entry. She had started to record the events of her days in St. Lucia shortly after Jason had come into her life and given her reason to have hope for the future. She had pondered and written for over an hour when the rain tapered off and she thought she heard music, wafting almost eerily, on the night breeze. Straining to listen, she arose, walked to the balcony and slid open the door. Beyond and behind the dripping trees, she heard it distinctly again, a rivulet of notes trilling in the distance.

A piano.

Seized with an excitement that she dared hardly entertain, she took a dry towel and draped it over her shoulders against the chill of the drizzle. With exaggerated stealth, she stole out of the cottage, pausing every few steps like a hunter sifting forest sounds, as she followed the spoor of the notes which led her back to the main villa.

During an earlier bout of depression, as a mood-altering strategy, she had trained her heart to soar on the melodic updrafts of classical composition. Now, as she began to feel the emotion of a recognizable theme, a fluttering in her chest promised an escape into rapture.

The music grew in volume as she approached the villa and she could easily discern the majestic ethereal strands of treble woven into the earthy basal tapestry of Wagner's 'Flight of the Valkyries'.

Her heart was beating in her throat as she opened the patio door silently and slipped inside the large reception hall from which the music sprang.

The storm clouds had hermetically sealed the heavens against the moon and not even a glimmer of light from the small lamps lining the paths outside penetrated the seamless darkness of the room.

As soon as she entered, she slid into a squat seeking to blend into the darkness. Through the silk of her pajamas she could feel the panes of the windows cool against her back.

An instant after she had settled herself into meditative attention, the music stopped abruptly. She held her breath not daring to stir, lest she be discovered.

All was silence within the room, the dark muffled solitude of the womb. The world outside had retreated, driven back by the mystical fantasy of the moment.

And suddenly the music began again. A geyser of notes crescendoing into the air to hang in luxurious suspension before settling mist-like upon her; feathering her brow, her lips, her skin, like a lover's caress. Her body slowly began to respond to the music's seductive force... absorbing, echoing, and, finally, vibrating in synchrony to the very sinews of her soul.

Within ten minutes, she had abandoned consciousness, fled into an esthetic swoon, freed from the awareness of anything but the sound which bathed her within and without.

Spared the awareness of time, she remained eyes closed, limbs folded upon themselves like rose petals in the dawn, lost to anything but the music and its magic. When the last note reverberated through the hall and silence fell, she remained huddled against the window, deeply asleep.

His kiss upon her forehead did not rouse her, and while he gathered her up from the floor and carried her in his arms to the cabin, she did not awaken.

The next morning, she awoke to sunlight pouring over the balcony ledge and streaming like quicksilver across the floor of her room. She sighed and stretched away the strands of sleep from her muscles. Her dreams had been sweet, overpowering and delicious.

As she threw off the coverlet of the bed, she stared in surprise at a halo of sand sprinkled on the bedsheet around her feet. She examined last evening in her mind. She could remember her shower clearly but her dream had claimed the rest of the night. No answer there... unless it had *really* been Jason at the piano. Had his playing woven the spell that had carried her away? The possibility that the events of the night had been real, and not fantasy, sent a tingle of excitement scampering squirrel-like up the rungs of her spine.

* * *

As she waited beside the van, forcing herself to admire the precise beauty of the lawns and gardens, she grew impatient for Jason's arrival. She was consumed with curiosity and anticipation, for she had never known anyone with musical talent equal to what she had witnessed last night.

Although blessed with the strong body of an athlete and graced with a quick and fertile intellect, Amy lamented the fact that she was bereft of any ability to create music. In spite of this deficit, she seemed to hear music everywhere with an appreciation and acuity that was purely instinctual... the ceaseless melody of the waves... the rumbling tumult of the distant storm behind the timpani of raindrops on leaves... an insect chorus burgeoning into the night air. And man's creations...the majestic imaginings of the composers who transformed the themes of nature into symphonies...had attracted, seduced and transported her beyond the boundaries of a desperate life.

Music had always been her escape... the summer storms of childhood... the symphonies, when she grew older.

For Amy, the very thought that this man, in whom she had been silently investing her emotions, might also be an accomplished musician filled her with intense excitement.

When, at last, Jason appeared in the villa's doorway she could no longer restrain herself and ran toward him. However, as she approached and saw his downcast eyes and measured step, she felt a sudden chill. Something seemed terribly wrong. His characteristic smile was gone and his features sagged in a frown. His eyes had a bruised look and his gaze seemed to be fixed on something far beyond her. He apparently took no notice of her excited demeanor and didn't look up to face her until she was literally upon him.

"Jason, what's wrong?"

She had grasped both of his hands and stood looking expectantly up into his face.

He attempted a smile, but it was wan and without energy, and failed to lighten the sadness she could see in his eyes. He squeezed her hands in a gesture of reassurance, wanting to dispel any suspicion she might be harboring that the source of his obvious concern had anything to do with her.

"I am glad you're here, Amy. I need to talk. I've just received bad news about a friend." He released her hand and turned her in a half circle, putting his arm across her shoulders.

"Let's go to your Banyan tree... I want to collect my thoughts... Things are still pretty much swirling about in my mind. I just got off the phone."

"The phone?" she asked quizzically, looking up at him again.

She knew calls to or from the outside were strictly forbidden. It was one of the clinic's fundamental rules.

"Yes. Brigham screened an emergency call late last night from the Albany police and suggested they call me early today."

"It's not the children..." she blurted.

"No, the kids are in Michigan with their grandparents... Just give me a few minutes... I'll try to explain it all, so you'll understand."

They struck out in silence along a path that cut across the lawn and then disappeared into the shade of a banana grove which hemmed one side of the property. A few broad tattered leaves had been torn by the force of the night's rain from the arching vault of vegetation that shaded the path, and now they lay wilting in the steamy heat that rose from the ground. They were unexpectedly slick and Jason almost fell when he stepped on one.

Ordinarily, he would have commented, perhaps a quip or a humorous remark, but he righted himself without a word.

His mind was struggling to process the implications of the news he'd received. He was being forced into decisions from which he wished to flee but, with the return of his sanity, had come a rediscovery of responsibilities. Things he could not ignore. Things that could not be reconciled easily with the new values in life that he had discovered here, away from the turmoil he'd left behind.

He was troubled.

Beyond the grove, the path had become serpentine, winding upwards to the heights of the promontory. Jason was breathing heavily from the exertion of the climb and perspiration circled his armpits and pasted the tissue of his shirt to his back. Amy had climbed almost effortlessly, ahead of him. They had made the short trip together before and he had enjoyed watching her leg muscles ripple into attractive relief as she climbed. But today, he had studied only the earth and rock of the pathway during its full length, as if some solution to the problems he pondered might be serendipitously found there, gleaming like a new coin.

They settled themselves on the soft grass below the Banyan's canopy which effectively shielded them from the sun's probing rays. Jason drew up his knees and hugged them while meditatively staring off into the endless blue before them. Below, the sound of the surf's muffled struggle with the rocks at the cliff base, barely reached them.

Amy sat quietly, a few feet from him, waiting.

Jason seemed to be painstakingly assembling his thoughts, as someone might piece together a shattered mirror that was the only means of seeing some essential reflected truth.

When he spoke, his tone was flat and detached, as if wringing all emotion from his voice was a stratagem that might make it easier to speak of difficult things.

"I've told you a little about the dissension that has torn our group of doctors at TurnerWest but, to understand the context in which it has occurred, you need more background information. Mark West and I, in the past, were as close as two grown men generally get... We were good friends, but this takeover struggle and changes in Mark's personality have decimated that relationship and put us at each other's throat. He can't see things my way any longer and, I admit, that I refuse to concede to his idea that we should grab the money from the takeover windfall, as if there were no wider consequences to our actions than those affecting us directly."

He paused, and when the silence became heavy, she interjected.

"What did he stand to gain from the takeover?"

Jason sighed.

"A great deal... I can understand his frustration with me. TurnerWest would be purchased as a corporation for over eleven million dollars and Mark and I, as senior partners, would split the bulk of that."

"Eleven million...," Amy repeated softly as she attempted to process the enormity of the sum.

"Yes, eleven million, and stock in CHC would be used to pay us. Their stock has been growing like Jack's beanstalk and Mark knows that, if we'd already signed six months ago, we'd each have about a million more by now as well."

"Does he need the money?" she interjected.

"No... Never has. WestWinds plantation is old money and, if he never earned a cent as a physician, Mark would still be a rich man. But he's developed a rabid obsession with power and the more money he has, the more powerful he becomes."

Jason paused in reflection for a moment, as if remembering the transformation of his friend that he was describing.

"I'd always seen his aggressive ambition but, a little over three years ago, he got mixed up with a very weird but gorgeous Creole woman from Martinique. She seemed to weave the same spell over Mark that her ancestor Josephine had wielded over Napoleon."

He continued, " They were only together for eight months or so, but he spent almost half that time with her in Europe. He must have blown almost a half million on her... jewels, a car, etc. She infected him with a taste for the life of the empty ultra-rich, and he's never recovered from it. Power and money are about all that matter to him anymore. There's none of his previous humanity left... He's become someone I almost despise, and that sentiment appears to be mutual."

Curiosity getting the better of her, Amy asked, "Where is the woman now?"

"Oh, after the eight months, she dropped Mark like he had AIDS and took up with some amputated scion of the Romanian royal family."

"How did he react to that turn of events?" she asked.

"Certainly no apparent depression, like you might have expected… He never talked about her or exactly what happened, at least never with me. He'd changed though, like I said. Medicine didn't seem to matter to him anymore. He was power mad, and our relationship really went into the toilet when I told him frankly what I saw happening in him." Jason paused and then went on.

" His father had been a federal senator and, at about that time, Mark began to see himself as a potential political player on the national scene. Through his financial backing, he already owned Senator Stephen Davlin, lock, stock, and barrel, but it wasn't enough to wield power from behind the scene, so, he actually toyed with the idea of running for the senate himself two years ago."

"What stopped him?"

"He had one enemy, an old democrat warhorse from Savannah whose family has locked horns with Mark's for the last century. It's a southern thing that we do almost as well as the Sicilians... a blood feud. Richard Shiver, that was the man's name, had been Mark's father's nemesis and would have opposed the WestWind political heir, to the death. It would have been a dirty fight and split the democratic party. Insiders convinced Mark not to risk the damage."

"So what happened?"

"Compromise candidate, single term. An interim solution."

"And now?" she asked.

"Shiver's gone. Suicide after he faced a scandal over an illegitimate daughter."

"Surely a kid, born on the wrong side of the blanket, wouldn't be reason enough to kill yourself there in the South?" Amy's tone of voice evinced a skeptical sarcasm.

Jason permitted himself a wry smile before he replied.

"His daughter had become the Madam of the largest escort service in Atlanta... When she pointed the finger at Shiver, who was an outspoken Southern Baptist, it created an uproar. But a lot of people, including me, were shocked when he killed himself... It didn't seem to be his style. Drove smack into a bridge abutment, just outside Savannah. Left a note on his office blotter apologizing to his family."

"So Mark's path is clear?"

"Would be, except he seems to be even more ambitious now and would like to secure a position as a captain of industry to prime the pump for politics. The senate has become small potatoes... He wants an ambassadorship, someplace in Europe."

"Is that where the CHC money comes in?"

"The money is important, but not as crucial to his plans as a seat on the board of CHC would be. Mark was trying to negotiate that side deal privately with CHC and he was outraged when I found out about it and told several other members of the staff. It was the strongest card I had to play in my hand. He's still working to pull it off and, once he's on the CHC board, he plans to worm or buy his way into the position of CEO. I'm convinced, that if he can get his foot in the door, he'd have a better than even chance of ending up in the CEO's chair."

"So, now you stand in his way. Is that it?"

"I hadn't thought of it that way," he said shrugging his shoulders.

"But it's true that CHC won't touch him without the TurnerWest takeover... However, I'm not his only adversary. Mark has opposition from other physicians in the group as well."

"Well, did the phone call say something happened to Mark?" asked Amy.

"No. I'm just telling you about him so you'll understand the impact of what happened to another friend, a man who is Mark's sworn enemy and my ally. In fact, Mark has had a rare turn of good fortune in the form of Cal Mellow's disappearance. That's what the phone call was about."

"Who is Cal in the business?" she asked.

"Cal is our vice president of surgery. His boat was found floating off the Florida coast two days ago and he's been presumed lost at sea. His wife Gloria called me after the police did. Apparently, the night before he disappeared, they had talked and he had been trying to contact me... It seems he was being blackmailed."

"Did he commit suicide, like Mark's other enemy?" Amy seemed a little incredulous.

"That's what it looks like, but I knew Cal very well and I can't imagine him choosing that option. He'd get angry, not depressed. If he'd killed someone, it would make more sense. Gloria agrees with me. She's convinced that if Cal really is dead, that it's murder... not suicide. His disappearance and the unanswered questions it raises have got my mind wading through a bog of very nasty implications."

He shook his head slowly from side to side and drew the spread fingers of one hand through his hair.

"There's been almost too much for me to handle ...Annette's death, and now Cal is gone… and none of it makes any sense. I feel so impotent when I even start trying to figure it out, let alone deal with it all, effectively. My mind may be almost back to normal functioning, but I can hardly summon the courage to face any more of this..."

She leaned toward him, slipping an arm about his bowed shoulders, and laid her cheek against his arm.

Above them, in the Banyan, the raucous squabbling of two parrots suddenly erupted and wings thrashed in the leaves. Neither of them looked up.

Several minutes passed in silence before he spoke again.

"Gloria seemed afraid to talk on the telephone. She sounded paranoid, almost irrational. I promised her I'd go back to help out, as soon as I could get a flight."

A leaden tone of resignation permeated his words.

His announcement struck Amy like a blow to the solar plexus and all she could manage to say was, "Go... now?"

She sat upright, suddenly rigid with apprehension.

Assessing her obvious dismay, his expression softened as he studied her. The tide of her breathing had quickened and a glimmer of a tear had appeared instantaneously in the corner of her eye. She was pleading with him to stay, without a word being spoken.

"I have to go, Amy. Cal was a good and loyal friend and Gloria and her children need me. Besides, if I don't get back quickly, Mark may maneuver in my absence to isolate me from the other doctors. Cal was my strongest ally. The situation at TurnerWest have been destabilized by his disappearance."

She said nothing, but grasped his arm with both hands and leaned closer in order to lay her face against his shoulder.

He opened his arms and folded her against his chest, nuzzling her hair.

"No choice for me, Amy… Staying isn't an option."

He caressed her neck with his fingers as he spoke softly into her hair.

Amy's heart was thundering against her ribs, her breath coming in staccato catches, as she sobbed silently and clung tighter to him. She was amazed at her own behavior. She tried by an effort of supreme will to pull back, if only internally, but her power to do so was gone.

Amy Davis was totally out of role and she could do nothing at all about it.

Her thoughts slalomed rapidly down the obstacle course that recent events had constructed in her mind. She slammed into the reality of her profound need for this man, into the potential freedom their relationship offered her… Then, she caromed off into her overwhelming fear of intimacy... of discovery... of potential rejection. The zigzag course of her ambivalence caused her to shudder, suddenly and violently.

Jason felt her shaking and pulled her tighter against him in reassurance.

Her sobbing became a soft stifled wail that rose from her constricted throat like a child's plea for succor from an invasive, possessive, fear.

Jason was shocked by the apparent force of her grief. His own thoughts were stumbling impulsively up the slope of strong emotion, as they struggled to be expressed in words. He stammered when he spoke.

"Amy... you could come with me... Would you consider it?"

She shuddered again and leaned even more heavily into him. '*What could she reply?... Did he truly realize what he was asking?... Could she make such a decision?*'

He slid his hand carefully under her chin and tipped her face back into his view. Her eyes were screwed shut like a child's in a nightmare. Her lips trembled, and her tears had soaked his shirtfront along with strands of her own hair which now clung to her face.

He started to speak... then reconsidered, recognizing that words couldn't adequately express what he felt. Tilting his face downwards he kissed her forehead with his lips slightly parted, tasting the salty savor of her fear.

When she didn't resist, he kissed her eyes, her cheeks, the slope of her nose, repeatedly and silently, as if to absorb her fears and her tears and remove them... share them. He brushed her lips with his... allowed the tip of his tongue to trace the outline of her mouth, and linger tentatively in invitation at the silky crevasse where her lips joined.

He stroked her hair, felt her rigidity melting into submission, felt the warmth as her lips opened and welcomed him... timidly, at first... then, hungrily. The accelerating passion and force of her response, like the release of a lifetime of tension and fear, seemed to spring from a coil of emotion wound tightly within her.

Amy had stopped thinking. She had given in, impulsively trusting him. She had succumbed to the seduction of dropping all pretense, of bursting the shell of restraint that had encased her all of her life like a steel shroud.

She felt a flush of warmth surging from some hidden visceral source and shivered in delightful liberation. She pushed against him, surprised by the instinctive force of her own aggression, and drove him backwards, bending him, slowly pinioning him between the soft grass and her pulsing desire.

Unconsciously, she drew herself up along the length of his body, swiveling herself into him, as if she wished to disappear within his very substance. No part of her body touched the earth. She had become part of *him*. Her decision was made. As his arms tightened around her, welcoming her surrender, she sighed and lay still while he rocked her gently.

Jason did not specifically understand the implications of what was happening.

But he knew that he wanted it to happen.

That he wanted her.

That he was *no longer alone.*

CH022: ALBANY, GEORGIA

The sun was sinking toward the western horizon and beginning to bleed crimson and orange into the clouds gathered there. Huge pines, planted with militaristic precision in exact rows by generations of hands now gnarled with age or already moldering in the grave, lined the road from the Albany airport. The air was thick with the scent of pine gum baking in the sun and Jason inhaled deeply through the open window of the cab. It was half respiration, half sigh. The tropics were gone and with them the lightness of heart he had rediscovered on the sands of St. Lucia in the company of Amy Davis.

She had left him in Miami to continue on to Atlanta. Her tears had replaced words when they held each other for a long minute before she exited through the gate to her plane. They'd had time during the St Lucia-Miami flight to clarify what they meant to each other and to agree that she would come to Albany as soon as she'd tended to her affairs in Atlanta.

"I can't promise anything, Jason. I know you can't understand yet, but this is all new to me. In a very real way, you are my *first* love and the feelings I'm experiencing are intimidating and novel... They scare me."

He didn't understand. But he sensed she was incapable of being more precise about what she felt.

"It's enough for me, Amy. I already owe you my sanity and I'm not greedy. I'm not asking for promises but I do want you to be part of my life, if you choose to."

"It will have to be day by day. I've still got a lot of changing to do and I'm not very good at it. I can promise you one thing, however, and for me it's a big thing... I won't lie to you and there'll never be any more games from me."

"What, no more stuff like you pulled on me in the clinic?" He looked a little disappointed.

She gave him a playful punch on the arm. "You know what I mean... We'll have fun together but there'll be no hidden agenda on my part. That's what I mean," and she looked up at him with softness in her eyes. "After a lifetime of closing myself off, I'm not good at opening up, so it'll only be a little at a time. I may even get scared and pull back on occasion, but it will all be real, no pretext, no dissimulation."

In response, he bent his head and kissed her on the forehead and she pulled herself closer, snuggling up against him.

He had to force his mind away from the memory of those moments and into the present.

The cab had passed the pine plantations and now, cotton fields, patrolled by huge mechanical irrigation sprinklers circling endlessly in plumes of windblown spray, filled the vista on both sides of the highway.

He was on his way to meet with Roger Atkins at Doublegate Country Club. The two men often dined together there and the meeting would arouse no suspicions.

Atkins had sounded worried when Jason had called him from the Miami airport. "Thank goodness you're back, Jason. You won't believe what's been going on around here since you left."

"Fill me in, Roger, I need to do some planning on the flight home," said Jason.

"Well, unless you've got an hour to listen, I can only give you a brief outline."

"That's all I need." Jason was becoming impatient.

"You know I've always assumed the role of peacemaker in our discussions in the merger committee. I hate controversy. It gives me gas..." and he laughed nervously at the other end of the line. "Get it, Jason... gives me gas... an anesthetist?"

"I got it, Roger, you just can't see me grinning," he replied dryly.

"Well, I'm finished with peacemaking. I'm firmly in your camp now. Since you left, Mark has stopped courting my vote. In fact, he's made my life a living hell. For example, last week he had Martin Howe call up the physician recruiters and place an order with them for *another* anesthetist."

"What? He initiated recruitment without my approval?" Jason was incredulous. Recruitment and other such major decisions always required prior consultation.

"Not only that, Martin came to me on the sly. He was as embarrassed as hell about it all and swore me to secrecy about where I heard the news. The poor fart is afraid Mark will have his head on a pole and I don't blame him for worrying."

"Did you confront Mark?" asked Jason.

"C'mon Jason, does that sound like something I'd do? ... But I did call Sheila at the office and ask to speak to him urgently on a personal matter."

"And...?" interrupted Jason

"...And I haven't heard a word from him since. I've called Sheila twice since then and she told me she passed on the message to Mark. She didn't know why he hadn't called back or given me an appointment. She was abrupt with me... not like her at all."

"So what else has happened?"

"Do you want the really nasty stuff?" Atkins sounded hesitant.

"Of course, I do. I need to get busy immediately and my hands are tied without the facts."

"You know about Cal disappearing or you wouldn't be on your way back, right?"

"Yes, Gloria called me in St Lucia and so did the police."

"Well, that's the worst that's happened, but Bobby Chen is on the warpath against you, and I guess that's a close second," said Atkins.

"Bobby? He and I have always gotten along. What's the problem?"

"Rumors, Jason. Rumors about Chen being a lousy radiologist and blind when it comes to detecting mammogram lesions. Believe it or not, I had one of the cashiers from the hospital cafeteria who I know from church, ask me whether she should have another mammogram because hers was read by Chen and she'd heard he ' *missed breast cancers as often as he found them*'. Those were her exact words."

"Damn!" said Jason, "Bobby's the best radiologist in town... in fact, in the region. Hell, when I recruited him he was touted as the best in the whole Bay area."

"That's not the worst of it, Jason. You're being cited as the originator of the slander."

Jason's heart sank, and then, he felt his anger boiling up like heated bile. He spoke quietly but firmly like he did when he was ready to explode. "Who's behind the rumors, Roger... Mark?"

"I don't think so, Jason, at least not directly. He's been in Atlanta every Monday and Tuesday since you left and all this crap about Chen seemed to surface when he was gone."

Jason wasn't satisfied. He knew it was West's work. "What else, Roger? Give it all to me."

"Our numbers, I mean the votes we have against the merger among the physicians are melting away like butter in hot skillet."

"Explain, Roger."

"We've had defections. Two before Cal disappeared and one more since, if Singh having lunch with West two days in a row is any measure of allegiance."

"Who else has bolted besides Singh?"

"Sol Goldman sent me a succinct note for forwarding to you. Something like '*don't count on me*' and Trang and Watson have both started booking out-patient procedures at Palm Grove which is a radical change for them."

"And, that's it?" fumed Jason.

"What?.. You were expecting more?" quipped Atkins.

Jason ignored the jibe.

"I need more details, Roger, and I don't want everyone to know I'm back in town. I want to examine what's going on before the instigators scuttle underground. Can you meet me at Doublegate this evening? I should be there by seven."

"Sure. I'll be there and I'll try to get the events in order so you'll be able to follow the flow of what's happened."

"Thanks, Rog, and remember I'm staying under cover as long as possible."

The cab was now on the outskirts of Albany and using back roads to come up on Doublegate from the south along the golf course itself. Carts still dotted the fairways and a wayward ball caromed off a stone barrier fence before pinging off the asphalt in front of the cab which braked abruptly.

"You'd think they'd be able to keep their balls inside the course," spat the cabby.

“You don’t play golf do you?” asked Jason, the irony in his voice undisguised.

“Naw, I’ve got better things to do with my money,” and a tattooed arm reached up to adjust the rearview mirror. “Side entrance to the club ok with you, sir?”

“Sure. I prefer it,” replied Jason.

* * *

Jason had requested a small side room away from the main dining area. He was savoring a tall iced coke and watching a waitress skillfully fold napkins into little fans to sit inside a series of wineglasses on a tray before her.

The aroma of prime rib permeated the room but he wasn’t hungry in the least and found the smell mildly unpleasant. He’d been there only ten minutes before Roger Atkins appeared in the doorway almost fully blocking it with his considerable bulk. He looked relieved to see Jason and started extending his hand in welcome as soon as he caught sight of his friend. Jason’s hand disappeared into Atkins’ palm like a ball inside a fielder’s glove.

“It’s great to see you, Jason,” and he literally beamed with pleasure... “You look great... How are you feeling?” he continued.

“If you mean the depression, Rog, it’s pretty much a thing of the past but I’m mad as hell about everything else.”

“Yea, I guess so. I’m pretty pissed, too, and it takes a lot to get me going.”

The big man sat down and the girl who’d been folding napkins came over to take his order for a drink. He turned his attention back to Jason.

"Mark's got the bit in his teeth, Jason, and he's running for all he's worth. Think he can be stopped?"

Jason averted his eyes in thought and swirled the half glass of coke as if it might contain some omen that would permit him to answer Atkins with certainty. He looked up and pursed his lips before answering.

"I'm Not sure, but I know this, I'm not going down without a fight and if I come to believe that Cal's disappearance is foul play, I'll move heaven and earth to discover who's behind it and see that he pays for it." Jason's eyes narrowed slightly and his face became stern. " If I'm going to have any chance of success, I'll need your cooperation and backing, Rog."

"For what it's worth, you've got it. I'm in for the long haul. It happened to Cal but after this last month, I'm convinced it could happen to any of us."

"What do you mean, Rog?"

"I mean that, if this business around the merger is linked to Cal's disappearance, anyone who opposes it could be next... anyone, Jason...and that includes you and me, too."

"Are you convinced Mark would go as far as murder?" Jason was a little taken aback by Atkins' statement. He hadn't allowed himself to come to that conclusion yet.

It was Atkins' turn to look away for a minute. He drummed his fingers nervously on the tabletop as he prepared his answer. "How much does the merger mean to Mark?"

"Conservatively, three million dollars and I already told you that he's been overheard in a bar when he was in his cups talking about a position as VP at Cumberland," replied Jason.

"And that's worth another seven hundred and fifty grand a year I'll bet," mused Atkins.

"At least that, in my opinion, Rog."

"People have killed for a lot less, Jason. You, Mark and I go back a long way. You always liked him more than I did. Remember in our senior year of high school there was a Mexican kid, Raoul Mercedes, muscular kid and well built... used to wrestle?"

"Yes, I think so," answered Jason.

"Ever wonder why he never graduated? Why he disappeared that March?"

"I heard his folks moved away and he went with them. Was there something more to it?"

"Yes, there was. It was hushed up by Mark's old man who paid off the kid and his parents and kept the police out of it."

"What happened?" asked Jason.

"It went down over in Grady County at a wrestling meet… I used to wrestle, remember?"

Jason nodded.

"Mark was there with the girl he was banging at the time, one of the cheerleaders...I think her name was Lacey something or other... A good looking blonde chick."

"Yes, I knew her... easy Lacey Lewis! And...?"

"Well, the meet was an all day affair and Mark left part way through to score some dope with a few of his friends. When he comes back, he learns that the Mexican and Lacey had been giving each other rubdowns out behind the weight-lifting building between matches."

Atkin's drink had come and he took a deep swallow before continuing.

"Mark went ballistic. He was outside of the gym with the guys smoking up in the parking lot when he got the news. He walked around in a circle cursing for a minute or two, then he goes to his truck and gets out a tire iron."

"Where were you?"

"I'd just lost a match and I was feeling kind of lousy. I went to hide out for a bit outside under a tree on the hill overlooking the parking lot where it happened. No one saw me. I'm sure of that because Mark sent away all the guys except Dennis Schirrah and the fat red-headed kid who always hung around with them. He didn't want witnesses."

Atkins took another swallow from his scotch.

"So, Mark sends Dennis and the fat kid to get the Mexican and he heads to an old rusty fence made of half inch iron rod built around a generator just off the cement of the parking lot. He studies it a bit and then starts prying at the fence with the tire iron. I couldn't see exactly what he was doing, but later I did. He pried out a six inch piece of bar bending it till it stood out at right angles to the fence, about belly height. Then he tests out the position of the spike, 'cause that's what it had become, by turning around and standing on the curb and measuring where it comes up to on his own back."

"You're sure of this, Roger?"

The question was more an expression of incredulity than doubt in the veracity of Atkins' account.

"Absolutely. I was there. Well, the Mexican kid is hustled out by Dennis and the fat guy and they push him toward Mark who is over by the fence. They yell a little bit at each other and then Mark gives the kid a shove. The guy pushes back and Mark gets Dennis and friend to hold the Mexican's arms and position him more or less in front of the spike on the fence.Mark turns his back like he's going to walk away from it all and the Mexican drops his hands and stops struggling. Mark just went a few yards back to get a good run at the guy. Anyway, he explodes into a run and drives his shoulder into the Mexican's chest literally lifting him up and backwards over the curb.You remember how good he was as a linebacker? Well, he put everything he had into this hit and the guy sails back and gets impaled on the spike. It took out one of his kidneys. Dennis and the other guy start to run away when they hear the guy start screaming but Mark got up, looked around and then gave him two sidekicks into the belly *even after he knew the guy was hung up on the spike!*"

Atkins' face contorted with disgust at the memory.

"But it isn't over. After he kicks, he punches the Mexican twice in the face and spits on him. About them, people start pouring out of the gym because of the God awful screaming and suddenly Mark goes into this act of horrible distress... As if the whole thing had been a tragic accident. He ran around apologizing to everyone."

"Crap," murmured Jason under his breath.

"Still want to know if I think Mark West would stop at murder to get what he wants?" Atkins downed the rest of his scotch in a single gulp and clacked the glass on the table. Neither man spoke for at least half a minute.

"Ever wonder what it would take for someone to kill another person, Jason," asked Atkins as he traced circles around the top of his empty glass with an index finger.

The question was unsettling and Jason sidestepped it. "I guess everybody speculates on that, at one time or another in their lives," he answered.

"I have," continued Atkins, "and I think it has something to do with why I hate conflict."

"How so?" asked Jason.

"I've been told all my life 'take it easy, you'll hurt someone' because I've always been bigger than others. People would tell me that even when I was a kid and was just fooling around. Then, one day some guy in a line-up for a bus after school, goosed my sister as she was getting on the bus. I saw it and just went nuts. I threw him up against the side of the bus and hit him hard in the mouth with my fist. He was down and out and people were pulling me away and leaning over him and screaming."

"I think I remember that, but he didn't die, right?"

"No. But he went to the hospital and was out of it for two days. The police charged me with assault. It was all pretty awful. In the end, the kid was ok but the whole thing scared the hell out of me. I was even afraid to tackle full out in football after that."

"And you still feel that way?"

"Yes. I don't think you ever outgrow something like that," answered Atkins.

"I've heard it said that every man's greatest fear is that he will kill someone and every woman's greatest fear is that she'll be killed," said Jason.

"Who said that?" asked Atkins.

"Can't remember... maybe I did," replied Jason a little sheepishly.

"So, you've thought about what it would be like to kill someone, too?"

Jason didn't answer. His eyes seemed to be focused on a spot in the air behind Atkins' head. He only shrugged in response.

Atkins pursued it. "What?... You've never thought about it?" he asked incredulously.

Jason's hands were on his knees under the table and he could feel his fingers tensing on the muscles of his thighs. "You mean have I thought that I might kill someone?"

"Yes."

"No, I haven't," he replied.

"Well, I'll be damned!" Atkins let out a low-pitched whistle. "You're one strange bird, Jason!"

"Why, because I don't think about killing people?"

"Yes. You said yourself that everybody must do it and then you immediately exclude yourself from the subset of 'everybody'!"

"I guess what concerns us right now is not whether I could kill or you could kill but whether Mark might kill or already *has* killed."

Jason wanted closure on the subject but Atkins didn't.

"That's what got me thinking about it Jason. I do believe that Mark could, maybe even would, kill and we have to deal with *him*. Seems to me that if you're going to deal with a murderer..."

"A potential murderer," interjected Jason.

"Ok, deal with a potential murderer, you'd better decide for yourself if you could kill. After all it might come down to *kill or be killed*, don't you agree?"

"I'm not much in the mood for theoretical philosophy right now, Rog, if you don't mind." Jason's palms were sweating.

"It's not all that theoretical anymore, Jason. We're into the death and disappearance scenario already. Remember?... Cal's gone."

"Ok," conceded Jason, "I have thought about it and I've decided that I couldn't kill."

"Under any circumstances?"

"I hope I couldn't, under any circumstances."

"How'd you come to that conclusion?" pursued Atkins.

"Well, it's kind of like you, only even more theoretical."

"How do you mean *more theoretical*?"

"I think I'm afraid like you are that, if I really got into a hassle with someone, I might just lose it and kill them. Since I was a kid, I've had nightmares, not about actually killing someone, but more about *having killed someone*. That's why it's more theoretical. Anyway, I dream that I hide the body in the family garden, then I live in fear that the body will be discovered."

He paused before continuing, " The dream used to come so often when I was a kid that it literally became a part of my reality. Every spring I'd get as nervous as a cat in a Chinese restaurant when it came time to till up the garden."

Jason smiled and shrugged his shoulders in embarrassment.

"Now, if you don't mind I'd like to drop the subject, please."

"Ok," agreed Atkins. "What's our next move?"

"I think we need to speak to one or more of the partners who've changed their minds. Find out why and see if we can get them back to our point of view. We've got to shore up our position."

"Agreed," said Atkins. "How do we go about it?"

"Trang is too closed-mouth and evasive to be an easy sell. If I see him, I'll do it but, if not, I'll wait till later. Goldman didn't even dare face you or me with his defection. He just sent a note. He's Jewish and I smell guilt. It may be a cliché but the guilt card usually works with my Jewish friends."

"Where and when?" asked Atkins.

"Tomorrow morning early. Seven a.m. If possible, before rounds. Let's do it at your office."

"Ok, how do I get him there?"

"He's your primary care physician, isn't he?"

"Hell, no, Jason. You are! Have you forgotten?"

Jason blushed. "Sorry, Rog, I guess all the depression's effects aren't gone. Tell him I'm away and you've got belly pain or something that you want him to look at. Just think of something he can't refuse to do."

"Ok, I've got an idea. I'll have him there at seven. None of my staff arrive till eight so we'll have a full hour if necessary."

"Good. Thanks Roger. I feel a lot less alone now and I appreciate your help."

"I don't mind, Jason. Secretly, I've had no use for Mark ever since high school. And by the way..."

"Yes?"

"I apologize for forcing this murder discussion. I didn't suspect it would get you going like it did."

"It's alright, Rog. I guess you never knew it, but my father died in unexplained circumstances and I guess I'm sensitive about murder and stuff like it."

CH023

Jason could feel the fatigue sloshing at the bottom of every cell in his body. The fragmented darkness of the early night had been populated with Annette, Amy and the children in brief distressing snatches of dreams but, by two a.m., sleep had fled. When dawn came, he was sitting listlessly beside the pool in his favorite lounge chair waiting for the night to end.

In front of him, the lawn sloped sharply downward from the pool and ran to a fringe of large oaks that marked the edge of the Flint river, some two hundred yards away. During the floods of '94 and '98 the water had risen almost to his pool and there were still a few pieces of flotsam in the tops of the oaks on the river flats that it was too dangerous to remove without a hydraulic lift basket.

Annette had chosen the house and, because she had redecorated it and landscaped the property, he had almost sold it all after her death. Everywhere he looked, he saw evidence of her handiwork and there were still rooms he didn't enter because of the memories they held that he couldn't face.

The dawn's ethereal fingers were feathering the sky beyond the river with a copper hue that promised another scorching South Georgia day. He'd always been struck by the fact that early dawn and late sunset seemed almost identical periods, at least for the sky, if not for the rest of nature.

The birds this morning were raucous and their noise had preceded the arrival of the sun by a good hour. One particularly aggressive mocking bird seemed irritated by his presence and had buzzed him within inches of his head, at least five times. Now, it was perched on a nearby chair scolding him loudly, with jutting tail and festooned wings that it beat against its body before it launched itself into another menacing circle around him. Twice, he had swung an open hand at it and narrowly missed, but the bird was not intimidated and, finally, it was the man who retreated to the empty house.

He breakfasted unenthusiastically on toast and orange juice and, at six thirty, left for Roger Atkins' office.

The traffic was light at that hour and he arrived before either Atkins or Goldman. He parked his BMW at the back of the lot and waited behind its tinted windows until both men had arrived and entered the building.

They were still in the lobby outside Atkins' suite when he stepped out of the elevator. Goldman's face fell. He was obviously disconcerted to see Turner.

He muttered, "Hello Jason. I didn't know you were back, yet," as Jason approached him but he didn't offer his hand in greeting.

"That's the point of this meeting, Sol. I don't want it known that I'm back, at least not just yet."

Goldman was a tall man, well over six feet and hefty, too, but tending towards fat. His body lacked any masculine definition and its ample curves gave him the appearance of an oversized woman in male drag. He was balding and always plastered a dozen or so long hairs from the right side of his head across his bald pate. It was a futile effort, much like a naked woman with large breasts trying vainly to hide them with spread fingers. Except for an oversize nose, he had blunt unremarkable facial features and lousy taste in tinted eyeglasses that drooped so low on his sagging cheeks that he looked like a bloodhound.

He frowned and said hesitantly, "I'm here to see Roger. He wanted me to check him for a hernia. What meeting are you referring to?"

Roger shrugged his shoulders before he spoke. "Sorry, Sol. That was just a ruse. We didn't think you'd come otherwise."

Goldman's face flushed crimson. He took two small steps toward the elevator and stammered, "If that's the case, I'm not staying. I'm due at rounds in twenty minutes and I think it's pretty low of you getting me here under false pretenses, Roger… I came as a favor to a friend."

Jason moved to stand between him and his path to the elevator. "You *are* here to do a friend a favor, Sol, only the friend couldn't ask you himself."

"If you are referring to yourself, Jason, you sure could have called me."

"Would you have come...?" asked Jason bluntly.

Goldman stammered a brief response Jason didn't clearly catch, so he followed up his own comment.

"Just like I thought, Sol," and he directed an arid smile at Goldman before continuing, "but the friend I'm referring to is *Cal Mellows*."

"Mellows... but he's..."

" Dead?" finished Jason.

"No, missing. I haven't heard that he's been found. But, what's that got to do with me?" Goldman had been glancing nervously at the elevator but he seemed to have understood Jason's resolve in blocking his way and he no longer looked like he was about to flee.

Jason stepped toward him and put a hand on his shoulder. "C'mon into the office, Sol. We only have a few questions for you and, if Cal meant anything to you as a colleague, you owe him at least that much."

Goldman still looked ill at ease but answered, "Sure, why not," and turned with Jason to follow Roger Atkins through the open office door.

Once inside, Jason and Sol sat around a small coffee table in Atkins' inner office.

“Coffee anyone?” asked Atkins, “It’ll just be instant but it’s not that bad.”

Goldman asked for his black, no sugar and Jason demurred. The two men sat in awkward silence until Atkins rejoined them.

“I put the kettle on so it shouldn’t be long.”

“Roger did you get the note?” asked Jason.

“Yes... here it is,” and Atkins withdrew a folded sheet from his pocket and opened it before putting it on the table.

Jason gestured toward the paper, “Sol, this is your note to Roger, could you enlighten us on what prompted you to write this?”

Goldman winced visibly. “First, what’s my note got to do with Cal? I have the right to know if I’m going to be grilled on my motives.”

“Seems fair, Sol. Let me explain,” began Jason.

A whistle sounded from the kitchen and Atkins excused himself to fetch the coffee.

Jason continued in his absence. “You couldn’t be expected to recognize a pattern when your part is just a single thread in the tissue of a larger conspiracy.”

“Now wait a minute, Jason, I’m not party to any conspiracy,” interrupted Goldman.

“Of course not… at least, not knowingly. Please, listen to what I have to say before you leap to any conclusions... Agreed?”

“Ok.”

Atkins came back with the coffee and rejoined them.

“During my absence, it’s become apparent that CHC agents and Mark West have been approaching partners in the firm attempting to reduce the opposition to the merger. At least four of you have reversed your previous positions as a result of their efforts... and...” he paused poignantly, “Cal has disappeared."

Goldman's hand was shaking visibly. He set down the coffee cup and clasped his hands together in an attempt to hide his obvious disarray. "Cal had problems, serious stuff, I heard. It didn't have anything to do with Mark or CHC."

"I'm not so sure, Sol. Someone did a lot of expensive digging into Cal's past, for some reason, and then this scandal about him breaks *two weeks after I'm out of the picture?* That's a lot of coincidence. When you consider, that next to me, Cal had the deepest objections to the merger going through, it starts to look like a lot more than simply coincidence."

"I never realized it was like that. You've got to believe me, Jason. I knew nothing about what had happened in Cal's case." Goldman was almost babbling as he began to appreciate the full picture of which *he* was a part.

"You and Cal weren't the only ones, Sol. There have been several others as well. You've surely heard the rumors about Bobby Chen?"

"Yes. I have but I don't believe any of them."

"They've done a lot of damage, nonetheless, and an excellent physician has been slandered... ostensibly by me, *but I was four thousand miles away at the time*. Is it starting to make sense?"

Goldman nodded affirmatively.

"What we need to know, Sol, to put this whole thing together is who spoke to you and what exactly happened?"

Goldman ran his open hand over his bald head and tousled the fringe of hair at the back of his head. A dew of perspiration had appeared on his upper lip and a sprinkling of the same seemed to be appearing in minuscule sparkles along the furrows of his forehead.

"Mark came to me about a month ago. He had an alumnus from Harvard with him. Somebody Smith, I think. Anyway, Mark had told Smith that my boy Eli was a football standout but still hadn't nailed down a university scholarship. Mark had borrowed some game tapes from Coach Jameson and Smith had been impressed. He said he just wanted to give my kid a chance."

"Did this fellow Smith mention CHC at all?" asked Atkins.

"No, not at all directly. But..."

"But what, Sol...?"

"Well, Mark did... He told me that CHC '*wanted to look after their docs*' and he asked me to withdraw my opposition to the merger."

"And did you?"

"Well, not immediately. I talked to Mark about my objections and he reassured me that CHC was ready to concede on most of the points I raised. He...", and Goldman hesitated... "told me that *you* were misleading us, Jason, and that you were just playing hard to get in order to drive up the takeover price."

"And did you believe him, Sol?"

Goldman palmed his scalp again. "Not really. But they got my kid a tryout with Harvard... did it in two weeks flat. Do you know what that means, a *tryout with Harvard for my kid?*"

By now, the sweat was literally running off his brow.

"Didn't you think that a little bit strange, Sol? Did Eli get tryouts anywhere else... even at a junior college?" asked Jason.

"No, but we really didn't push it. No one has ever looked at his films before..."

"C'mon Sol. You *knew* what was happening," interrupted Atkins brusquely. "He was *bribing you!*"

"No! I swear I never saw it that way! Not for a minute! I just took him at his word that CHC looked after their own."

"And, how do you see it now, Sol?" Jason softened his tone doing his best to remove any hint of sarcasm.

Goldman shook his head, shrugged his shoulders and ran his hand over his scalp a third time before stammering, "I see it differently, now..." Then he looked up at Jason with a mixture of sadness and dread in his eyes, "Jason, do you really believe CHC was behind Cal's troubles?"

"Do you see a more plausible explanation, Sol?" Jason asked.

"No, I guess not."

The three men sat in silence for a long minute.

Jason spoke first. "We want to thank you, Sol. We don't blame you for what you did but we want to get to the bottom of this thing. Since it stretches well beyond you, and we're still digging, we're asking you to keep this meeting a secret."

"You've got it, Jason. My lips are sewn shut."

"One last thing, Sol..."

"Yes?"

"This Smith fellow, do you know where he is now?"

"Not right now, but I did see him at the hospital last Friday. He said 'hello' when we passed in the hall. I just thought he was here on CHC business."

"Undoubtedly he is. What's he look like?" queried Jason.

"Weird-looking guy, only 'bout five nine but heavy, I mean heavier than me if you can believe that..." and Goldman laughed nervously. " His hands are huge, real hams, and he talks like a Texan. That's about all I can tell you..." and his voice dwindled off lamely.

"Thanks. It helps, Sol. And remember... nothing to anyone, please."

"Of course."

Atkins looked at his watch. "It's only seven-thirty, Sol. You can still catch rounds if you hurry."

"Thanks, guys..." said Goldman and he disappeared out of the office.

Jason looked at Roger.

"That dots a lot of 'i's and crosses a few 't's as well. We need to catch them in the act, and then, expose what they're doing to all the partners," said Jason

"Don't we know enough to talk to everybody now, Jason?"

"Our case isn't strong enough. We might not convince everyone. I think Cal's story is the one that will bring everyone onside... Maybe even the law. This guy Smith seems to have a key role in this someplace, I'm sure of it. We need to find him."

"Cal's nurse has disappeared, too. She probably knows a big chunk of the truth. We need to go after her, too," added Atkins.

"Good idea," said Jason who had pulled an agenda out of his pocket and was scribbling in it.

"I'll get on that if you'll try to sniff out Smith. I don't want to be seen yet."

"Jason, remember the story I told you about Mark and the Mexican… Watch your back."

"You too, Rog. I'll be in touch."

CH024: ALBANY, GEORGIA

The light turned orange and, uncharacteristically, Jason slowed to a stop rather than accelerating through the intersection. He was in no hurry to meet with Gloria Mellows but he knew it had to be done, not only for the sake of decency, but also because he needed to know what had transpired between Cal and Mark West.

He would be seeing Mark the next morning when West returned from Atlanta. The conversation yesterday with Dr. Roger Atkins had filled in many of the blanks for him but he still had no proof to back his suspicions that West was behind the defections of Singh, Goldman, Chen and Trang. Perhaps Cal's story would provide the evidence.

The Mellows' home was an imposing colonnaded antebellum mansion well beyond the means of a simple surgeon. The `Gravely House' had been built in the 1830's as the home of a lieutenant governor who entertained extensively. Gloria's father had purchased the mansion for his daughter as a gift on the occasion of the birth of his first grandchild. Cal had enjoyed the prestige that came along with owning a local landmark.

On the carpeted lawns behind the main house, Cal had constructed a driving range, putting green and a single par-three hole. He had also installed a pool table and several pinball machines in the apartment above the carriage house that, on occasion, he had used as a retreat. Otherwise, the estate house and grounds reflected his wife's tastes and not his.

As Jason turned into the tree-lined entrance, he saw that the huge black iron gates were closed although they began to swing ponderously open even as he approached. Cal used to leave them open. Gloria was more formal and the closed gates were the first sign of Cal's absence Jason had encountered. As he passed the surveillance camera he concluded that Gloria must have been watching the monitor for the gates to open so readily. She had been expecting him.

The overarching boughs of the live oaks lining the approach to the mansion provided a verdant canopy against the southern sun. Streamers of gray Spanish moss hung from the branches lending the oaks the appearance of tattered centenarian confederate sentinels guarding a stately symbol of southern glory. Random shards of sunlight penetrating the overhead greenery shattered strobe-like against his windshield as he drove down the corridor toward the great home. He squinted to minimize the effect of the bursts of blinding light.

He parked his BMW in front of the carriage house and was crossing the courtyard to the side entrance of the great house when Gloria called to him from the ballroom-sized balcony which ran the full length of the front of the mansion.

"Jason, I'm up here. Use the outside steps."

Jason had never been on the balcony before but easily found the stairway alongside of which hibiscus bushes had been planted. A profusion of crimson blooms hid the actual stairway until he was literally on the stairs. A low droning was audible from the dozens of bees attending to the flowers. He'd never felt comfortable around large numbers of bees and he mounted the stairs taking care to stay close to the wall and as far away from the blooms as possible.

He'd been intending to rehearse his first words to her but the bees and her appearance on the balcony distracted him.

She waited at the head of the stairs. Her corn-silk blond hair cascading over her shoulders made the black satin of the conservative pantsuit she wore seem even darker. Her eyes were red-rimmed and her face bereft of makeup. He could see sadness graven in heavy almost puffy lines around her eyes and across her brow. Her grief had transformed her.

Her arms were open and he stepped into her embrace wordlessly. He could feel her shudder as the sobbing began. Withdrawing from the hug, she mumbled, "I apologize. I just can't seem to keep it together."

"No excuse necessary, Gloria. I'm sorry that I took so long to come."

She was dabbing at her eyes with a crumpled Kleenex but motioned him to a chair. A Bible sat open on a small round table, a scarlet ribbon marking the page. She sat down opposite him and did her best to put on a smile.

"I'm glad to see you Jason. You were a good friend to Cal and I'm afraid that I need someone I can trust with the whole mystery."

"Tell me what happened. I've only heard bits and pieces and I imagine even that has been distorted. When was the last time you saw him?"

She sniffed, cleared her throat, then she drew herself up in the chair as if the more formal posture would prove an effective barricade against her tears.

"He came home drunk the night before he disappeared."

"Drunk? I didn't think he drank," said Jason in surprise.

"Cal had a serious drinking problem in the past but, with the Lord's help, he had put it behind him. Once or twice over the years since Nicaragua he's fallen off the wagon... Usually, it was at times of high stress but, even then, he'd hide it if he could. I think God and I may have been the only ones to share that secret with Cal." She smiled bleakly.

"Is that how you knew he was stressed this time?"

"Pretty much. There'd been other signs, insomnia... more distracted than usual, but he said nothing to me about what was bothering him 'till that night."

"Did you have the impression he'd been worried for long?"

"Not really. He'd stormed around bad mouthing Mark West a little more emphatically than he'd done in the past but nothing more sinister than that. Cal has no use for the man..." She looked up at Jason for some confirmation that he might share Cal's opinion of West.

"I don't see eye to eye with Mark on anything anymore," volunteered Jason. "I can understand Cal's frustration ... Did he talk about what Mark had done to get him going?"

"Cal didn't do much but grumble about incidents at the clinic at first, but that night he told me that he felt Mark was one of '*them*'. He sounded more than mildly paranoid but part of that I took to be the effect of the alcohol."

"Who did he name?"

"Besides Mark, no one specific but he felt like someone from his past was out to destroy him and had joined forces with Mark."

Jason echoed, "From his past?... What exactly was he referring to in his past?"

"I assume you may know even more than I do. Cal hid the details from me, and I understand why, but I know that he confided in you."

'Actually, he didn't,' thought Jason but he allowed her illusion to persist.

Gloria continued, "He'd been blackmailed before when he practiced in Oregon... His partners and his ex-wife conspired to create a scandal. Cal was cornered. He was forced out of the practice, deprived of his children's love and eventually left the country... I met him when he was working in Nicaragua and that's the story behind how he came to be there in the first place."

Jason had known nothing of the blackmail and wanted more information but he felt that if he told her he knew nothing, she might conclude that he wasn't as close to Cal as she'd thought and decide to whitewash or even stop the story.

"And so what had him frightened and stressed was *more* blackmail?" He asked almost cautiously.

"Yes, the same sort of trash... Lies about him sexually molesting patients..." She hesitated... "touching their breasts!" Her expression was a mixture of anger and sadness and Jason guessed that she might have doubts about her husband's behavior.

"I can't believe Cal would ever overstep the bounds of propriety," Jason blurted out trying to sound indignant on behalf of his absent friend.

Gloria looked relieved.

"Neither can I," she said "but they apparently corrupted his nurse too and she was prepared to go public with lies about his patients and claims that he sexually harassed her."

"Jenny Watson sexually harassed by Cal?" Jason's voice was laced with incredulity. "Cal could hardly tolerate the woman. He'd complained to me about her on a dozen occasions. No one in their right mind would lend credence to such a story!"

"Mark West did." she replied matter of factly. "He came to Cal accompanied by some administrator..."

"Wallace Makin?" interjected Jason.

"I'm not sure... but that could have been the name. They told him that the nurse had filed a complaint with them and with the police. She didn't show up at the clinic the day they came to see him... I think that's when Cal cancelled his patients and began to drink. He didn't come home 'till the following night."

"Was there any warning? Anything leading up to their visit?"

"Cal told me he got a threatening phone call... maybe a week before. It was a man's voice threatening him... Cal told me the guy was going to sue."

"Did the man attempt to blackmail him?"

"He may have. I'm not sure. But Cal did use the term '*blackmail*', however, I think he was referring to Mark's visit."

Jason was silent for a moment, his mind whirling to process the information and fit it into the pattern of defection of the other doctors that he had learned about yesterday from Roger Atkins.

"Gloria, this is important... When I heard that Cal was missing and suicide was suspected, I couldn't believe it. It didn't seem like Cal... *Was he suicidal in your opinion?"*

Gloria Mellows had begun shaking her head emphatically before he had even finished his question. "No... angry, frustrated... '*damn angry,*' he would have said... He seemed depressed but not suicidal. That's what makes the note he left so cryptic... It *reads like a suicide note* but I can't believe it. Cal wouldn't... couldn't take his own life. He would never have risked God's disapproval like that."

They both seemed deep in thought and many seconds passed before Jason asked, "Gloria... was there anything else about all this that didn't add up to you?"

"Yes," she said, then she hesitated. "Two things: first he took his .45 cal. revolver and a hunting rifle but he also took all the boxes of ammo he had for them. If you're going to shoot yourself, you don't need all that ammo. I checked all the gun safes. Only he and I have the combinations. The second thing seems more trivial but it doesn't make any sense to me. Cal had two favorite fishing rigs. He worried so much about them that he didn't dare leave them locked in the boat. Every trip he'd bring them home, wash, polish, oil them and they had a place of prominence in his closet."

"And?" asked Jason.

"Well," she replied "they're still there… there in the closet. He *never* went fishing without them and the police said there were trolling lines rigged to the boat..."

"Then Cal wasn't really fishing... Is that what you are telling me?" questioned Jason.

"What I'm saying," replied Gloria, "is that *if you're planning suicide you don't bother to put out trolling lines...* but, if *Cal* had really decided to go fishing, those poles wouldn't still be in his closet."

CH025

Jason hadn't slept again. It was the third time in as many nights since he'd returned from St Lucia, that sleep had eluded him. He'd told no one at TurnerWest, except his secretary, that he had returned, but he knew that the fact of his conversations with Gloria Mellows and Dr. Atkins would soon reach Mark West's ears. Besides, Albany, was a small city, really no more than a large town, and he'd already been recognized by at least a half dozen patients and acquaintances as he'd moved discreetly about. If he hesitated in contacting West and gave him time to concoct excuses or alibis, any confrontation he'd planned would lose its shock value.

He set down his steaming mug of Ovaltine on the kitchen table, reached for the phone and dialed Mark West's office.

"Hello, Dr. West's office, may I help you?" came a woman's voice

"Sheila, it's just me, Jason... Is Mark in yet this morning?"

There was a moment's hesitation before she replied with a question, "Dr. Turner, I thought you were still on leave?"

"The Mellow affair cut short my trip... Is Mark in?"

"I haven't seen him, Dr. Turner, but he may have come into his office the back way. Please hold a moment."

The line clicked and suddenly Jason was plunged into a local newscaster's preview of the significant daily events in Albany. One non-fatal shooting. A rape. A four-car collision on the bypass and the federal government was threatening again to slash the peanut subsidy. The announcer had begun to provide details of the shooting when he himself was abruptly snipped out of existence as West's secretary came back on the line.

"He's not in his office, Dr. Turner, and I have nothing on his agenda until noon. Do you wish to leave a message?"

Jason pursed his lips and cursed inwardly. He'd wanted to challenge Mark this morning on some of the things he had heard from Atkins and Goldman. He felt a cold anger rising at the possibility he wouldn't get to him that soon.

"Yes... I do. Now listen carefully to me, Sheila, because I won't repeat myself... *You find him...* I don't care what you have to do to get it done, but *find him."* The edge in his voice was deliberate and he spoke slowly emphasizing every word. "And when you do, tell him to get his ass down to the Fish Factory restaurant at noon sharp. He's to come alone... Is there anything I said that isn't clear?"

There was a pause and Jason pictured the curvaceous 'Sheila of the constant cleavage' squirming uncomfortably as she listened to him. She had never been exposed to this side of his nature.

"Yes, sir... noon at the Fish Factory... I understand."

Jason put down the phone without another word. He wanted the message delivered with all its emotional wrapping intact. Any sign of conventional courtesy in delivering it to the secretary would have risked blunting its effect when she told West.

He pulled the mug of Ovaltine closer and clasped it in both hands feeling the warmth of the porcelain as he silently squeezed till his nail beds blanched.

* * *

The Fish Factory restaurant on Oglethorpe Avenue actually didn't serve seafood. The proprietor, a rotund florid-faced Italian had lost a wager with a friend when he bought the place and, as his reward, the friend had facetiously named the eatery. The story of the name was condensed into a one-paragraph explanation on the back of the menu in the form of an apology to disappointed seafood seekers. Their pasta, however, was the best to be found between Macon and Tallahassee.

Jason had positioned himself in the corner of a booth, which, because of its poor lighting, was usually occupied by young couples seeking a little privacy along with their food. His hands were now clasped around a Heineken bottle which he gripped with the same ferocity he had used on the Ovaltine mug earlier that morning. His red-rimmed eyes were riveted on the restaurant's entrance. He was feeling the effect of sleepless nights and his mood had not improved. A knot of muscle worked rhythmically at the corner of his jaw as he clenched and unclenched his teeth.

Inside his head, his thoughts snarled like battling toms in a catfight. The more he had worked things through in his mind, the more convinced he had become that West was directly responsible for the defections of Trang, Chen and Singh and he already had the proof about Goldman. His anger was further fueled by the knowledge that, if West could pull just three more associates to his side of the equation, TurnerWest would disappear into the maw of CHC and he would be powerless to prevent it. He couldn't let that happen and he had to convince West that it never would. The battle lines had been drawn for months but, during his medical leave, West had clearly outflanked him and the outcome of the conflict was once again in question.

He glanced at his watch. Twenty past twelve.

Jason knew that Sheila Clark had found Mark. She and Mark had shared a sporadic sexual dalliance for the past four years that Sheila skillfully kept from her husband, an influential member of the board of Albany General Hospital. She knew West's habits, his hideouts and all the numbers to get hold of him. If West didn't show, or if he came late, it was deliberate. Either way, his absence simply stoked Turner's agitation.

Over the past twenty-four hours, Jason had been evaluating the leverage he held over Mark West. He knew details of all of West's multiple episodes with women, including the wives of colleagues and other movers and shakers in Albany and environs. His information was dated, however, since Mark had ceased to brag about his conquests to Jason after they fell out over Mark's infatuation with the Creole woman.

West had an obsessive penchant for seducing the women of powerful men. It was as if cuckolding the men, by subverting the loyalties of their wives, fed a twisted need to feel superior to his peers. It was a perilous habit but West appeared to have practiced it without detriment, although Jason suspected that one murder-suicide several years ago among the couples of his conquests may have been linked to his predations.

Jason suddenly longed for his dead wife. He needed to talk through his options and Annette had always been able to help him unravel the complexities of any challenge and choose a course of action confidently. He thought of Amy and wished she had already arrived from Atlanta.

Left to himself, he feared that the pressure of needing to act would lead him to choose precipitously, without precision, like a hunter firing into a covey of quail hoping to hit at least one… and missing them all. He was certain of only one thing... he had to stop West and, if blackmail seemed viable, he'd use it.

The restaurant door opened and the noon sun blazed in, an explosion of blinding light against which a tall figure was outlined in blurred strokes like an oversized alien emerging from the cauldron of his spaceship. As it closed against the light, the door dragged the shadows of the interior across the features of the man who had entered but not before Jason recognized Mark West.

He stood to signal his presence and West started toward him, ignoring the waitress who bustled up to him.

Jason was seated when Mark West slid onto the bench across the table. No word of greeting had been spoken. Even in the poor light, Jason could see the set of West's jaw and sensed the aggression he sought to convey. Both men sat for a moment grappling silently for some mental advantage, seeking some sign of the other's intimidation.

West spoke first. "*Get my ass over to the Fish Factory*", was that *your* message, Jason?"

Anger was arm-wrestling with caution for control of Turner's voice and silence hung between the partners for a long frozen moment before caution won out and Jason answered, "Couldn't risk you not coming, Mark."

Another moment's pause.

"Well, here I am."

"*And where is Cal,* Mark? ....And why do I have to hear of his disappearance from the police and *not* from you?"

"I guess this is where I'm supposed to ask: '*Am I my brother's keeper*?' Is that how you've got this figured? Cal takes a header off his boat and it's suddenly my hand shoving him in the back?"

"That's about it, Mark. Your fingerprints are all over the place, in this thing."

Jason's words were flint against steel. He had been expecting profanity, an indignant explosion, even in this public place and had been ready for that with his own verbal broadside. He almost needed the decompression of a raging argument, even a brawl, in which they could slug out their mutual animosity. It had gotten to that point inside him.

Abruptly, West laughed out loud, a gut-driven guffaw that startled his partner and echoed through the restaurant turning heads for several moments before Jason recovered his wits.

"What'd you expect, partner? You accuse me of murder and I'm supposed to deliver myself from the burden of my guilt and confess... You're more messed up now than you were when you left," said West derisively.

Jason's vision blurred suddenly out of focus and a surge of hissing tinnitus blocked out the sounds of the room and West's voice.

He felt all his muscles tighten as his hands slipped under the table's edge. He was holding his breath as he tensed, then lunged upward and forward driving the table into West's abdomen before lifting it to slam the surface against his torso. A spray of saliva was driven out of West's mouth by the force of the blow and his eyes widened in pain and surprise.

Before he could recover, Jason grabbed a handful of his hair and pounded his face twice into the table. Blood gushed from his nose and mouth and he coughed convulsively.

Never releasing the hair, Jason braced his foot against the edge of the booth and yanked as hard as he could dragging West down and out to collapse on the floor.

In an instant, he was astride him, his hands around his neck driving his thumbs deep into the cracking cartilage of the trachea which crumpled like a huge plastic straw under the pressure. West's face flushed red, then quickly purple, and his eyes bulged like they were about to pop from his face. His mouth was smeared with a crimson froth and the little air that passed between his pouting lips produced only the faintest wheeze. Jason drove his thumbs deeper, the muscles of his forearms beginning to burn with the effort.

"...Worse than when you left, Jason... You can't be trusted with TurnerWest's interests and sitting there breathing hard and squeezing the crap out of that Heineken bottle is proof enough that you've slipped over the edge...." West's voice seemed to echo at first, intruding from far away, but it became clearer as his face swam into focus and Jason returned slowly from his rage.

With a chilling rush of awareness, Jason realized what had happened. He'd hallucinated the attack! "*God, I've lost my mind... I'm crazy!*"

He blinked twice, crimping his eyelids shut for a few seconds each time, but he could still clearly see *that West was sitting across the table from him and not on the floor under him.*

He slowly relaxed his stranglehold on the Heineken bottle and drew in a shuddering breath. He tried to speak, but his mouth was tinder-dry and his words seemed strangled, "Screw you, Mark… Screw you... You won't win," was all he could manage to get out.

West laughed again and stood up. "We'll see about that, partner. The state medical board already has an incident report on your stay in the brain bin... Give it up, Jason. *You don't have any idea of what you're up against.*"

Jason simply glared, still enormously distraught at the terrifying dissociation he'd just experienced. He had no more words.

"Oh, and the next time you want to see me... get an appointment for the clinic like all the other sickies," West hurled over his shoulder as he strode toward the door.

* * *

Every evidence of mental disarray carries its own level of alarm but this afternoon's vivid and waking hallucination terrified Jason far beyond the effects of any panic attack. Losing control of reality like that had happened to him only twice before, both times during his childhood.

Once his drunken father had been slapping at his mother's cowering form in their bedroom when he'd burst in and begun attacking his father with blunderbuss blows that had leveled the brute.

That time, when Jason swam back to reality in stages, like a diver decompressing, he'd finally opened his eyes to see his mother hovering over him as he lay on the bedroom floor. Her eyes were red and puffy. Her cheeks, over which her tears coursed, were swollen. She was holding an ice pack to the side of *his* face and, when he tried to speak, an electric shaft of pain drove upward from his broken jaw into his head and he'd passed out again.

He obviously hadn't attacked his father, as he'd hallucinated, *but his father* had *attacked him*.

The second instance had been almost a year later. His father had again been beating his mother. Between delivering blows to the side of her head, he'd been holding her by the shoulders and shaking her. Jason had stumbled out of his bedroom, awakened by his mother's screams. His vision had blurred and the roaring had erupted in his ears, then, he'd flung himself again at his father, feeling omnipotent in his own rage, more powerful than a giant, despite his eight years.

When he'd come to on that occasion, his mother had been on her knees pressing him into her bosom shuddering sobs. His father lay in a crumpled heap at the foot of the stairs, his head lolling at an unnatural angle to the rest of his body. The ambulance came and took him away and Jason never saw him again. He and his mother had left Atlanta for Albany shortly thereafter.

Over the intervening years, Jason had often pleaded with his mother to tell him what had happened to his father but she had never spoken a single word about the brute's death except to say that he'd been drunk and fallen downstairs. She had made him promise never to consult the police reports.

He never had.

CH026

Jason had come into his office early to go through the stack of papers and letters that had accumulated during his absence. As he began the task, the telephone rang and he picked it up. The conversation was brief, no more than a minute. He wasn't officially in the office and had answered on impulse. He stopped short of calling the impulse intuition, but, since his experiences in St Lucia, he had recognized the wisdom of paying closer attention to information arising from someplace other than his rational intellect.

A Mr. Meake had left a message. It had been succinct, "I need to talk to you about the accident. Your wife's automobile accident. It's important."

Jason had agreed to meet with the owner of the Mercedes franchise in Albany, immediately.Now, to fill the minutes the fellow would need to travel from the dealership, less than a mile down Jackson Street, he speculated on what the man might want.

Perhaps he was conducting some study trying to decide how Mercedes could entice previous owners, who'd experienced disastrous accidents in their vehicles, back into the purchasing fold. Or, maybe he was coming to discreetly discuss some mechanical fault that had been discovered in the type of vehicle Annette had been driving.

As he speculated, he turned his attention to the pile of mail and documents and began to sort through them looking for the letter Meake said he had sent. It was in the very bottom layer of his inundated 'in' tray. He slit it open and unfolded the heavy embossed velum and read.

Dear Dr. Turner,

Please accept my condolences on the tragic passing of your wife. I had met her once or twice when we both sat on the advisory board for the symphony. She was a charming and talented woman and our whole community has been impoverished by your loss.

I dare to contact you so soon after her death because I have information which only recently came to my attention that I feel I should share with you first before speaking to the police.

To the police!

It has been my custom, for many years, to personally examine any vehicle I have sold that has been involved in a fatal accident. Perhaps, it is my background as an engineer that pushes me to see if any mechanical flaw in our vehicles' construction contributed to the fatality.

I recently went over your wife's vehicle which is now in the possession of a specialty wrecker in Jonesboro. I discovered what I believe may be evidence of foul play. I am obligated to inform the authorities of my findings but not before we talk privately.

Please examine the photos of the automobile that I have attached, if you feel up to it. What I have discovered is not difficult to identify and I am surprised that the police examination of the car didn't detect it.

I look forward to your response.

Sincerely,

Arnold Meake

Jason tipped the envelope up with some trepidation. He had attempted to expunge from his memory all images of the crumpled vehicle in which Annette had drowned. He had seen the car only momentarily in the early dawn after divers had located it and it had been winched to the surface, but the sight of it had immediately been impressed eternally into his mind. By the time he'd been called to the scene, his wife's body had already been placed on an EMS gurney.

In death, Annette had retained her beauty, pale but still radiant with her lustrous ruby tresses lying diagonally across her forehead, then wrapping wreath like along her cheek. Her eyes had been thoughtfully closed and no marks of trauma beyond two flakes of glass, sitting like diamond splinters on her right cheek, were visible on her face. He had expected, in fact had braced himself, to see the horror of her last moments etched indelibly on her features but there had been no betrayal of any emotion but peaceful resignation.

The autopsy had revealed that her lungs had been full of water, confirming his worst fear: *she had been alive and trapped in the Mercedes when it sank.*

They had often spoken of death. Her hazardous pastimes had stimulated his fears for her where she seemed to have none. She had always laughed off his concerns by stating her intention never to die in bed.

She'd once said, "Look, sweetheart, I could be knocked over by a truck, some perfectly ordinary afternoon, when I step off a curb coming back from the courthouse. Think of it... whisked off to meet your maker with your mind intent upon such mundane concerns as the croissant you had waiting at the office… That'll never be me. When I finally meet St. Peter, I'll have a story to tell him about how I got there."

In spite of his nervousness, he smiled at the recollection.

Maybe during her final moments, she'd been preparing the story for St. Peter, emphasizing her excitement at beginning a new adventure rather than her abrupt departure from earth. Or perhaps, she'd even been thinking of him... attempting a smile even as she died, knowing that he would be among the first to see her body. It would have been in character for her to think, even in extremis, of what he would have to face. After all, she had recorded several videotapes for the children to be played in the event of her death and on the occasion of special events in their lives thereafter. Although it had been heart-rending to watch, her message to them in the first tape had been a miracle of consolation.

Jason was an astute observer. His ability was not a gift conferred by nature like the eyesight of the hawk, but acquired, cherished and developed during years of conscientious practice. It was the reason why he was an excellent medical diagnostician.

During this apprenticeship, he had learned that the appreciation of details, and not broad strokes, was the key to divining the essence of anything, especially things camouflaged. He'd discovered that the senses, like the mind itself, were intuitively reductionistic. The senses sought comprehension through the evaluation of the obvious and sacrificed precision by preferring the simplicity of closure to the tedium and effort of thorough examination... The senses would see only the wall upon which the chameleon lies in plain sight with neither outline nor shape, invisible... until it blinks.

The glossy surfaces of the three photos that slipped from the envelope did not picture the whole vehicle. Rather the photos had been confined to the right front of the vehicle, the point of first impact with the guardrail, and the rest of the same side up to the door. He was studying them carefully when the secretary notified him of Mr. Meake's arrival.

He'd been expecting someone rather shuffling, perhaps almost professorial, high forehead, disheveled hair and thick glasses. He'd been wrong. Arnold Meake was over six feet tall, around forty-five with a square face, heavy brows and an expansive mouth. He was wearing a generous smile and impeccable gray slacks and blazer. He entered the office with his hand outstretched in greeting.

"Dr. Turner, I appreciate your willingness to meet with me..."

"Mr. Meake," replied Jason, "I've seen the photos you sent and, while I don't like thinking about what happened, I want to hear why you suspect foul play. No one has suggested it before."

"Well, let's move right to the problem, if you're ready. Do you have the photos?" replied Meake, without hesitation.

There was a coffee table and a sofa at one side of the office and Jason motioned Meake to be seated while he brought the photos from his desk.

Meake took them and laid them out in a sequence side by side and Jason could see that each photo moved in succession from the front of the vehicle to its right side. From his pocket, the car dealer took out a pen which he used as a pointer indicating the first photo.

"Here is the first clue. Notice how the upper portion of the front fender is relatively undamaged, although, when a car is careening heavily to one side in a curve, the chassis is normally pulled lower on the inside edge of the vehicle by the centrifugal force, thereby, exposing the upper area of the fender to any potential hit."

He looked up from the photo before continuing.

" I've examined the road where the accident occurred. There is no concrete lip at the edge of the pavement to carry away rainwater like we sometimes see on curves. In fact, the shoulder, which is four feet wide from pavement to barrier, sloped down and away from the asphalt."

He looked up at Jason as if he expected a nod of comprehension or a glimmer of understanding.

Jason did understand, but he gave no indication of his comprehension. He asked instead. "Please go over that again for me, if you don't mind."

Meake nodded.

"Well, think of it this way, the force of the car on the outside curve plus the slope of the shoulder of the road should have carried the chassis *lower* than the mark of impact shown on the fender. There should be no sparing of the upper portion of the fender. We should see damage, heavy damage up to the full height of the barrier, reflected on the car with no concrete lip or any other obstacle to lift the vehicle higher in the air."

Using his pen he pointed to the fender.

"The lack of damage to the top foot or so of the fender just doesn't fit."

Jason studied the photo again carefully. "But there *is* some damage at the top, it's dented and the paint is chipped."

"Yes, but notice the dirt and bits of grass still visible around the top of the headlight casing even after it was submerged in the water, "said Meake.

"I see, and I have an idea what it means, but please continue."

"Compare the damage, relatively superficial to the upper fender, small dents, paint chips and not much more. Now, look lower," he pointed again with his pen, "See how contact with the heavy structure of the barrier crushed the very form of the metal further down. It has been totally flattened, distorted, even caved in. Only a few streaks of paint remain on the portion of the metal that actually slammed into the barrier. The damage above this point," and he drew an imaginary line with his pen, "came from contact with soft earth, not metal. The car hit the barrier with the front of it much higher than it should have been, given the circumstances of the curve and the shoulder of the road. Cars do not jump off flat surfaces... yet, it appears this one did."

Jason had been following Meake's logic. He nodded.

"And, here," continued Meake, pointing again at the second photo, "is the second clue. Where is the wheel?... Pushed down and under the car, as we would expect?... No, it's *bent up*, almost sideways, with the rim twisted at an apparent right angle to the barricade."

He paused for effect... "Impossible, under the presumptive circumstances of the accident."

His face became grave and he spoke more deliberately. "Something happened to lift the front end of the car and force the wheel to come up sideways *before* the car slammed into the safety railing..."

"What could do that... a blowout?" asked Jason, although he had already divined the real answer with a churning of his gut.

"No, no blowout could ever generate such force. The vehicle weighed over a ton. It was hurtling along at nearly one hundred miles per hour. It would take enormous power to lift its front end off the road..."

Meake was watching Jason's face and he stopped talking, halted abruptly by what he saw there.

Horror had contorted Jason's features. He felt as if he had been slammed full in the gut by a speeding wrecking ball. He was literally thrown back bodily into the pillows of the sofa by the realization that leapt from the photos. He gasped to get his breath and struggled slowly to his feet, then staggered to the edge of the sofa where he could turn his back to Meake and partially hide his shock and grief.

From deep in his chest, he could feel a coarse vibration beginning to rise into his throat. He felt the stifled creak from his larynx that signaled the arrival of a visceral scream of horror and rage. He fought it back, his elbows locked tight and his hands now digging into the armrest of the sofa.

Meake watched the transformation in stunned silence. He knew that there was nothing more he could say or do and his own throat tightened sympathetically. For a moment, he wondered if he had done the right thing in coming first to show the photos to Turner, rather than to the police.

Several minutes past and Jason's disarray began to wane under the imperious commands of his intellect. *Annette had been murdered. He would find those responsible for her death and he would* kill them.

With an effort that required every element of control his mind and body could manage, Jason turned back to Meake and sat down once more on the sofa.

Silence.

Meake squirmed in discomfort.

Finally.

"Mr. Meake, is it your own conclusion that an explosive device was placed on the front right suspension of my wife's car?"

"On the axle itself, Dr. Turner..."

"... And that this explosive device caused the crash and the death..." Jason's voice broke, and tears began to stream profusely down his cheeks, but he kept looking directly at Meake, his eye contact never wavering"... of my... my wife, Annette Turner?"

"That is what I believe, Doctor."

Meake continued to fidget nervously, twisting his pen in his fingers.

"So," went on Jason, still with a quivering voice, "... in your opinion, *my wife was* murdered?"

Meake nodded his head affirmatively.

A long shuddering sigh escaped Jason's lips and he began to tap his temples rapidly with the fingers of both hands while staring at the photos on the table. Finally, he spoke again and he seemed to have recovered a measure of his composure.

"Then, Mr. Meake, I obviously have work to do."

"And the police, too, Doctor."

"Yes... Well, maybe not just yet, if you'll bear with me for one more minute please, Mr. Meake."

"I'm sorry, Dr. Turner, but I don't understand..."

"Of course not. I'm not at liberty to reveal a great deal to you, at the moment, but you deserve to see the bigger picture..."

"*Bigger* picture, Doctor?..." queried Meake with obvious surprise.

"Yes, Mr. Meake. If I'm correct, my wife's murder is the centerpiece of a much larger conspiracy. Other crimes have been committed and it goes well beyond our little town of Albany. Many police jurisdictions would be involved. There would be bickering, skepticism and turf wars among the enforcement agencies and the waters might be irrevocably muddied. The criminals could be warned by all the activity and they may well escape detection, if they can cover their tracks effectively."

Meake blushed nervously. "I understand better now, but I'm afraid it may already have begun."

"What has already begun, Mr. Meake?" asked Jason, almost wearily.

"Why, the covering of tracks, of course."

"What do you mean?"

"The vehicle. It's gone. The week after I took my photos at the wreckers in Jonesboro, I went back to see if I could dismantle the front end of the car and bring back the axle to show to you and the police. But it was gone already." He looked apologetic.

Jason was suddenly alert. "Where did it go?"

"That, I don't know. Wrecks of expensive cars like yours are highly sought after by certain unscrupulous colleagues of mine. As soon as they are released by the insurance company, they're snapped up." He paused and pursed his lips as if to say '*it takes all kinds*'. "They, that is the dealers, dismantle the cars and sell the parts as new... It enlarges the margins of profit."

"So, you think a dealer has the wreck?" asked Jason.

"It's probable, but that raises another problem. The wreck would almost certainly have been purchased through a third party since Mercedes monitors such deals. Both the purchaser and the wrecking yard will be highly motivated to conceal the details of the transaction. It won't be easy to trace..."

"But you said Mercedes monitors such deals, didn't you?" Jason was obviously irritated at the potential setback.

"Yes, I did, but I meant that the company monitors purchases *by its dealers*. Most dealers, who buy wrecks, can easily and effectively disguise their end of such transactions."

"Mr. Meake, you've seen what I've gone through here this morning. I need your help. My wife has been murdered, one of my friends and colleagues has disappeared and is probably dead as well. Over the years, I've had enough dealings with the police to have no confidence at all in their methods or abilities..."

"That has been my sad experience as well, Doctor, and part of the reason why I came to you first," interrupted Meake.

"So, you'll help me?" Jason was almost pleading with the man.

Meake let the tip of his tongue protrude between his lips for a moment as if he were almost chewing on it while considering the proposal Turner was making. If the police became involved eventually, the whole process was not without danger for him. But, he fancied himself a bit of a detective and his full sympathy lay with Turner.

He spoke slowly, "Doctor, I will commit to keeping our secret so that you can pursue the criminals as you choose. Additionally, I promise you that I will do my best to find out where the wrecked Mercedes is currently and purchase it without leaving any trace of where it disappears to," and he winked knowingly at Jason and extended his hand to seal the agreement.

Jason took his hand readily, "Thank you, Mr. Meake… Thank you."

As Meake got up and crossed the office toward the door, he said, "Please keep the photos, Doctor. They are copies."

When Meake was gone, Jason returned to the table and examined the photos again. As he did so, he was overcome again with grief. He crumpled sideways upon the sofa and, grabbing up a throw pillow, pushed his face deep into it and screamed out his loss until he lay soaked in perspiration, exhausted but drained of the sadness.

Now, nothing was left but his undiluted, blood-red rage.

CH027: ATLANTA, GEORGIA

Amy adjusted the volume and fiddled with the earpieces of her I-pod until the strains of Ravel's Bolero were fully stereo and her ears didn't ache. It would have been more comfortable to wear the larger external headset she used when at home, but she was still too aware of her appearance to permit comfort to be her primary concern. The little earplug- type speakers were hard plastic torture items that she could barely tolerate for an hour and she had already been here in Olympic park for over two hours.

She'd come to the park to kill time and to sunbathe because she was going crazy trying to fill the four days it was taking for Mayflower movers to free up a van and schedule her furniture pick-up. It was the shortest delay she'd been able to negotiate from any moving firm, and now, she better understood people who stuffed all their belongings into U-Haul trucks and just hit the road without formality. As it was, she'd already packed everything she owned and her apartment was window-high in boxes. Only the large pieces of furniture remained to be packed.

Adding to her impatience at having to stay in Atlanta, was the tremendous longing she felt for Jason. It had been only a little over seventy-two hours since they parted and yet it seemed as if she hadn't seen him in a month. If he had not asked her not to call him for the first five days to avoid the possibility of his presence in Albany being revealed prematurely, she would have been on the phone every ten minutes like a lovesick teen.

All these sentiments were new and exhilarating for her. In the past, when she'd been involved with men, it had been the game and her playacting that had provided the excitement, but, with Jason... It was just Jason. No game. No more pretending. She ached to be near him again, to begin a life where pretense, if it existed, would be only an accoutrement to, and not the essence of, her existence.

Two high-school kids in cut-off jeans and T-shirts were in-line skating along the meandering paths that wound through the park. She had watched them earlier as they had raced, jostled each other and practiced jumping onto, and then off of, the cement platform of a drinking fountain alongside one of the paths well below her.

She had staked out a sunbathing spot under a tall palm on the top of the highest knoll in the park. The tree reminded her of St. Lucia, and the approaches to the little hill were steep enough to discourage the majority of wanderers in the park from passing too close to her. Thus sequestered, while blocking out the city's noise with her music, she could lie on her blanket, watch the clouds and pretend she were still in St Lucia. Still close to Jason.

She was wearing a bikini modest enough to be appropriate for the park but it had obviously attracted the attention of the boys with the in-line skates. They were pumping their way up the steep track which passed within ten yards of where she lay for the third time. She'd become aware that they had abbreviated their larger circuit around the park in favor of a much briefer route that brought them to the top of her hill about every five minutes.

Once there, they would make a great display of how tired they were from the climb, despite the fact that they appeared to be as fit as tri-athletes. They would collapse for five or ten minutes on the grass... always in a position where they could surreptitiously glance at her and probably stare greedily whenever she was in a position where she wouldn't see them. They couldn't have been more than fifteen years old.

At present, they were huffing and puffing and talking loudly about how tough the climb was while they looked for a place to lie down. She smiled in amusement and something devilish inside her made her lie on her stomach and unhook the back of her bra, ostensibly to get more sun, although she already had a honey-amber tan all over her body.

She turned her head sideways where she could spy upon the boys from behind her sunglasses and pretended to doze off.

When they thought she couldn't see them, they rolled on their sides and gave each other a 'high-five' then settled in to unabashedly stare at her and undoubtedly fantasize that she might somehow, inexplicably, roll onto her back and send them both to teenage Nirvana.

As the minutes passed, she *did* almost doze off and the boys never did resume their skating. Amy didn't mind being the object of their innocent voyeurism. There were many worse sexual activities for teenage boys to indulge in. This bit of skating and 'girl-watching' were, by comparison, pretty wholesome pursuits for these young men.

Her ears had started to throb again from the earpieces and she re-hooked her bra before sitting up and removing the small speakers for a minute of two of careful ear massage. She looked over at the boys and caught them looking at her. She stared directly back and, in a few moments, they both flushed beet red, got up and went whizzing down the hill.

The sweltering sun was baking the tops of the high-rises that formed the western horizon and shadows were lengthening. She began to gather up her things and place them in the beach bag she'd brought with her.

She was thinking about the two teenage boys and smiling at their embarrassment when it suddenly occurred to her that she had slipped back into the mode of deriving pleasure and excitement from game playing. She felt a flush of guilt burn in her *own* cheeks and she chastised herself for having permitted a relapse into bad habits.

She was still scolding herself and re-formulating new resolves to purge all pretense from her activities, if it were possible.

She had reached the bottom of the hill where the walking path forked. One branch went out to the main street and then paralleled the sidewalk. The other went off to the right and into a graffiti-spackled tunnel about fifty feet long that provided a shorter access to the parking lot where she'd left her Toyota.

She'd slipped on a pair of jeans, runners and a sweatshirt and her bag hung on her shoulder by its long strap. Her wallet was in it but she wasn't wearing any jewelry. All these facts were quickly processed and weighed, as she stood at the fork deciding which way to go. *'Hell, I could outrun any would-be assailant and the worst I'd have to do is drop my bag,'* she reasoned. She was enough of an inner-city dweller to be ever vigilant.When they'd built this park years ago for the Olympic Games, they'd bulldozed whole blocs of crime infested 'projects' to obtain the land.

In doing so, they'd pushed back the putrefying center of Atlanta just far enough that a sizeable number of suburbanites used the park for a break when they came downtown. The area would be surrendered to the crack dealers and pimps after dark, but it was still light, and so Amy set off toward the tunnel.

Clumps of azalea bushes had been planted on both sides of the entrance but the abuse of the graffiti artists' feet and bodies had reduced them to a few nearly bare stalks and one or two anemic blooms that paled against the acrylic colors of the graffiti.

Nature eclipsed again, thought Amy sadly as she remembered the tumultuous blooms of St. Lucia.

As a final precaution before entering the huge culvert-like structure, Amy looked around her but no one was in sight except the two skaters who were preoccupied again with their jumps from the fountain platform. She stopped squarely in the entrance to the tunnel and stared into the darker interior lit only by a few ceiling-mounted lights that gave off a sour inefficient yellow light. Nobody was in the length of the tunnel, or even beyond it, based on what she could see.

She quickened her pace and ignored a prickly feeling on the back of her neck that, she knew from experience, afflicted her whenever she sensed the possibility of danger. She was about halfway through the tunnel when she heard a scraping sound behind and above her. She turned just in time to see a tall black man drop out of a cavity that must have existed in the roof of the tunnel.

Landing lightly on all fours in a crouch on the floor, he quickly sprang up. He wore a tie-dye T-shirt, blue jeans and had long thick dread locks that draped Medusa-like over both his shoulders. He looked menacing.

As she stared at him, he began to laugh and the sound was grotesquely distorted by the tunnel.

Amy froze for a moment, then bunched her muscles to sprint ahead, but when she turned back around to face the far end of the tunnel, two more black men were advancing slowly toward her.

She cursed her stupidity and started to lower her bag from her shoulder while backing up against the nearest wall of the tunnel where she could keep all three men in view.

The first man spoke. He had a heavy Caribbean accent. "Well, me pretty lidda sistah, yer come back from dee island at last and us bin waiting so long tuh meet yuh... Miss *Davis,* ain't it, naw?"

Amy's heart thudded in panic against her chest wall but her mind was alert. "How do you know my name?" she demanded trying to sound as ferocious and unaffected by events as possible.

In the pocket of her jeans she always carried a whistle. The lanyard it was attached to drooped in a loop that her fingers found as she lowered her bag to the ground. In the periphery of her visual field, she could see that the other two men had stopped advancing as if their assignment were to block her retreat and perhaps keep others from entering the tunnel as well.

"Oh, ah knows yuh well, lidda sistah. Ah bin watchin' yuh careful like, cuz yuh means money tuh me."

"If it's money you want, I'll give you all I have. My wallet is in the bag, so just back off, you ape!"

He laughed again. His voice was deep, intimidating, bass. "Oh, it's not *yuh* money ah'm bein' paid wit, lidda sistah. It's big, big money ah'll be gittin' for dis job. But yuh do have somet'ing ah wants..." and he continued advancing as she siddled away from him along the tunnel wall.

"Nah, doen' be runnin' away, lidda sistah, cuz dat jes gunna make it hurt all dee mor'" and, having spoken, he opened his right hand and snapped out a switch-blade knife that looked to Amy as if it were a foot long.

"What do you want?" she demanded, now with an edge of panic in her voice.

"Why it's *you* ah wants, lidda sistah. Ain't no one but a pow'ful lawyah cud hep yuh naw, an' yuh dun trowed away yuh own lawyuh, didn' yuh naw?"

"My lawyer? What are you saying?" Amy was getting closer to the two other men as she kept edging down the tunnel. The man with the knife had already passed by the bag she'd set on the ground. He was close enough now that shc could see his milk-white teeth, as he grinned.

She had to make her move without delay.

Yanking out the whistle, she put it to her lips and blew a sustained blast at the same time that she spun on her heels and ran as fast as she could toward the two men at the closer end of the tunnel. One of them seemed shocked by the noise and recoiled a step or two, as if he were prepared to bolt, but the other one held his ground.

Amy aborted her rush stopping within the reach of the closer man. She was still blowing the whistle desperately when an arm locked around her face from the back and knocked it from her mouth, cutting her lip in the process. She could taste the blood and smell the acrid ganja odor of her first assailant as he tried to put his other arm around her waist and lift her from the ground.

She twisted violently in his grip and felt the knife blade in his hand slice into her left shoulder. The knife cut seemed unintentional, occurring when he grasped around her neck and she knew the wound wasn't deep.

With all her strength, she drove backward with her right elbow into her assailant's chest and simultaneously swung her right leg ferociously back and upwards. Her elbow thudded into bone with little effect but her leg had driven up between the man's own legs and delivered a crushing blow to his scrotum. He cried out releasing his grip on her and both of them stumbled forward slamming into the man ahead of her with enough force to carry all three of them to the ground.

The third man bolted.

Serendipitously, when she fell forward, sandwiched between the two men's bodies, her forearm had been across the second man's throat. When the man behind her rolled off her holding his crotch, she saw the second assailant grab at his throat in pain, his eyes wide in surprise.

She had no more that a split second to escape.

With lightening speed, she drove two fingers into the eyes of the man lying under her. She registered surprise at how hard the eyeballs felt to her jab. He screamed in pain, and, at the same instant, she knelt upon his chest and regained her feet.

The first man was up on his knees and rising. He cursed and flung out an arm landing a glancing blow on the back of her right calf just as she drove off her left leg starting to sprint toward the end to the tunnel where she'd entered. Her right leg came forward for her second step but, having been pushed out of alignment, it drove into the back of her left calf and she stumbled and fell forward onto her hands and knees. She was screaming for help as she scrambled back to her feet and started sprinting again.

She felt a hand on her right shoulder as her assailant grabbed at her sweatshirt pulling her to the right. She slammed into the wall going forward but so did her attacker and his grip loosened, then his fingers slipped away.

Amy pistoned her legs toward the entrance screaming. She could hear the man cursing as he pursued her. He seemed literally to be at her back when she burst out of the tunnel and into the sunlight. She felt the fingers of his hand close again on her shoulder.

Suddenly a figure rocketed around the corner of the path and whooshed past her. She heard a collision behind her and, an instant later, a second body rounded the curve and flashed past. It was the two skaters.

Amy tried to turn her head to see what was happening but she stumbled on the grass at the side of the path and fell to the ground. The force of her momentum sent her skidding a couple of yards along the grass.

When she looked up, the black man was behind her on the ground. One skater was on his knees beside the guy pummeling him with his fists while the man tried to ward off the blows with an upraised arm. Her attacker was still cursing but the knife was nowhere to be seen. The second skater was landing repeated kicks with his skate boot into the man's sides.

It was only a few seconds before her assailant scrambled to his hands and knees, still being beaten by the boys, and ran staggering across the grass where they couldn't follow him in their skates and then back onto the path and into the tunnel.

The boys were skating toward where she sat on the grass.

"Are you ok, miss? Should we get the police?"

Amy was trembling but her breath was no longer coming in gasps. She held out her hand and the taller boy, who'd been kicking at her attacker, pulled her up. She leaned forward at the waist with both hands on her knees for a few moments trying to orient herself.

When she stood up, she instinctively touched the wound on her left shoulder..

"Hey, you're bleeding," said the other skater.

She shook her head. "It's nothing boys, believe me. I'm ok, just a few scrapes and this little cut. Thank God you came when you did. I think they would have killed me."

She was still shaking visibly.

The taller boy asked again, "Should we get a cop, there's always one sitting down at the park entrance," and he pointed off somewhere behind him.

"No please, don't get the cops. I'm embarrassed enough as it is and those pricks are long gone by now."

"Yeah, one of them will be aching tonight," said the smaller skater, "Look what I did to my knuckles on his face," and he held out hands that were contused and scraped.

"Thank you again, guys... Like I said, I think you saved my life," repeated Amy.

Then she remembered her bag. "Could one of you check to see if they left my bag in the tunnel, please. I dropped it, when they jumped me... Be careful," she added.

The taller boy sped away to the tunnel, didn't hesitate at the entrance, and in less than a minute came out carrying her bag.

"Got it, miss," he called as he rushed up. She took it from him gratefully and unzipped it searching for her wallet.

"They steal anything?" asked one of the boys.

“No, I don’t think so. It all seems to be here,” she replied searching in the wallet and pulling out a twenty-dollar bill which she proffered to her two rescuers.

Both boys simultaneously held up their hands in protest and started to skate backwards to emphasize their refusal. “No, m’am. We don’t want no money. We were happy to help you… So, if you’re alright, we’ll be going.”

“I’m fine boys... I just want to say thanks, again.”

The smaller boy had a gleam in his eye as the two rolled backwards and, when he was about ten feet away and felt bold enough, he called out, “Besides, miss, we’re the guys from the hill... *You already paid us well.*”

“Big time!” shouted out the second boy. Then, they gave each other double high-fives, laughed and skated rapidly away.

Amy left for Albany within the hour after leaving the key to her apartment with the custodian of the building and telling Mayflower to pick up her stuff and take it to storage.

CH028

Jason had been back from St. Lucia for five days and was expecting to hear from Amy. He hadn't resumed office visits with patients because of the urgency of other things he needed to do since he'd learned that Annette had been murdered. Besides, he'd made arrangements for a replacement physician to cover the practice for two months and that period would extend until the end of next week.

The sun was high and brazen in a cloudless sky and the temperature so torrid that the air smelled like heated copper when he stepped into the street.

He'd only been in the police station for twenty minutes but their air conditioning wasn't working properly and his shirt was already pasted to his back with perspiration. After sitting in the sun, the interior of the BMW was a furnace and he swore a steady stream of mild epithets as he got in, started it up, then rolled down all the windows to create a draft until the air conditioning overcame the heat.

He knew that GM had built a remote ignition device into their Cadillac so that heaters or AC's could be turned on from a distance. "Ugly as they are, almost makes you want to buy a Cadillac," he murmured to himself when he'd stopped swearing and the cool air from the AC vents was pouring out. He closed the windows and sat in the parking lot contemplating his next move.

At his ankle, he could feel the unfamiliar weight of his snub-nosed .38. He'd been in to see Willie Travisol, the police chief, to commiserate over the disappearance of Cal, which Jason pretended to believe was a tragic accident, and to renew his permit to carry a concealed handgun. Travisol was a decent man but he was kept so busy tiptoeing along the razor's edge of the thorny race-relations in Albany that he rarely got to do any real police work. The same was unfortunately true of all his subordinates, as well.

Roger had phoned Jason earlier to tell him that the CHC's man was called Randall Smith and that he was still in town and staying at the Ramada Inn. Jason had informed Roger that he'd met with Mark West and the gloves were off. Jason also recommended that Roger carry a gun and told him that he was strapping on his own piece. He'd said nothing about Annette's murder. He would keep that information to himself for reasons he would share with no one but Amy.

The kids didn't know he was back yet and that was just as well. Although he missed them dearly, since he'd learned that Annette had been murdered, he had sufficient reason to be thankful that the children were safe in Michigan.

As he sat and pondered developments, he decided that he would pay Dr.Trang a visit after all. It was time to start reinforcing his own support or at least attacking West's allies. Jason had never much liked the Vietnamese but the guy was a good dermatologist and he worked hard. Every year, even after bonuses were paid out, Trang produced a lot of money for TurnerWest.

Whereas Jason had gone easy on Goldman, he was prepared to play hardball with Trang since he sensed that the Vietnamese might not respond favorably to anything but threats. He pulled out of the parking lot headed for the TurnerWest building mentally mapping out a strategy when his cell phone buzzed.

When he touched the phone, he withdrew his hand immediately. The plastic casing was hot enough to burn his fingers. He'd left it on the dashboard while he'd been in the police station. Pulling a Kleenex from the dispenser beside the phone, he gingerly picked it up being careful not to place it fully against his ear. As a result, he could barely hear and couldn't understand the voice. He shouted for the party to hold on for a minute. Thrusting the cell phone into the cold airflow from the AC vent he kept driving with his left hand. When he put the cooler phone to his ear, his heart leapt. It was Amy.

"Oh, Jason, you can't believe what it means to me to hear your voice again."

His pulse quickening, he answered, "I might be able to imagine it, darling, because I've been wishing for these four past days that I hadn't asked you not to call. It was a stupid, useless precaution and I'm sorry I even thought of it. Where are you now and how are you?"

There was a pause and then she said, "I'm in my room at the Ramada."

"The Ramada? Have you already cleared out your apartment and gone to a hotel?"

"Jason, I'm *here* in Albany. I've been here since yesterday afternoon. I drove down Wednesday night from Atlanta and stopped in Macon, then came on to Albany in the morning."

"This is wonderful Amy. I'm only five minutes away. What's your room number?"

"Room 411. Are you coming over now?"

"Coming?... I'm almost at your doorstep," he enthused.

"No, wait, Jason. Stop for some coffee or something, please. I'm a mess. I just came up from the exercise room and I'm all sweaty."

"You know you're turning me on, don't you, with all that talk about your sweaty body. If you think *you're* bad, my back is plastered to my leather seat with perspiration and it looks like I dumped a pitcher of water under each arm. I'm coming right up," he said, his spirit suddenly soaring, and he clicked the phone off before she could object again.

Jason knew the Ramada Inn well. It was one of the few places in Albany decent enough to house guests and most visitors to TurnerWest stayed there. He pulled his BMW into an empty parking slot at the far end of the building where he knew room 411 would be found. He literally ran past the soft drink and the ice machine inside the back door and flew up the stairway taking two steps at a time to the fourth floor. He was breathless when he knocked impatiently at her door.

When it opened, Amy was standing there trying desperately to pin up her hair. Her mouth was full of bobby pins.

He rushed in and kicked the door shut with his foot, walking her backwards with his hands on her shoulders as she objected unintelligibly through the mouthful of pins. Just before she fell backwards onto the bed, she spat out the pins and called out, "Jason... Jason..." But his mouth cut short her protest and she surrendered to his searching tongue.

She was wearing a black spandex exercise jumper and gym socks. Her hair fountained over the bedcovers and he took two handfuls of it and held on. She clasped him to her tightly and drew her legs up so high around him that he could feel her heels on his buttocks. He kissed her forcefully for almost a minute, then suddenly thrust himself up on his arms, took a deep desperate gasp of air and started laughing. She released him and looked up into his face.

"I just ran up... four flights of stairs," he puffed, " and nearly asphyxiated myself... because I needed to kiss you... so badly."

His chest was still heaving and he slid down along her body twisting as he went until he was sitting on the floor between her legs with his back against the bed, panting.

"I'm sorry... sorry, sorry... how utterly unromantic... you must think I am."

She slid closer to the edge of the bed so she could cradle his head in one arm against her stomach. "You are romantic… crazy romantic, and just like I've always dreamed of..." She kissed his sweat-soaked forehead, "and I do *so* love you," she murmured.

He reached up and took her hand in his and kissed it gently. They stayed that way for at least ten minutes while she stroked his hair with her free hand and he toyed with her sock, massaging her foot gently.

When he finally pulled himself up with a groan, he joked, "I'm slowing down, woman... all creaks and groans. Can't even run up four flights of stairs to the woman I love without almost suffering a coronary. Are you sure you still want me?"

"What floor is your bedroom on in your house?" she asked coyly.

"Ground floor, why?" he queried a little perplexed.

"Then... I'll keep you," she said playfully and slipped into his arms and they kissed again, long and languorously.

When she stepped back from him, she said, "Jason, I wasn't kidding. I really *do* need a shower. Just give me a few minutes and I'll be brand new. I'm sure you'll approve."

He hesitated to release her hand, but she had turned toward the bathroom door and pulled down her bodysuit showing him her bare back before she closed the door behind her.

Jason sat on the bed a little crestfallen, looking about the room trying to take in every detail, trying to assimilate everything about her. He heard the shower sizzle on and, in a few moments, was lost in reverie reliving the last few minutes over again.

Only five minutes had passed when he heard her calling.

"Jason, can you hear me?"

He stood up, crossed to the closed door and called back.

"I can hear you, Amy."

"Then open the door and please come in ... I need someone to wash my back!"

* * *

The next morning Jason felt refreshed. He had slept at last. He marveled at how the simple fact of being able to reach out his hand and touch Amy sleeping beside him could be so beneficial for his emotional health. A wry smile curled his lips as he reflected that Brigham Landry would have seen in his miraculous restoration even further proof of his dependency. No matter, whatever the source of peace and vitality that he'd found with Amy, he welcomed it.

He raised himself up on one elbow and watched her as she slept. She lay on her back and the sheet was draped across the right side of her body only, leaving her exposed from the waist up on the left. Her smooth unblemished skin was the hue of burnt amber. She was thin enough that the profile of her pelvis was clearly visible at the edge of the sheet with the flawless expense of her flank and abdomen sloping gently up and away from it. Her chest rose and fell rhythmically raising one exquisite breast into sharper profile with each inspiration.

Her left arm was raised above her head, the forearm and hand lost under the munificence of her hair. A tress of hair lay incongruously over her face covering one eye and falling haphazardly across her cheek to nestle in a glistening coil between her chin and raised arm. He reached carefully across and lifted it, spreading it out and straightening it until it flared along the outer edge of her cheek and trailed down onto the upper curve of her breast. Studying his handiwork for a moment, he took the end of the tress and divided it so that half fell on one side of the nipple and half on the other.

Pleased at the result, he continued to retrieve more locks of her hair and arrange them about her face and torso. He next began to configure the sheet so that it lay smoothly in easy swaths across her body. His portrait of a Celtic goddess lost in slumber was slowly taking form.

Intrigued with his task, he slipped silently off the bed being careful not to disturb her, and stood at the foot of it to better appreciate the canvas he was creating. While there, he again rearranged the sheet and covered one of her feet that had been partially uncovered. Moving to the right side of the bed, he busied himself again with elements of her hair that he hadn't been able to reach before.

Finally, after studying his subject again for several moments, he gently drew down the right side of the sheet to uncover her other breast. It was while he was arranging more of her hair upon this breast that she opened her eyes, watched him surreptitiously for a moment with amusement glinting in her eyes, then she spoke softly.

"Jason if you wanted to see my breasts there was no need to steal about uncovering them while I slept… All you had to do was ask." There was no reproach in her tone.

Literally startled by her voice, he had jumped back from the bed like a child caught stealing cookies, but he recovered his poise almost instantly.

"Amy, don't move... not even a hair... now, give me just a half-smile with something sultry and a little pouty in it."

"Jason what *are* you doing?" she laughed and began to stir.

"Stop!" he cried, "Please, no movement at all for just a minute," he pleaded, "and give me that seductive expression I asked for... Do it, and I promise you a wonderful surprise for breakfast."

"Oh, alright," she said, "how's this?" And she assumed a sultry, sinful expression. She also moved her leg into a more provocative pose but the sheet ended up too disturbed for his taste.

He straightened the sheet while he spoke, "I like the leg... nice touch..." and then in a teasing tone, "I see you've done this before."

He stood back again to survey the scene. Raising his thumb and forefinger curved into a small circle he pronounced it, "Almost perfect! A Celtic goddess seducing a king of the mortals into her bed."

"*Almost* perfect?" pouted Amy petulantly.

"Yes, almost... one more detail and it's finished, but you must promise not to move *no matter what happens*," and he raised a forefinger in admonishment.

He moved up to the right side of the bed and sat on the edge of it pretending to critically assess what he saw. "Your right nipple just doesn't want to get into the spirit of things, it's still lying down snoozing." He bent forward lowering his lips to her breast, "but I have just the thing to wake it up..." he murmured.

She shivered deliciously then lowered her arms and enfolded him to her.

* * *

"This is the *wonderful surprise* you promised?"

Amy's nose was wrinkled in distaste and she poked at the glistening greasy omelet on her plate like it was some repulsive dead rodent that a child might prod with a stick.

"Yup, says so right here," and Jason pointed to an item on the stained IHOP menu, "*morning surprise omelette.*" He was grinning broadly.

Amy winced, pushing her plate away from her while tentatively tasting a gluey-looking glass of orange juice. She put the glass down without drinking and leaned forward across the table toward Jason who was chewing a mouthful of *his* 'surprise omelette' with exaggerated gusto, still grinning.

"Why are we here, Jason? The restaurant at the Ramada was quite a decent place. Is this your idea of a joke?"

Jason quickly lost his grin and his expression sobered. He swallowed and put his fork down. To reassure Amy, he reached across the table and took her hand in both of his.

"No joke, darling. I don't want to be seen by anyone *yet,*" he paused "and I don't want anyone to see us *together*, for the present. I need you to do something important for me and you'd be compromised if anyone knew we were together."

"I don't understand, Jason. Please explain."

"There's a man, a Texan, staying at the Ramada Inn by the name of Smith, Randall Smith, if I remember correctly. He's an agent of Cumberland Health Care and I believe he's responsible for some pretty awful things... I have no proof however, and that's where you come in."

"What do I need to do, Jason?"

"I've got an old Jeep Cherokee at home that Annette used to use for off-road driving. It has local plates and won't stand out. I want you to follow Smith. Find out what he's up to, but be very careful. The man may be a murderer."

"*A murderer*!" she repeated in a forced whisper. "Who did he kill?"

Jason blinked twice, sat up straight and pinched his nose with his left hand, thought for a moment, and then answered, leaning forward again. His voice was husky with emotion.

"Since I saw you last, I've learned that Annette didn't die in an accident," he paused and cleared his throat. "...She was murdered, Amy. There was a bomb in the car that caused it to crash."

Amy now sat up straight. She put her hand silently over her mouth and her eyes widened in dismay.

Jason continued, "Until I know differently, I've got to assume that Annette's murderers are among *my* enemies."

His voice became flinty and his eyes hardened, "But I *will* find them. They won't escape me... I've already promised that to Annette."

Confusion flitted through Amy's eyes at the mention of a promise to Annette, then compassion flooded her face and she reached for his hands. "Oh, Jason, I'm so terribly sorry". Any more words would have been superfluous.

His grief had caught up with him again and he lowered his face to gain a private moment in order to deal with it. When he looked up, his eyes were clearing of the sadness.

"This whole mess is like a terrible nightmare in ten acts that keeps getting worse each day," he said quietly.

"I know what you mean, Jason. I've had my own little nightmare this week, too..."

He looked suddenly quizzical, asking for details with his eyes.

"I was attacked by three men in a park in Atlanta, two days ago. That's why I came down here so quickly. Jason, *they knew my name, who I was and they'd been following me.* That's how I got what I told you was a little 'scrape from a fall' here, on my shoulder."

She indicated the spot where the Band-Aid was visible beneath her blouse.

"It's a knife cut."

"A knife cut, Amy? Good Lord! What's happening?... Who were they? What did they want?"

"They were strangers to me, from the Caribbean judging by their accent, but the one with the knife was pretty clear he'd been paid to murder me or at least do me serious harm."

"Who paid him? Did he tell you that?"

"Not exactly, but he talked about me '*throwing away my own lawyer*' which, after I thought about it, I took to mean my ex-husband... He's about the only lawyer I know."

"Has Davis got it in for you, Amy?"

"I knew he was angry but I never suspected he'd go that far. He has assault charges pending because of an attack on me. If he's convicted, he'll probably be disbarred which will mean the end of his filthy little world." She almost spat out the last few words.

"Do you think he was behind the attack?"

"It's about the only explanation that makes sense. About two months ago, he asked for a meeting with me in which he pressured me to refuse to testify. I said 'no'... If I had backed down it would have been like betraying myself... again."

She had a distant look in her eyes that hinted at a world of pain which she kept to herself.

"Does anyone know where you are now, Amy?"

With his question, she seemed to snap back to the booth where they both sat. She paused, then replied, "Only the movers. I told no one else."

"You'd better call this morning, as soon as possible, and tell them to store your belongings in Atlanta until further notice. If it was Davis, no sense leaving a trail to be followed."

"Ok. But where will I stay?"

"For now, we need you at the Ramada to follow Smith. Later," and he took her hand, "you can stay with me at the house, if you wish."

"But that's Annette's home, Jason," she protested.

Jason's face became somber again and he seemed to be listening to a voice inside his head for a moment, then he spoke slowly and deliberately. "Amy, Annette's dead, but I know clearly what she would have wanted for me."

CH029

The intercom beeped and Cheryl Montfort's voice said, "Dr. Turner, you have two visitors to see you, a Mr. Gallo and a Mr. Rossi."

Jason pushed on the intercom button, "Please pick up, Cheryl."

He didn't want his comments broadcast to the visitors.

When his receptionist answered, he asked, "Do I have anyone booked to see me this morning?"

"No, sir. You told me to put Dr. Atkins or Ms. Davis through, if they called, but I have no one booked."

"Then who are these two Italian guys with names that belong in a wine commercial?"

"Mr. Gallo is a lawyer from Detroit and Mr. Rossi is his companion."

She paused, as if she were listening to someone, then came back on the line. "Mr. Gallo says he has a court order to deliver to you, personally."

Jason hesitated. A *court order from Detroit*?

"Send them in, please," and he got up from his desk and crossed partway to the door from the outer office.

The receptionist ushered in two obviously Mediterranean types and, indicating the younger one said, "Dr. Turner, this is Mr. Gallo."

Michael Gallo moved closer to Jason while Rossi, who walked with a pronounced limp and was carrying a briefcase, was a step behind. Gallo almost extended his hand in greeting but, when Turner didn't budge, he lowered it and reached behind him for the briefcase that Rossi held out to him.

Michael Gallo was about thirty-three, thought Jason. He was almost handsome with chiseled Roman features that were just a bit too heavy guaranteeing that they'd age poorly. Based on a quick appraisal of broad shoulders, tapered torso and fireplug neck, he was trim but powerful. He had dark aquiline eyes and expressive brows.

For the moment, he was smiling. Rossi on the other hand was frowning.

He was a much older man, squat, with a top-heavy body that was three quarters belly and seemed to be teetering on badly bowed legs. His nose and ears had a rubbery, swollen quality that looked like he'd had a disappointing ring career before assuming his current duties as briefcase carrier for a Detroit lawyer in a two thousand dollar suit. Even at a distance, he stank of stale tobacco smoke; a poster boy for at least three deadly habits.

"May we sit down, Dr. Turner? Our business may be quite lengthy," inquired Gallo, politely.

"And, again, it might be quite brief, Mr. Gallo," responded Jason aggressively, giving the lawyer a venomous glare. "State your business and then I'll decide if we sit down or not in *my* office."

Gallo opened the briefcase and withdrew a sheaf of documents on legal length sheets.

"This is a court order, quite lengthy actually," and he turned it sideways for inspection, "from the Wilkinson County court in Grosse Pointe, Michigan."

Jason held out his hand for the papers but said nothing.

"There is quite a lot to cover here. We could discuss it more easily sitting down," repeated Gallo.

"I have no difficulty reading while standing," said Jason tersely, leaving his hand out.

"As you wish," shrugged Gallo and passed the papers to him.

Jason read with a pounding heart.

'Order of Interim custody in the matter of the custody of the minor children:

Michael Adam Turner

And

Caroline Michele Turner

Jason felt suddenly weak but, not wanting the two men opposite him to detect his reaction to the document, he gestured brusquely to a group of chairs around a small conference table at the far side of his office. "We can sit there."

He preceded the two Italians to the table and sat at one end of it. Gallo took the chair to his immediate left but Rossi remained standing while leaning on a chair back after placing the briefcase on the table.

Gallo spoke. "Alberto has an old war wound. His right knee doesn't bend anymore, so, if you don't mind, he'll pull a chair back from the table."

"Suit yourself," replied Jason who was already perusing the second page of the court order.

After a moment, he looked up at Gallo. "Are you acting for my father-in-law?"

"Yes. I've been retained by Judge McLean. But," pursued Gallo, "I'd prefer to deal with these matters amicably, and out of court, if possible."

Jason's eyes flashed at the impertinence of the young lawyer. "Well, Mr. Gallo, you can '*prefer*' all you want but forget about '*amicable*' and consider yourself lucky that you and your gimp," he gestured rudely at Rossi, "don't get tossed out of my office on your asses," growled Jason, his hands clenching until the papers he held crackled and bent.

Gallo looked nonplussed by the outburst.

"I'll assume that the natural affection of a father for his children is behind your threat and disregard it as an understandable reaction, Dr. Turner."

He spoke levelly and without apparent malice.

"Assume that at your peril, if you will, Gallo," snapped Jason.

At that, Gallo's eyes clouded over, his brows knitted and his lips became thin with obvious menace. He glared silently at Jason for a full twenty seconds and then spoke through partially clenched teeth.

"I came here to try and talk to you. It *is* in your best interest to listen. That court order is not the only reason for my visit... If you refuse to listen, we'll go, but *don't ever threaten me again.*"

The men continued to glare at each other until Jason broke gaze, sat up, and leaned back in his chair. "So talk, Gallo," he growled again.

Gallo immediately resumed his previous professional demeanor and began.

"Your mother-in-law nearly died of grief when your wife was killed. At the present time, her doctors, who were in almost daily attendance upon her, have been dismissed. I have personally seen her playing with your children as if she were thirty years old, full of energy, life, and pure joy."

"Why are you telling me this?"

"Because I don't want you to mistakenly assume that this court action is being undertaken in a punitive mode toward you," said Gallo.

"Do you assume, Mr. Gallo, that depriving me of my children's love and companionship is, by some facile reasoning, '*not punitive toward me*'?"

"No one is proposing depriving you of your children's affection. Neither you nor the children would ever be prohibited from frequent and liberal visitation. You could see them whenever you wished to. We're not proposing anything more than what happens daily in thousands of American families when a wife leaves her husband, for example."

"Need I remind you, Mr. Gallo, that my wife *left me*, as you put it, by dying?" Jason's words were sated with sarcasm.

"I guess I need to repeat that the custody of the children is not being pursued in order to injure anyone. In fact, there are compelling grounds to believe that the children might be better off with their grandparents, as primary caregivers, than they would be with you."

"Are you suggesting I'm a pervert, a child abuser or, in some other elemental way, unfit to parent my own children, Mr. Gallo?"

"Not in the least, although I am aware of the understandable depression that you suffered at the loss of your wife."

Gallo was being particularly careful about how he broached the subject of depression.

"Please set your mind at ease on that point, counselor. I've been treated and have fully recovered. I sought medical help, received it, and my depression is a thing of the past. Undoubtedly, if you could observe me playing with my children, you would agree that *my* doctors as well could be dismissed."

"When you had the children with you, you were still very depressed. In fact, you requested that Judge and Mrs. McLean care for your children temporarily. This implies their acceptability to you as custodians or parental surrogates..."

"It doesn't," interrupted Jason, "imply that I would choose them over myself when I was no longer depressed."

"Of course not, Dr. Turner," and Gallo paused, "But there is another major consideration we haven't mentioned yet."

"And what is that?" asked Jason.

"The children's safety," replied Gallo, flatly.

Jason felt a chill trickle through his bones. "And what is the danger to them, in your opinion, Mr. Gallo?"

The sarcasm was gone from his voice.

Gallo didn't respond immediately but signaled Rossi to bring him the briefcase. Rossi levered himself up from his chair and brought the case. Opening it, Gallo withdrew a large manila envelope which he placed on the table between them.

"If you'd please examine the contents of the envelope, Dr. Turner."

The envelope contained a four-page report, complete with photo attachments, from a company named, 'Forensic Incorporated'. The subject of the report was an examination of Annette's Mercedes. It was both comprehensive and detailed. The conclusions were that an explosive device, utilizing military grade C-4 plastic explosive, had been detonated remotely causing the crash of the Mercedes and the death, by subsequent drowning, of Annette Annelise Turner.

Emotion washed through him as he read the report and he deliberately extended his examination of it to allow him to rein in his internal disarray before he commented.

"So, *you* have the car and you know that my wife was murdered, *too?*" asked Jason with as much composure as he could muster.

Gallo looked taken aback by Jason's comment and nodded his head almost imperceptibly while stroking his mustache.

"I must admit, I'm surprised that you were already aware of thefacts in the report, Doctor," he said cautiously.

"Why would you be surprised?... Did you think that I wouldn't have had my own wife's death investigated? My own investigator was about to run a series of tests on the car wreck when it disappeared. And, incidentally... when we traced the purchasers, we learned that '*an auto body firm in Bloomfield Hills, Michigan with ties to organized crime*' had gone to considerable lengths to buy the vehicle."

Gallo smiled. Turner was much brighter than he had been led to believe.

Jason continued, "But you'll be pleased to learn, Mr. Gallo that your visit and the source of this report answers a few questions for me about Judge McLean's business associations. Associations I might add that I'm certain most judges, ruling in a custody case, would take into consideration."

"Touché, Dr. Turner… but let me just say, that if I were seriously concerned about embarrassing skeletons falling out of family closets at discovery, I wouldn't have taken on the case. And, as you can see, I have."

There was silence in the room again for several moments before Gallo spoke again.

"Do you understand, Dr. Turner, how your parents-in-law might fear for the safety of your children if they remained in the same area where their mother was *murdered*?"

After a moment's reflection, Jason decided that further antagonism, at that point, would be counterproductive.

"Yes, of course, I do, Mr. Gallo. Regrettably, I've been stalked by the same horrifying fears, so I have a proposition for you to take back to the judge."

"I'm listening, Doctor."

"If Judge McLean will suspend any action on this court order, agree to keep all these proceedings hidden from my children and assist me in tracking down Annette's murderer, I will leave the children with their grandparents until this whole business is cleared up."

"I'm certain he will agree," said Gallo. "My recommendation will be that he agree."

Jason smiled skeptically, "You obviously don't know the old judge that well. He does what he wants and, very often, logic isn't a big part of his deliberations... I know, because I lived with and loved his daughter... and she wasn't his daughter for nothing. She had certain family traits."

"Well, let me rephrase myself, I'll do my utmost to convince the old judge that you share his love and concern for the children and are prepared to do whatever is in their best interests, now and in the future, and that you trust he will do the same... How's that?"

"Better, but don't ever believe that I won't have my children back, Mr. Gallo," said Jason evenly.

"I wouldn't expect to hear anything different from a good father, Dr. Turner," and he was smiling again as they stood up from the table.

"By the way, it may help to explain future events if you know that *your* enemies become *our* enemies if our joint purpose in all of this is to protect the children."

"*Our enemies*?"... repeated Jason with a quizzical look. "Mr. Gallo, just who exactly *is* protecting my children, right now?"

"*Mi famiglia*," replied Gallo and the two men shook hands.

CH030

Dr. Nguyan Trang had just finished with his last patient when his nurse came into his office where he was dictating. He put down the recorder and asked, "Yes, Miss King?"

"Dr. Turner is here asking to see you, Doctor."

Trang's expression was unperturbed by the news. "Well, send him in Miss King...No, wait … I'll come out."

He rose from his desk and followed her down the hall to where Jason was sitting in the waiting room. Trang appeared pleased to see him and extended his hand in greeting. "Jason, it's good to have you back. Please come into my office."

Inside, Trang went back behind his desk and Jason pulled a chair up beside it and sat down.

"How are you feeling, Jason?"

Trang's concern sounded genuine, although Jason had learned, from dealing with the man through the years, that Trang's tone of voice and facial expression rarely changed no matter what was being discussed. He was truly the inscrutable oriental and Jason was ill at ease when deprived of the multiple non-verbal clues that a doctor instinctively seeks in order to detect emotions or dissimulation.

"I'm well, Nguyen. My trip was fruitful and my grief is now in check. It was good to be away."

"And, is it as good to be back, Jason?"

Nguyen's question was an obvious probe to discover the reason for the unannounced visit.

"Not entirely. I've learned things since my return that concern me a great deal."

"Such as my '*getting into the same bed with Mark*'... Is that how you English speakers say it?" interrupted Trang.

The frankness surprised Jason but it wasn't unwelcome.

"I couldn't have said it better myself, Nguyen."

"I suspected as much when I saw you, Jason... Excuse me please for a moment."

Trang got up and walked to a counter beside his desk where a delicate tea set with miniature cups was standing on a silver tray. He poured himself a cupful and then asked over his shoulder. "Tea, Jason? Business is always conducted over tea in my country but Mark West and the CHC man, Smith I think, they let me drink alone. I didn't appreciate it."

"Since you put it that way Nguyen, I'd love some tea."

"Wonderful, Jason, I thought you might."

Trang returned to his desk and set the two cups down between them. He was smiling.

"And what do you want to know about me, and all these '*goings on?*... How am I doing on my colloquialisms? Miss King teaches me one new expression every day."

"That one was *right on the money*, Nguyen."

Despite his joking, Jason was thoroughly nonplussed. He didn't know what to think and he said so. "I'm not sure how to go about this, Nguyen."

"Why not simply ask me what you need to know?" suggested the dermatologist.

"Ok," said Jason. "Have you changed your mind about the desirability of the merger with CHC?"

"You're doing very well... That was, how should I say it, ' *right on the nail's head*'?"

Jason chuckled.

Trang said, "I guess that one needs more work."

"A little," said Jason.

"Well, the short answer to your question is 'no', I have not changed my opinion on the *desirability* of the merger."

"I'd heard differently."

"But not from me. And I assure you, no one else has ever heard me say that I changed my mind on the question, although," and he paused and winked at Jason over his teacup as he quipped, "if it became the expedient thing to do, I may *say* that I have had a change of mind."

"Nguyen, you've lost me entirely."

"Jason, have you ever tried to blow over a reed?"

"Do you mean have I ever tried to play a reed instrument?" asked Jason obviously perplexed.

It was Trang's turn to laugh. "No, I mean *blow down* a reed like the wolf did to the tower of the three pigs."

"You mean 'house' don't you?"

"For the pigs?"

"Yes, for the pigs."

"Well, then *house* if that makes it any easier to understand what I'm saying about the reed," said Trang.

"It does."

"Well, have you?"

"Have I what?" asked Jason.

"Tried to blow down a reed?" Trang repeated but he was having difficulty keeping a straight face.

"You mean like a bullrush?" rejoined Jason.

Now, Trang looked perplexed.

"I did not say anything about bulls, I was speaking of a reed."

"A bullrush is a type of reed, Trang."

"I didn't know that."

"Be patient, it'll come up one day in Miss King's lessons," Jason said without a hint of sarcasm.

"But we do not speak of reeds, she teaches me euph.. umum.. euphemisms," and Trang stumbled over the word several times before pronouncing it correctly.

Jason broke out laughing and, to his relief, so did Trang. They both kept laughing as they finished their cups of tea. Then Jason spoke.

"Listen, Nguyen, what were you trying to tell me about West and Smith and reeds."

Trang gathered himself, but it took a few moments before he spoke. "I simply meant, Jason, that I am a reed and they were the wind. They came to see me, both of them huffing and puffing and promising something I wanted desperately which they could do, but I could not."

"And?"

Jason was fully composed now.

"I am a reed, Jason, I bent before the wind. The wind passed and I am back where I was before. Do you see?"

"So you accepted what they would do for you, listened to what they had to say and *didn't change your mind?*" asked Jason.

"Precisely."

"Did you make any promises?"

"No. They assumed that I saw things their way because I agreed that I wanted very much for them to use their influence on my behalf and do what I could not." Trang's expression had resumed its opaque quality.

Jason pondered the response for a moment, then asked, "Nguyen, am I the wind too?"

"Yes, you are Jason. But I am a reed and my roots are deep in the soil of TurnerWest and they will not be easily removed."

"Should I be pleased with that as an answer, Nguyen?"

"If I were you, Jason, my answer would be *your cat's meow*."

"Ok, I think I understand," smiled Jason as he got up and was shown out by the dermatologist.

CH031

Jason was reading a fax he'd received that morning on the machine at his home. The lunchtime crowd at Blackbeard's Cafeteria was unusually large for the middle of the week, so he had skipped the serving line, and was nursing a coke at a table in the darkest corner of the dining room. He expected Amy's arrival at any moment.

The fax had come as a result of his call to an old law school classmate of Annette's who worked at the FBI office in Manhattan. Jason had met the woman once at a class reunion and she had impressed him as intelligent and shrewd.

As Annette had once said, "Darling, when you see a woman who has men as peers in her workplace, you can be damned sure she's the brightest one in the shop."

Julia Watson had been one of only a few of Annette's old friends that Jason had called after her death. When she heard that information on Randall Smith's background was needed to investigate Annette's death, she had agreed to his request without asking any embarrassing questions. The information she had sent was succinct, but useful.

He felt a hand on his shoulder. It was Amy. She bent to kiss him on the cheek but he twisted away and waved her to a chair.

"Careful, sweetheart, this place is crawling with my patients and rumors spread like wildfire in this town."

"Well, I could just hike up my skirt and pretend that I was a prostitute and we were getting it on under the table. If president Clinton can get away with it, who's going to condemn you?"

In response, he grimaced and stuck out his tongue at her.

"Look at this. It's Smith's FBI sheet!"

She quietly perused the fax. '*Known associate of* ...'must appear here ten times, although I don't recognize any of the names."

"He has slimy friends, Amy. That's all we need to know, but look down at his own arrest record."

She read quietly, then blew her breath out between pursed lips.

"This guy's a slug... a *violent* slug."

"Yes. Four extortion arrests over ten years, but no convictions. Assault with a deadly weapon twice, also thrown out of court. And he was kicked off the police force in El Paso for use of excessive force *repeatedly*. What has he been doing since you started following him?"

"Nothing incriminating. Yesterday, he spent an hour inside the Dougherty County Medical Society office, but it was so small that I didn't go in..."

"He had to be checking out the docs in town. All of our curriculum vitae are kept there. Other than that, there is nothing much else of interest that he could access there," commented Jason.

"He has made about six trips to an insurance office over on Jackson near the hospital. Again, it was too small to follow him in, but I peeked in the window and he was in one of the back offices."

"Was the place called Williams and Williams?" he asked.

"Yes, I'm sure of it."

"They act as the primary agents for CHC's managed care product, 'CareDixie'. I'll bet that's where he does his faxing and phone calling from. Nothing would look out of the ordinary because they are in touch with CHC legitimately on a daily basis. What else?"

Amy consulted her agenda.

"Yesterday, he had lunch with Emily Tyson in the St. Luke's hospital cafeteria. I think she was a nurse."

"She's *the nurse* at St. Luke's. Nursing director in fact. I wonder what they were up to?"

"Don't know, but he gave her a large envelope, must have been 8 by 12 inches... Oh, and he spends a lot of time keeping track of you. I was two cars behind you three times yesterday. And, when you went to see Trang, he sat across the street until you came out. Made about four calls on his cell phone while he waited."

"Damn," said Jason grimacing. "I should have been more careful."

"That's about all I have. How'd your meeting go last night with Roger?"

"We actually played nine holes of golf and I enjoyed myself. He's keeping tabs on the other docs at TurnerWest who may be targeted by Mark. Roger's having lunch with Tim Watson tomorrow. He's our podiatrist and he's started scheduling outpatient surgery at Palm Grove. We think it's because he's been intimidated or bribed by Mark and Smith."

"Have you seen any of the other defectors besides Trang?" asked Amy.

"Yes, in fact, I've talked to them all and only Singh is being a dickhead and denying any contact or pressure. Says he *just changed his mind* and that's it. The others aren't that far gone, but I wouldn't want to see a vote on the merger yet because I really don't know everybody they've corrupted. We don't have another staff meeting until late next month because we drop the August meeting every year and Mark can't call an extraordinary session without my agreement."

"Well, what's next on the agenda," she asked.

He looked at his watch and then teased her. "Too bad you need to keep tailing Smith 'cause I have a little afternoon tryst arranged with a luscious blond over at the Ramada. We could have made it a ménage a trois... Ouch!" he winced as she kicked him firmly in the shin. "That hurt, Amy."

"I intended it to, Jason. Please, don't joke about stuff like that. I have silly fears that cause me enough anxiety without that."

"Sorry," he apologized, while rubbing his damaged shin. "You have my word... Listen Amy, leave Smith at seven p.m. no matter what he's doing and I'll meet you at your room."

"What if he's into something heavy at seven p.m.?"

"Use your discretion, but at least call me. I've still got your room key. I'll be waiting... Now, you leave first, I'll hang around a bit longer so we don't go out together."

CH032

Well before seven p.m. that evening, Jason was at Amy's suite. He was loaded down with bags of Styrofoam takeout containers and, not having eaten at lunch, he was famished. The food had come from the Fish Factory and smelled wonderful.

He heated two plates in the microwave, set the table with two candelabra he'd brought from his place, opened a bottle of Chianti and waited.

At eight o'clock, he took the food and put it in the small refrigerator in the kitchenette. He was worried and began walking the floor. At eight thirty he wrote a note to Amy asking her to call him on his cell phone should she return while he was out looking for her.

Before he left, he walked by Smith's room and put his ear to the door. Hearing nothing, he went to the lobby and used a house phone to ring the room. No answer.

Albany was not a large town but it was extensive enough to be frustrating to search. He went first to the offices of Williams and Williams and then covered both hospitals' parking lots looking for his Jeep before he began to cruise the main thoroughfare of the town.

By nine thirty, he knew his search was an exercise in futility and turned back toward the Ramada. About five minutes out, his phone rang. He grabbed for it with such force that he stubbed his thumb ferociously against the armrest trying to get it.

"Hello!" he fairly shouted.

"Jason?"

"Yes, Amy, where are you?"

"I'm at the room. I read your message... *and,* I smelled the food. I'm sorry darling."

"The food doesn't matter. Are you alright I was worried sick."

"I'm ok. Are you coming back?"

"As fast as I can."

"Slow down and drive carefully. I'm alright, I'm just going to have a shower," she said wearily.

"Something happened. Didn't it?" he pushed.

"Yes. Something went wrong but I'm alright and we'll talk about it when you get here."

Only about ten minutes later, Jason was at the suite door using his own key to get in. He could hear the shower sounds as soon as the door shut behind him and he went directly to the bathroom. He knocked, then went in and said hello.

"It's amazing how good a shower can make you feel" she called out almost cheerily.

Surveying the steam that filled the upper half of the room, he commented, "Are you sure that you're not scalding away your skin?"

"Sure I'm not what...?" she called back.

"Scalding away your skin," he repeated.

"*Scalding away my skin?...* Why would you say that?"

"Say what? I couldn't hear you very well," he said.

"Scalding away my skin..."

"Yes, that's what I asked."

"Yes. ...but why?"

"Why what?"…

"Why did you..." suddenly she broke off speaking and the door of the shower enclosure slid open. Amy stuck out her head.

"I've got to admit that I've seen some pretty convoluted schemes cooked up by men to get at naked women but this *talking gibberish* so that I have to invite you into my shower takes the cake."

He grinned broadly and fairly ripped off his clothes.

* * *

Amy was sitting on the floor in front of the sofa and Jason was toweling her hair dry. When he had used up all the absorptive capacity of the towel in his hand, he asked, "Got another towel?"

"Just the one around your waist... There is only supposed to be one person staying here you know and they really ration the towels."

"Well this couch has a wool weave to it and I'm not going to subject my bare bottom to the torture I've avoided since I stopped wearing wool knee socks thirty years ago in cub scouts."

"What on earth did you say?" she asked turning partially around trying to see his face.

"I said, I'm allergic to wool and I can't use *my* towel to finish your hair..."

"Oh, I thought you said something about 'cub scouts'."

" Not a word. It must be the echo in here," he joked, then added, "How about using the towel *you're* wearing?"

"Now, you want *my* towel," she said playfully.

"Want your hair dried?"

"Yes... but does that mean I have to put *my* bare bottom on this *wool* carpet?"

"Amy, the carpet is not wool... This is the *Ramada Inn*, not the *Inn on the Park,"* he scoffed sarcastically.

"Well, monsieur," she said standing up to face him with one hand on each end of her towel, "Voila!" and she yanked the towel open exposing herself to his view.

He'd been smiling impishly when she stood up but, when she pulled the towel open, his smile faded and he got up from the sofa and moved toward her.

"What's this Amy?" he asked with concern.

She was puzzled by his reaction. "It's my breast, silly man."

"No, I mean *these,"* he said and taking his index and first fingers he traced along two angry red gouges that went from the lower inner quadrant of her breast up past the inside of the nipple and almost to the top of her breast.

She looked down in surprise.

"Oh, I didn't know they were there. He hurt me when he grabbed my breast but I didn't think he left marks."

"Amy, when *who* grabbed your breast?" Jason asked gravely.

"That Smith guy."

"Is that what you had to tell me about when you said *something went wrong?"*

"Yes," she replied in a subdued voice and closed the towel. "I guess now's as good a time as ever."

"Take your time," he encouraged.

"It's pretty straight forward. I guess maybe Smith got wise to having the same Jeep behind him for two days straight. Anyway, he made me. I think it was because he drove out of the city to a little town south of here to some real foul smelling chicken plant. I tried to keep my distance on the highway without losing him but it's hard to tail someone when you don't have the distraction of other traffic.

"I know where he went but I'm not sure why," said Jason.

"Could he have been talking to the chicken people about his CareDixie insurance product. That's what I thought he was doing. There had to be a hundred cars in that parking lot. They have a lot of employees," Amy suggested.

"Yep, they sure do. They employ everybody in Mitchell County and a lot of the surrounding counties who have no more than an eighth grade education. Of course, you're right, it had to be about CareDixie." He said, pursing his lips and nodding his head to emphasize the correctness of her deduction.

"I watched where he parked and let him go inside for about ten minutes or so. Then, I sat off to the side at an outdoor lunch area with picnic tables waiting for him to come out. But he didn't and it was getting to be a quarter of seven."

"He was still inside when you got ready to leave?"

"I *thought* he was because I hadn't seen him come out but *he* must have been watching me. Anyway, when I got back to the Jeep I just crawled in. Did you know the automatic four-way locks don't work?"

"I didn't know that."

"Well they don't and Smith was in the vehicle. I guess he was hidden on the floor of the back seat. I didn't see him until he grabbed me. I'd clipped the seat belt and he just yanked it up and around my throat. If there were marks on my throat instead of my breast I wouldn't have been surprised. It seemed like he was intent on choking the life out of me."

"Did you say anything..." asked Jason.

"Not at that point, but I tried to scream. I'd been digging my nails into his arms but it did no good and he put a hand over my mouth. The filthy thing was as big as a catcher's mitt and covered my eyes too, blinding me. That's when he said something like 'If you want to live, bitch... no screaming!' Then he squeezed my face till I thought my eyes would pop out."

She worked her jaw, briefly massaging a spot midway between her chin and ear. "It still throbs."

"Did he have a weapon, Amy?"

"At the time, I was afraid he might have but, when I think about it now, I can account for both his hands so I don't think he did have a weapon except those monstrous hands of his which were weapons enough."

"How did you get away?" Jason could feel the bile rising in his throat as each detail of the incident stoked his anger.

"Don't you want to know what he asked me?"

"Yes, tell me, please."

"He wanted to know who I was and who I worked for..."

"I told him I was a reporter doing a story on the chicken plant and I begged him not to hurt me. But he saw through my ruse and told me I was lying. Then he asked me the same question again. That's when he ripped open my blouse and shoved his damn hand in to grab my breast. He told me he'd rip it off if I lied to him again."

"Then what happened?" Jason's voice was hoarse and his fists were clenched.

"The darndest thing. You'll have trouble believing it. I know I did and so did Smith. Right in the middle of his threats and squeezing there was a sudden blaring of a horn and a green Explorer with heavily tinted windows banged right into the back right corner of the Jeep and the person in the Explorer just kept leaning on the horn. Did you know that the seat belt release in the driver's seat sticks?"

"No, I didn't."

"Well, it does. Look at this" and when she held out her right hand Jason could see that the nails on her index and second fingers were trimmed short. "I broke them pushing on the seatbelt release. I thought it would never click off… It seemed like an eternity."

"Where was Smith?"

"He was still in the back seat, at this point, and he'd let go of me but the Explorer was burning rubber and literally *pushing the Jeep sideways.* I got loose and jumped out the driver's door and ran like hell for the factory. People were beginning to come out to see what was going on and a security guard was standing like a useless dork by the factory door just watching everything."

She shook her head in disgust before continuing.

"When I was safely away from the Jeep, I looked back. That fat turd Smith was running toward his car and the Explorer was literally following him as he ran, flashing its lights and blowing its horn. Smith screeched out of the lot on two wheels and the Explorer stopped blowing its horn and took off after him back in the direction of Albany. They were both really moving."

"You never saw the Explorer's driver?"

"Not a glimpse. I thought, at first, it might have been a woman worker who just happened by and saw him attack me but, when the Explorer pursued him and *I mean pursued* because it was so close behind Smith's car it looked like it was being towed, I had my doubts. A woman might have stayed inside her car to be safe and still scare him away but no woman would go after him. I believe it was a man in the Explorer. Maybe he didn't get out because he didn't want to be recognized."

Jason's face was livid by now but he forced himself to sit down and mull things through for a minute. Amy looked more worried by his reaction than by her adventure. Suddenly her face brightened.

"Oh, Jason. There is something else. I almost forgot," and she got up and moved to the counter by the entryway and picked up a large manila envelope which she handed to him.

He turned it over. In black ink marker and clumsy cursive lettering was scrawled, '*Jason*'.

"This was sticking out from under the Jeep's driver's seat when I got back in. I think I would have noticed it if it had been there before I left the Jeep at the chicken place because it was too large to fit unnoticed under the seat. I tried to slip it back under to see if it fit but it didn't."

Jason stared at the handwritten name for several seconds. Then he leaned forward over the coffee table and tore open the end and poured out the contents onto the table.

The envelope contained four enlarged photos of the same woman, two in a business suit and two in a nurse's uniform. They appeared to have been taken without her knowledge as she wasn't looking toward the camera in any of them. One had been snapped as she was leaving a hospital the name of which was clearly visible in letters graven into the stone sill above the door. Jason read aloud "Good Samaritan Hospital 1966".

"Do you know her, Jason?" asked Amy.

Jason looked puzzled and was searching the empty envelope for any further clues but there were none. He looked at the back of the photos but all he found was a date and three words scrawled in the same careless hand as the name on the envelope. The date was September 2nd '07. One week ago. The words were '*director of nursing.*'

"Her name is Jenny Watson and up until I left for St Lucia, she was Cal Mellows' nurse. I've been looking for her," said Jason.

"Was she the one who accused him of sexual harassment?"

"Yes, she's the one. She made the accusations in camera to Mark and then disappeared about the day after Cal had gone missing."

"What's the significance of all this, Jason and who sent you the pictures?"

"I'll know the answer at least to one of those questions as soon as I've done a computer search on hospitals named after the Good Samaritan. I'd bet money that this one is owned by CHC"

He slipped the photos back into the envelope and crossed to the bathroom where she could see him dressing through the partially open door. When he came out, he put his right foot on the edge of the bed, pulled up his pant leg and began putting on the ankle holster with his gun in it.

Amy was worried and it showed on her face. "Where are you going? It's too late to do anything more tonight."

He flashed a thin smile at her. "The Internet never sleeps, sweetheart."

"You know what I mean, Jason. Are you going after Smith?"

He didn't look up from tying his shoes. "I'm going to drop by and see if he's in his room if that's what you mean."

"Then let me come with you. I want to see his face," she lied.

"No, Amy. I'm going alone." There was an edge in his tone that should have warned her off but she was too afraid for him.

"You're not a cop or a gunman, Jason. What could you do to this criminal?"

"Well, since I *am* a physician, I guess I could take his medical history and do a physical exam," he replied mirthlessly.

"I didn't mean you were incompetent. I meant I'm afraid for you," she apologized, coming up to him and sliding her arms around his neck.

"I'll be fine, Amy. Please let me go. This little discussion is finished and I'll see you in the morning," he said emphatically and kissed her cheek when she turned her lips away from him.

When the door closed behind him, a flood of regret that she hadn't kissed him rushed over her.

CH033

Damned screwed up roads," cursed Randall Smith squinting at the map under the feeble yellow light of the inadequate bulb of the glove compartment of his rented car. It had quickly become dark after the incident in the processing plant parking lot and his dome light wasn't working.

That madman who had pursued him at breakneck speed for twenty minutes had nearly run him off the road twice. If they hadn't overtaken the Mitchell County Sheriff's vehicle on a side road, Smith knew he might be lying somewhere in a ditch, at this very moment, with shattered glass and bent metal around him. The Explorer had swung down the first cutoff they'd come to after encountering the police vehicle. Smith had stayed close to the cruiser for another fifteen minutes as it proceeded across the county until it finally stopped in the driveway of a double wide trailer and the officer got out.

Smith had continued on for more than a mile and now, he was lost on a back country dirt road in South Georgia where no roads went in predictable straight lines.

"Looks like a damn handful of red wrigglers crawled across this paper and made a map," he mumbled to himself.

After five minutes of fruitless searching for his position, he decided to backtrack in hopes of finding a blacktop road with a sign that had a name or a number on it. Once he knew where he was, he could use his cell phone to ask for directions even if he couldn't read the map.

He started the car and looked at the fuel gauge. Less than a quarter tank. He'd have to find that blacktop soon.

It was a cloudy night and the heavens were sealed. As Smith drove along dodging potholes and anticipating unmarked curves, his eyes began to sting with the effort of the constant vigilance on unknown roads. Ten minutes later, he came to a paved road but there were no identifying signs. It had to be county and not state maintained because the yellow dividing center stripes had been worn virtually away by years of rain, sun and tires.

Shutting off his headlights, he got out of the car and climbed puffing up onto its trunk. From that vantage point, he circumferentially scanned the clouds above the surrounding pines. In what he thought was a northerly direction, and off a little to the right, he was convinced he saw the lights of a fair-sized town or city reflected off the lowering clouds.

"Albany that way," he announced to himself, quite proud of his problem solving. He hummed as he drove along. His strategy proved to be sound and, after another ten minutes of driving, he came to a larger highway. Off in the distance, he could clearly see the clouds lit up over the city. Now, he just needed some gas, a good meal and a bed.

Tomorrow, he'd tell West about the girl tailing him and the madman in the SUV. They were supposed to meet at ten at Williams and Williams. There would be time enough to go through all of tonight's details. West might know who the woman was because he could describe her clearly. The guy in the Explorer would have to remain a mystery.

Although he was quite certain that he had completely lost the Explorer, Smith still surveyed the view in the rear mirror every few minutes and, each time a pair of high-set headlights approached, he felt the anxiety ants burrowing under his skin until the taillights disappeared. Once, a pick-up truck pulled onto the paved road from a side road and followed him until he hit US 19 north. He heaved a sigh of relief when the vehicle finally turned south.

At the first stop light off the freeway in Albany, Smith reached over and picked up the Berretta automatic he had hauled from his document case during the pursuit by the Explorer, and stuffed it back inside. Wouldn't do to have a cop pull along side him and accidentally notice the pistol lying in the seat.

Five uneventful minutes later, during which he continued feeling the ants each time he saw an Explorer, no matter what the color, he pulled into the parking lot of the Ramada. Cautiously, he drove completely around the building squeezing past the dumpster bins in the back to make a full circuit. He saw nothing to arouse his suspicions and he returned to his habitual parking spot. It was five minutes past ten. He'd have a shower and then order in a pizza as the hotel's restaurant was already closed.

The meeting at Cagle Foods had been worthwhile. The benefits manager had liked the medical insurance plan he'd laid out. And this was before he even suggested the kickback. The bribe offer had been indirect enough to deny if he were ever to be challenged. After the moment in the conversation where he'd mentioned that he had a well-equipped bass boat he needed '*to fire sale out*' to '*someone who will care for it with the same affection I've lavished on it in the short year that's she's been mine*', the manager had been all smiles. The guy had asked four or five overt questions about how the boat was outfitted and trailed.

The insurance business was lucrative. The four thousand covered lives at the Cagle processing plant at ten bucks a pop for commission was a helluva good contract and would allow him to pick up a good used boat for the manager and still do very well on the transaction.

Suddenly, he smiled and slapped the steering wheel almost in glee. What a goof he was! He had plenty of funds in the bribery account for the TurnerWest docs. He could easily dip into that for the boat and no one would ever know the difference. Well, it looked like a day that had turned to crap up until a few minutes ago, might just finish up not badly at all.

He got out of his car, document case in hand, and entered the hotel. Five minutes later, he unlocked the door of his room and turned on the lights. As he was setting the safety chain and dead bolt, something exploded in the back of his head. The lights in the entryway surged to flashbulb intensity and then suddenly went out, even before he slumped to the floor.

When Smith opened his eyes, the first thing he was aware of was the spot in the back of his head where the dynamite had gone off. Rhythmic, seismic surges of excruciating pain, timed to his heartbeat, caused him to cry out. The second thing he noticed was that he *couldn't cry out* because of the duct tape over his mouth. He couldn't reach up to pull it off either because both his arms and legs had been effectively taped, with multiple passes, to the arms and legs of the chair in which he was sitting. There were also several wraps of tape fastening his chest and thighs to the chair as well. He was very effectively secured.

As he slowly realized the peril of his predicament, he looked around him for his attacker but could see no one. The lancing pain in his head was blindingly fierce and he rocked his head from side to side seeking any measure of relief, no matter how small. However, he noted to his horror that even the agitation of these minimal efforts caused an increase in his respiration rate incompatible with the limited amount of air he could easily draw in and expel from his nostrils. A flash of pure panic twisted his gut as he experienced the paralyzing fear of partial asphyxia. He settled quietly and began to repeat, mantra-like, under his breath. "Calm and comfortable... calm and comfortable," till his lungs finally got the message.

He sat quietly for about five minutes assessing his situation and wondering where his assailant had gone. Suddenly, he heard a match striking somewhere behind him and the acrid smell of burning sulphur stung his flaring nostrils. He tried to turn his head but someone slapped sharply on the side of his head with an open hand.

A voice said, "Welcome back, Mr. Smith."

Then without warning, the man grabbed his hair firmly and shoved the burning match deep into the canal of the ear that was still ringing from the recent blow. The hot sharp stick, against the sensitive flesh of the inner canal, felt like a red-hot ice pick had been jabbed into his brain.

He became immediately nauseated and saliva began to pour copiously into his mouth. He swallowed repeatedly, attempting to stifle any gagging, knowing that if he retched into his taped mouth, he would strangle on his own vomit.

The voice came again. "Your ear is smoking, Mr. Smith... Don't you know that smoking in any orifice of your body is bad for your health?"

The voice stopped and, horrified, he heard a second match strike. He tried to turtle his neck into his chest but succeeded only in flexing it low upon his sternum.

"You can't get away, Mr. Smith... I can still get hold of your ear," and his assailant laughed briefly before continuing. "If you promise to play the game by the rules, which means no yelling or talking loudly, I'll unzip your mouth so we can have a meaningful exchange of information. Would you like that?"

Smith nodded his head vigorously.

"Very well, we'll begin by establishing clearly that *any* infraction of the rules will be punishable immediately by death... because the game is called '*life and death*'. From what I know of you, Randall, you've played the game before... but *you* were always the dealer. However, tonight, *I'm the dealer* and you're just a simple player. So let's get started."

A hand grabbed hold of the masking tape over the fat man's mouth and ripped it off in a single motion. Smith gasped deeply twice and then began coughing.

"Two minute time out for coughing, Mr. Smith and then we begin the game."

Smith stopped coughing and spat out a small piece of adhesive from the tape that had become sodden and stuck to his lip.

"Who are you?" he sputtered, "and what do you want?"

"Oops, I apologize. I forgot to tell you abut the rule that allows only *the dealer* to ask questions... *Players* only get to answer."

"If it's money you want..."

A match lit behind him and his hair was grabbed, his head bent back...

"No! No!.. Ok!... Ok! Whaddya want to know?... I'll tell you..." The terror in his voice was palpable.

"Nasty little old fat man, you've pissed yourself," came the voice. "Lucky this is your *own* room,"... and the man laughed again, this time more harshly.

Without warning, he jabbed the smoldering match against Smith's neck and the fat man startled, jerking his head sideways, and almost cried out.

"Whew! That was close, you almost shouted and that would have meant lights out..."

There was silence for several beats, then Smith heard a click and the man behind asked, "Who do you work for?"

"Milton Kleinberg, CEO for Cumberland Health Care."

"Do you take your orders directly from him?"

"Yes," Smith mumbled.

"Speak up! This is being recorded," snapped the voice in obvious irritation.

"Ok! Yes," he repeated more loudly.

"Who pays you and how?"

"I'm an insurance salesman for CareDixie and I draw a check each month from them... salary and commissions."

"Does CareDixie habitually offer kickbacks to employers who switch insurance to their services?"

"If it looks like a kickback will help, we offer one."

"Do you receive other remuneration from CHC?"

"I get occasional cash payments for special assignments."

"Like the one that brought you to Albany...?"

"Yes."

"What is your assignment here?"

"I told you, I sell insurance."

At that response, Smith heard a click as the tape recorder was switched off.

"What the ..."But he was cut off abruptly as the piece of tape which had been hanging off the side of his cheek was pulled tight again across his mouth. Two fingers pinched his nose and Smith began to make strangling sounds in his throat.

After only twenty seconds or so, the tape was ripped back off his mouth and his nose was released.

"A warning, Mr. Smith," and the voice rasped like fingernails on a blackboard. "*Do not toy with me.* I could kill you with about the same regret I experience stomping on a cockroach! We'll begin again."

The tape recorder clicked on again.

"What is your assignment here?"

"I'm supposed to subvert the resistance to the CHC takeover of TurnerWest..."

"What methods are you employing?"

"Bribery, blackmail, rumors..."

"By rumors you mean character assassination?"

"Yes."

"Extortion?..." the voice asked.

"Yes, extortion, too... *whatever it takes...*"

"Does that include kidnapping and murder?"

"No!" said Smith emphatically. "I never did anyone out here..."

"And elsewhere, Mr. Smith?... Remember I know a lot about you and the penalty for lying is...?" and he yanked on Smith's ear hard.

"Death... ouch!... death!" whimpered Smith.

"Well... elsewhere Mr. Smith?"

"I've been in this business a long time..." and he hesitated.

A hand took his ear and the voice asked gruffly, "And...?"

"Yes, I've had to kill someone... Nothing else was working..."

"How many people have you killed in the course of your employment at CHC?"

"Two."

"Did Kleinberg know about the murders *before* they happened?"

"Only one... The other was a spur of the moment thing... him or me."

"So, Kleinberg sanctioned the first murder."

"Yes. He agreed the guy had to go."

"Where did this happen and when?"

"Philadelphia... Last year in the summer sometime... maybe July."

"Did you kill Dr. Cal Mellows?"

The question was unexpected and Smith panicked.

"No, we went at him through his nurse and one of his patients... He got depressed or something and offed himself... You gotta believe me... I didn't lay so much as a finger on him!"

"Oh, you laid *a lot more than a finger* on him," spat the voice, "but I know *you* didn't kill him. It might have been better for you, if you had."

Then it continued, "Did Kleinberg know what happened to Mellows?"

"I gave him a full report."

"And he *still* ordered you to continue?"

"Yes, he was angry... Said the job was only halfway finished and behind schedule... He told us to get off our asses."

"*Us*, Mr. Smith... who is working with you on this assignment?"

"Mark West..."

"You mean Mark West, the VP of TurnerWest, the target organization?"

There was hesitation and a match flared.

"Yes... yes... Dr. Mark West..."

"What is his interest in all this?"

"We already greased his palm once and he'll get a lot more from the merger... and I think Kleinberg promised him something high up in CHC."

"So, West knows everything you've done...?"

"Yes. We planned it together..."

"Has he gotten his hands dirty, too...?"

"Yes, up to his eyeballs."

There was another click then the sound of a small hand held recorder rewinding.

"Are we done?" asked Smith.

"Oh dear, Mr. Smith!... No questions!... Remember?... You just broke the rules!" The voice was hard. Gravel in a sink.

"No! No!..." yelled Smith frantically, as the tape went back across his mouth.

He wriggled his whole body causing the chair to creak. His muffled cries could be easily heard through the tape.

"More tape needed..." came the voice now almost dispassionately, and the man behind Smith began to unwind the tape directly off the roll around the mouth and *up the face* of Randall Smith.

Air and blood-tinged mucous whistled from his nostrils and his eyes were jammed open in surprise and horror.

"One last trip around the old schnoze and I'm off, Mr. Smith. I thank you for your cooperation."

The hand moved more slowly, positioning the tape carefully, as he covered one ear and dipped down to draw the two-inch band over Smith's nose. Smith pivoted his head madly side to side, but to no avail. The tape passed over his nose... once, and the wheezing could still be heard between the constricting strips... twice... and the wheezing was much diminished ... Finally, with a firm pinch of the nose under the tape to close the gaps, *the wheezing stopped altogether.*

Smith bucked and struggled against his bands while his executioner wrote a short note clumsily with his left hand using a black marker on a newspaper lying on the table.

It read: *Mark West is next.*

CH034: CHICAGO, ILLINOIS

The street outside the Sears tower was jammed with vehicles, two deep, jostling for curb space like antelope at a desert watering hole. West's taxi driver stopped the cab and said something in a singsong voice that West couldn't decipher. West pushed a twenty-dollar bill at the man who beamed when he realized no change was expected and began unintelligibly babbling his thanks.

Inside the building, several large banks of elevators efficiently coughed out boluses of humanity that quickly disintegrated into individuals scurrying intently toward the exits or other elevators. West glanced at the information display and headed for the express elevators serving floors thirty-five to the top. CHC's corporate offices were on the seventy-second floor but Kleinberg had set their meeting for a private conference room on the seventy third.

He joined a group of people coalescing into a knot outside three of the express elevators. Like brokers watching the stock board, everyone craned his neck to follow the silent blinking race of the descending cars and, as it became apparent which would win, they shifted as one toward that door taking great care not to speak to, or even brush against their fellow passengers.

Once inside, they whooshed upward in silence, all eyes riveted on the floor display that spun like the dial on a gasoline pump until the first stop at the forty-second floor. By the time the elevator reached the seventy-third floor, West and two other men who acted as if they were totally alone, were the only passengers. He left them still staring at the floor indicator, mesmerized.

Outside, an oriental woman who had been standing across from the elevator approached him smiling efficiently, "Dr. West, I presume?"

"Yes."

"Please follow me, sir. Mr. Kleinberg is waiting for you."

As they approached an imposing dark oak door, she spoke over her shoulder, "Doctor, there is coffee and tea inside. Would you care for anything else?"

"No, thank you very much, coffee will be fine."

She had opened the door and Kleinberg, who had been seated at the far side of a round table reading from a sheaf of papers, got to his feet. His face was appropriately grim.

"Mark, how was your trip?" he said, gesturing with a wave of his hand to any one of the chairs around the table.

"Lots of time to think. We circled O'Hare for as long as it took to fly from Atlanta. Apparently inefficiency increases as the airline industry expands, but that was the least of my concerns, Milton," he replied as he pulled out a chair across from Kleinberg and sat down.

"I brought this to show you," and he fished a photocopy of the threat left on the table by Smith's murderer and slid it across to Kleinberg who studied it silently as West watched.

"I've had two death threats before in my career, both from disgruntled patients, but I knew who they were and I discounted them as hasty words spoken in anger. But this," he pointed to the sheet, "is different. It was found on the table next to Smith's body and the crazy who wrote it is a sadist... I saw *how* he killed Smith."

Kleinberg put down the sheet and picked up the papers he'd been reading. "I know. This is the police report. I was just re-reading it to see if I could gain anymore insight into what happened. What's your take on all this?"

"I know the medical examiner. He walked me through the salient points of the autopsy. Smith's lungs were filled with vomit and the M.E. thinks he asphyxiated over about four to six minutes. Apparently, he could still get a whiff of air in through the folds of the tape that covered his mouth and nose. Just enough to die scared crapless... and I mean that quite literally."

"Anything that might give us a clue about who did it?"

"I didn't like Smith, no sense pretending otherwise, but no one deserves to go out like he did," said West shaking his head. "The M.E. believes the sadism of the act means the killer *knew* Smith and hated him. He said there was vengeance written all over the murder. He thinks that's a pretty good indication it wasn't a professional hit."

"But there was no evidence left behind. The place was squeaky clean of even forensic clues if the police report is accurate. That doesn't sound like an amateur," said Kleinberg.

"Not a stupid or sloppy amateur, at least," added West. "We're definitely dealing with someone who knows how to cover his tracks."

"Smith had a way of irritating people. I know at least four or five guys from his past who could want him dead. Who do you think is behind it?" asked Kleinberg.

"I'm not sure. The fact that the killer obviously wants me as well, makes me think he's tied into our business with TurnerWest and what's happening in Albany. But the sadism doesn't fit anyone I can think of."

"Could Turner do something like this?"

Mark West pursed his lips and wagged his head before answering. "I doubt it. He hasn't got it in him. Whoever killed Smith tortured him with burning matches in the ear canal, according to the autopsy. Turner has a tough time even shooting quail. I've watched him deliberately miss after he'd shot fifteen birds, and he once told me that shooting any more than that was just waste, not sport."

"But we're not talking quail here, Mark. People get real bent out of shape when close friends or family get snuffed."

"What do you mean? Are you alluding to Mellows?"

"Yes," and Kleinberg hesitated purposefully before continuing, "and Turner's *wife* as well."

West blanched in spite of himself. "Why? Do you think she was murdered?"

"Don't you?" asked Kleinberg.

West had recovered his composure in a few short seconds. He shrugged his shoulders and answered, almost nonchalantly, "Maybe."

"If a man loved his wife and she's murdered, that could turn most of men into sadists."

"I still don't think Turner could do it... On the other hand, that hothead Mellows had a mean streak, if *he* were still around."

"Could he still be alive?" Kleinberg's eyebrows were raised. "They never found the body and we need to consider every possibility... By the way, I didn't give Smith the green light to eliminate him." He paused. "Did you have a hand in his disappearance?"

"If you mean did I have him killed, the answer is no. I was glad to see him gone, but I had nothing to do with his disappearance or death."

"But is that what Turner believes, Mark?"

West became suddenly reflective and his eyes rolled up toward his left temple as he accessed the memory images of Jason Turner during the incident in the restaurant. When he spoke, he was still pensive.

"Turner almost attacked me during a meeting in a restaurant about three weeks ago, just after he got back from the Caribbean. He was angry as hell and he was really spaced out... almost like he was having a seizure. He was bent out of shape about Mellows, but about a lot of other stuff, as well."

"Still think he isn't our man?... Has he got any history of violence?" asked Kleinberg.

West was shaking his head again.

"No... none that I know of... except," and his eyes were up accessing memory again, "once, he said something when we were at medical school, after his mother died and he was depressed. He'd been drinking, and he told me that he had recurring nightmares of pushing his old man down a flight of stairs and killing him when he was just a kid… His father died after a fall down a flight of stairs when Turner was about nine years old."

Kleinberg's eyes brightened and he leaned forward on the table. "If he killed his *own father*, he's got the seed for murder in him, and besides, *we* need a place to start."

"Start?" repeated West.

"Yes, we've got to act soon or everything in Albany goes down the tubes... and *we* go with it. Aren't you worried about your own safety?"

West leaned back and held open his jacket far enough for Kleinberg to see the butt of a nine millimeter pistol. "Of course. And I've had someone watching my back in Albany since the morning they found Smith," he replied.

"Well," rejoined Kleinberg, "much as I detest extreme solutions, I'm about convinced that Turner has to go, but I'm not going to put my neck on the block without you beside me, Mark."

West was thoughtful and he sucked in his lip bottom as he contemplated an answer. "I guess, there's no other way... but," and he paused for emphasis, "I'm not prepared to do it myself. That would just be stupid."

"I agree," said Kleinberg, "and I wasn't suggesting that. I have contacts but we'll need your help."

"How?"

"We need to make this look like an accident. Give that some thought to that and get back to me as soon as you think you have an angle."

"And in the meantime, you'll replace Smith?" asked West.

Kleinberg smiled. "Smith was never alone. We've had someone else there, off and on, but he'll stay put from now on. I'm sending a second man as well. I'll have him contact you as soon as you get back to Albany."

West felt a hiccup of irritation when he realized that Kleinberg had kept him out of the loop on Smith's accomplice but he felt it would be unwise to show his displeasure right now. "Alright, Milton... I hope the new guy has more on the ball than Smith did. I want someone competent between me and the madman who killed Smith."

"You'll like my choice, Mark. Trust me," said Kleinberg, as he stood up from the table and headed to a silver decanter sitting beside some cups on a tray.

"Coffee?"

CH035

Overnight there had been an energetic thunderstorm and the waters of the Flint roiled with the aftereffects. Never clear, the river's effluent was now so laden with silty runoff that the consistency of the swirling eddies near shore seemed as thick as cake batter. Branches and leaves flecked the surface and, further out into midstream, the carcass of a large brown dog rolled and dipped along the curls of the central current.

Among the straggling clouds limping off to the west after the storm, a pale sun made tentative forays, feebly attempting to reassert control over the heavens.

The slope they had chosen for their picnic site was steep enough that little of the night's rain had seeped into the thick grass covering it and, the blanket they'd spread had only the occasional damp patch showing through. It wasn't exactly the romantic scene Jason had imagined the previous day when he'd arranged to be with Amy on his afternoon off.

She'd been very withdrawn and distant for the past week, and he had planned to use the time to reconnect with her in the catalyzing presence of nature's beauty. Twice in the past three days, she'd made excuses after dinner and retired early, and alone, to her suite at the Ramada. He hadn't pushed, remembering what she'd said about how difficult it was for her to open up and remain open. But he was worried.

He'd been back working with his patients at the clinic since Monday and had been reassured to discover that the vault doors of his memory banks, which had been bolted shut by depression, were now fully open. He was back into a familiar routine at the office but nothing seemed to be going well elsewhere.

He'd also spoken regularly with the children, who hadn't asked to come home but who had pleaded for him to come to Detroit. They'd agreed that he would fly up on the weekend.

He knew that he would have to tell them about Amy and he worried about their reaction. In short, pressures were building on several fronts and he'd hoped to simplify things today by resolving Amy's obvious malaise, if possible.

Jason was under no illusion as to the cause of Amy's distress. He'd been there at her suite the morning that Smith's body was found and he'd used his influence with the EMS crew and the police to gain access to the crime scene. He'd spoken with the coroner who had been present, and learned that the time of death was estimated to be between ten and midnight, the night before.

When he'd returned to find Amy standing outside Smith's room, he'd been shocked by the transformation that had come over her. It was as if a door had been closed behind her eyes and something essential shut off. He'd tried to initiate conversation, speculate on what he'd seen and been told, but it was like she had drifted away inside herself.

Ever since, although her voice was the same and she even smiled at the jokes he attempted, the spontaneous touching, the liveliness, and the spiritual connection they'd had between them had been severed... turned off, as if a switch had been pulled.

The alienation he felt was experienced as physical discomfort, a heaviness and aching in his chest that he'd felt before, although much more severely, at the death of his mother and Annette. He recognized the symptoms as harbingers of worse things to come and, hence, had made the hasty arrangements to be with her today before more time passed and their relationship deteriorated even further.

They'd packed sandwiches and champagne, but the basket sat beside them on the blanket, unopened. Amy was wearing a brightly patterned yellow sundress and had tied a ribbon in her hair, so he knew she was trying to contribute positively to the moment. She was sitting below him on the slope, leaning back against his belly, her hair fragrant and billowing upon his chest. He had his arms around her shoulders and his face was buried in her hair.

"You smell so good, sweetheart," he said. "I'm sorry that the weather is so contrary."

"Maybe it isn't, Jason. Did you ever think that perhaps *we* bring on the weather as a reflection of our internal environment? I used to think that as a child. Storms, as frightening as they were, weren't awful things for me, just externalizations of what I was experiencing inside." Her voice was lackluster, and though he waited for her to continue on, she didn't.

"Is that what you're feeling inside now, Amy?" he asked, hesitantly. "Stormy, you mean?" she asked.

"Yes."

"No. Not at all... *after the storm*."

"What, like right now... like here?" he asked.

"Yes, like here and now... no storm, *but* no sun. Transition."

"That could be good," he offered, "... No sun *yet*, but fighting through the clouds?" and he pointed to the confused sky.

"An optimist's interpretation, Jason... Things could go the other way, you know. Those distant thunderheads could suddenly wheel around and turn on us again. *That* scenario would be more in keeping with my experience of life." She sighed audibly.

"Tell me more about your feelings, darling. I want to understand what's come over you." His tone was imploring, but hopeful.

There was a long pause and he wondered if she were retreating further inside herself. A clock began ticking inside his mind. Anticipation. Explosion or release of tension.

She raised one of her hands, which had been lying in her lap, and placed it gently upon his forearm. He sighed in relief, and the clock stopped ticking, although she still remained silent for yet another moment.

"Smith," she said simply.

He waited, but she didn't say anything more.

"I don't understand, Amy."

"Smith and death... the horror of reality. The world and all its ugliness crashing in on us. It's like the craziness of my life is starting all over again. I'm in the middle of conflict I'd rather flee. Conflict that I thought, at least partially, I'd escaped... But it comes bubbling back up like a plugged toilet. People trying to hurt us and people dying."

"He was an evil man, Amy. Evil people come to evil ends." He'd been trying to sound matter of fact about Smith.

"Don't you believe *we all* have some evil in us, Jason?... Maybe that's why we can never seem to get away from it for long. We draw it to us, just like the storms."

As she spoke, she turned her face sideways to look up at him and he sensed that this was a loaded question. He was full of trepidation and would have chosen to ignore a response but he had to keep her talking. "Do you mean '*we*' as in *you* and *me?*" he asked, almost timidly.

She sat up and turned around to face him, kneeling between his legs and looking up directly into his eyes. Her eyes were no longer hooded, there was a hopeful connection reestablished. But there was also something challenging, almost aggressive about what he saw there. "Exactly, Jason, *you and me*... Is there evil in us? Deep down, or at the surface, hidden or overt... Do we have evil in us... *innately* in us?"

He couldn't match the intensity of her gaze and dropped his eyes while he pondered. When he spoke, he asked a question. "I'm not trying to be simplistic or evasive, Amy, but what do you mean by *evil*?"

"Evil like Smith, Jason. You called him evil... He's a liar, he's violent, he hurts people..." and she paused, "Maybe he's even killed... Are we like him in any way?" She was studying his face as she spoke, cornering his gaze, corralling the evasive movements of his eyes with her own eyes.

He shrugged, and she reached up to hold him by both upper arms in an attempt at preventing him from turning his face away.

"What about *me*, Jason... *What if I were capable of killing someone*? How would you feel about me?"

"Killing, isn't necessarily evil, Amy."

"Isn't it, Jason? Just how is becoming so angry that you could take another person's life, not evil?"

"I truly don't know," he replied simply, no longer seeking to evade her inquisitional stare.

She shrugged, let her hands fall from his arms and broke gaze with him by looking past him... past the edge of the earth and out into space itself. "I think killing in anger is evil. I've tried to rationalize it away, deny it... but in the end, I'm quite certain that *it is indeed evil*."

She stopped speaking and continued to stare into space.

"Then", said Jason quietly, "I guess we all have the capacity for becoming evil within us... At least, I know that *I* have it."

Her question, although she continued looking away, skewered him with its directness. "Did you kill Smith, Jason?"

He was shocked and it showed in his voice. "Is that what all this distress is about, Amy? Whether I killed that scumbag or not? ..." Then, without waiting for her response, he said emphatically, "No, I wanted to, but I didn't kill him."

And he took her by the arms to pull her back from her detachment and force her to engage with him again.

She met his eyes and there was no surprise in her gaze. "No, it's not really about that. I was sure you hadn't, but I did need to hear you say it. Smith was a piece of garbage and I don't regret the fact that he's dead... In fact, I'm a little relieved after what happened the other night."

"Then *why* would you ask me that?" queried Jason, with true perplexity showing on his face.

"Because, if you *had killed him*, although I could have understood your motives, it would have forced me to revise my impression of you... of us... of the overall balance of good and evil that exists in our couple."

"How's that?"

"Well, frankly, I see you as a reservoir of *goodness*... call it righteousness, humanity... it can have a hundred names... in our couple. You sort of cancel out *my own evil.* You bring balance to our unit. Ying and yang, I suppose, in some macabre calculation. Does it sound that crazy?"

She seemed anxious that he understand.

He hesitated before answering with a question of his own, "*Are you saying that you're evil?*"

"Using my own definition of evil, meaning that I am capable of killing in anger?" she asked.

"Sure... ok," he answered.

Her response was matter of fact, devoid of intense emotion, but sober.

"Yes... I *know* I could kill in anger," but despite the lack of emotion, her gaze drifted away again from him, defocusing on anything external, as if she were fixing upon images hidden within her mind.

There was a long pause before he spoke. "Have you killed someone, Amy?" His voice was pregnant with apprehension.

Suddenly, she turned to look right at him again, as if she'd just come running up to him from a distance, and she smiled.

"No, Jason, I'm not a murderer... but I know that there is something, *someone* I should say, hiding deep inside me who could kill and do it without remorse under the right circumstances. I've met her. She's real and, though I'm not comfortable with her presence within me, I'm realistic about her existence."

Jason sighed audibly and Amy, who had been studying his face closely, unexpectedly laughed. "No, I'm not the black widow or the devil's agent, but I carry around my share... more than my share of evil. Believe me. And I'm not proud of it."

He said nothing, but he was looking at her with relief written all over his face.

"You know, Jason. I'd swear... and it really means a lot to me, that you just heard me tell you my foulest secret about myself, and yet, you *actually look relieved*!"

"Oh, I am. You wouldn't believe *how relieved* I am," Jason fairly gushed.

"Why, this is wonderful, you big goof..."

Her face was suddenly transformed, emptied of all the strain he'd seen, just moments before. She pushed him back upon the blanket and fairly climbed up onto him, burying her face in his chest, her arms pulling him into her with all her strength.

He stroked her hair and they lay in silence for what seemed like an eternity, before she finally spoke. "If you only knew how much I feared telling you that about me, Jason. I really thought it might be the secret I'd have to *finally* divulge to you on the night of our fiftieth wedding anniversary."

"*Anniversary?*" he echoed. "Were you planning on proposing to me?" he asked with amusement clearly evident in his voice.

She looked up at him, bright-eyed now, and full of impish glee.

"Of course, you big goof... I've slept with you *already*. I consider us *more than engaged*. The only reason I haven't proposed is because I didn't want to steal your male thunder, emasculate you, or whatever locker room term you men use to describe the actions of aggressive women."

"'*Bust my balls*', you mean?"

"I'm not up on the jargon," she chided.

He put his arms under hers and pulled her up fully onto him and kissed her passionately. As she lay upon him, looking into his eyes and toying with a lock of his hair which she curled, and then uncurled where it lay on his forehead, she said in a little girl's voice, "I have another secret I'd like to share, Jason."

"What is it?" and his brow furrowed a little, quizzically.

"I'm starved... I haven't had an appetite for four days, and now, I feel like I could eat a horse."

"Well, keep watching the river. We've already had a dog float past, the horse can't be far behind."

She yanked on his hair and he yelled, and they rolled over together both struggling to be the first to get at the sandwiches in the basket.

* * *

They had eaten and made love, oblivious of their exposed position on the hillside, although a few disinterested cattle in a nearby field were the only possible voyeurs. The sun had finally triumphed over the clouds, and the air was heating up until it was almost too hot to stay lying unprotected from its rays on the blanket.

"Let's go to my place and get in the pool," Jason proposed.

She had been tracing the features of his face with a wisp of grass and lingered with it on his lips, as he spoke.

"Not yet, Jason. The house is still Annette's and I'm not ready for that. We'll go to the pool at the Ramada... I'd like that."

He reached up with one hand and smoothed back a lock of her hair from her face, as he asked earnestly. "Look me in the eye then, darling, because I want you to promise me something important."

"Ok," she said and squared her face up directly over his with their eyes locked.

"Promise me that you'll give the house a try when we get back from St. Lucia, next month."

She looked frankly puzzled, and repeated "*Back from St. Lucia, next month?* Why would we be going to St. Lucia, Jason?"

"Why to get married, of course, darling."

Confusion churned through her eyes for an instant, and then they cleared and fairly glittered, as tears began to well up from the joy she felt rushing outward from her heart.

"Oh, Jason..."

CH036

Jason lay alone in his bed. The sliding doors to the patio were open and birds that hadn't yet begun to sing were already flitting about in the shadows of the morning. Crickets rasped their chirping calls from a dozen crevasses outside and one of their kind answered from the corner of the bedroom.

The ceiling of the room was alive with swatches of shifting shadows that his imagination had been morphing into scenes from the past all night long. He'd spoken to Annette in husky tear-sodden tones, replayed the mental tapes of St. Lucia with Amy, studied and restudied the faces of his children and reflected upon his dependency on women.

Jason had always felt that he was not quite like other men. He had been marked indelibly by his childhood bonding to his mother …both marked *and maimed.* Other men grew up and left their mothers, gradually tying off, one by one, the arteries of the emotional vasculature linking them to their maternal origins. In place of these ties, adult to adult bonds, much less intense than the mother-child transfusions of feelings, developed naturally during the son's maturation. And, eventually, the process of growth emancipated the child while guaranteeing an attenuated but adequate attachment between mother and son.

But it had not been that way for him and, because it hadn't, his relationships with his wife and children had been tainted.

Mysteriously, there had been no healthy closure to his dependency upon his mother. Even her death had not freed him from his need for her. And when he'd attached to Annette after his mother's death, it had been with a neurotic limpet-like clasp of desperation driven by the need to rediscover his wholeness in the bond with a woman.

As a result of the strength of his attachment to her, when the children had been born, they'd been much more hers than his. His ties to them had been more fraternal than paternal, more sibling than sire. Like electrons jostling in the magnetic field of the mother-wife, they clustered alongside him. He had related to the kids largely *through her.*

However, this fact implied no measure of indifference toward his children. His attachment to them was profound, far surpassing anything he experienced outside the family, but it paled in comparison to the intensity that bound him to the woman who was their mother.

And now she was gone. With the nucleus destroyed, her satellites orbited aimlessly about a void unable to find sufficient attraction in their sameness to recreate even an imitation of a family. He was neither father nor independent male and he was failing both his children because of it.

As he thought about it, he realized that he would feel somewhat better about his flaw if it were shared with all his gender rather than being simply a solitary burden. Was it this way for other men? He knew the morbid statistics about widowers dying within the year following their spouses' deaths.

In his medical practice, he'd watched old men, as desperate as asthmatics struggling for breath, frantically searching for partners to replace their dead wives. As elderly parents, these men couldn't be satisfied just living with their grown children or grandchildren as widows did. Long past the age of sexual activity, they still needed a woman and, without one, *they simply died.*

And he was convinced that he would have died too, if he had not found Amy.

She had given him the binding site he needed to reattach and survive. Her love had been enough to pull him back from the brink of dissolution. She had not displaced Annette in his life but had simply moved into the vacuum created by her death. Amy was now where Annette had been without anyone trying consciously to replace his dead wife.

But while this was true for him, how could it ever be true for his children? In his love for Amy would they see him as betraying Annette or betraying them? Would they reject Amy out of loyalty to their dead mother? Would they force him to face an impossible choice?

He had proposed to Amy yesterday in an act of uncharacteristic impetuosity, but now, he needed to tell the children of his decision. However, the prospect of doing so filled him with profound apprehension. Telling them what he'd done was not just a duty but an obligation he owed them and yet, despite the benefit of a night's reflection and hours of rehearsal, he lay uneasily on the spikes of a piercing awareness that he didn't know how to even approach the topic with them. He'd been prepared to talk to them *about* Amy, but marriage to her was an entirely different thing.

Jason knew that a child's heart has nothing in common with a boat dock where fathers and mothers tie up temporarily and then pull away to be replaced by the next arrival. His own experience of childhood had taught him that maternal bonds were immutable attachments that transcended even death. Yet, in some undeniable manner, the woman married to a father or the man married to a mother *became* a parent in spite of a child's wishes. And so, his choice of Amy was a choice he was making for Michael and Caroline as well and, as yet, they knew nothing of it.

Regrettably, because yesterday's proposal was a fait accompli, there was no time or opportunity to allow them to warm up to her, the way he had hoped they would, before the marriage. How could it not seem to them that the arbitrary fact of their mother's death was being followed so quickly by his dictatorial announcement of her replacement by a stranger?

He shuddered as the thoughts formed in his mind.

He had no answers and the nocturnal pleas he'd addressed to Annette had borne no fruit. He was trapped within the confines of a dilemma that encased him, body and soul, like an emotional sarcophagus. A shot of terrible sympathy for his children swept through him and hot tears of shame and betrayal burned his cheeks. He felt utterly lost.

Then, to his amazement, in the midst of his despair and sadness, he heard Annette's voice so clearly that he turned his head toward her accustomed resting place beside him on the pillows, fully expecting to see her lying there breathtakingly beautiful.

"*Use the tapes I made for the children...*"

He was as surprised at the emptiness of the bed as he had been by the sound of her voice.

From the open doors, the indigo tones of dawn diffused softly into the room and the cadence of the moment gave him the permission to accept the gift without understanding how it came to him.

* * *

"Michael, I'll be there tomorrow at noon and you and Caroline are to meet me at the yacht club pier. Grandma knows all about it."

"Are you coming to stay with us, dad?" The child's enthusiasm literally bubbled through the phone line.

"No, son. In fact, I have to leave the next morning because of business problems down here but we'll have a good time. I promise you. You'll be staying at the hotel with me. The one with the waterslide that you liked."

"Will you go down it this time, dad? You chickened out last time."

"I'll go down it, Mikey... as many times as you want... Now, please put your sister on. I love you."

"Me too, dad. Here she is."

Caroline's voice lacked the excitement that had infected Michael's tone. He sensed her reserve as soon as she said 'hello' and imagined the look of sober anticipation on her face. She was old enough to appreciate the gravity of circumstances that separated parents from children and Jason worried that perhaps her grandfather had hinted at the custody proceedings despite the agreement with his lawyer.

"How are you darling? I miss you so much."

"Me too, daddy. I'm fine, I guess," she replied hesitantly.

"I guess?" he parroted back.

"Well, I love grandma and we have a lot of fun together, but I still miss mom so much that my stomach aches when I think of her... and I miss you, too."

Jason bit his lower lip fiercely to hold back the tide of emotion that was lapping at the seawall of his composure. "Me too, sweetheart. I spent the whole night, pretty much thinking about you kids and her. I even spoke to her and asked for help with my problems."

"Are you cured now, dad... the depression, I mean?"

"Maybe not cured, darling, but well on the way to it. I'm back at work and handling things much better than I did."

"Then what are the problems you told mom about?"

"Lots of stuff, kiddo. Not the kind of things we need to get into over the phone but I'll tell you all about it tomorrow when we're together. I'm really anxious to see you guys. You don't know how much I've missed you."

"Wanna bet? It couldn't be more than we missed you, daddy." Her tone of voice had lightened considerably and he breathed a heavy sigh of relief.

"Darling, do you know how good it makes me feel to hear you say that? I was pretty lousy company for a long time before I went to St. Lucia and I'm so sorry for that." An accent of emotion, soft and deep within his throat, almost betrayed itself as a quaver in his voice.

"What was it mom used to say, daddy 'what's past is done'?"

He smiled in pleasant recollection, "I remember her saying that often, kitten."

"Well, 'what's past is done', daddy. We get a new start tomorrow."

"Yes, darling, a new start"... he echoed.

"What did she answer you, dad?"

"Who, mom?"

"Yes, you said you talked with her last night."

He paused uncertain of the words he should use to describe what had happened, or if he should tell his daughter anything at all about his continuing relationship with her dead mother. When he spoke, he stuttered initially as if his thoughts were stumbling about in his mind. "Yes, y...yes, darling, she did answer me."

The line remained silent.

"She spoke very clearly and told me what I should do," he continued.

"Did you *see* her, daddy?"

Her voice seemed to be curling tightly around a nucleus of expectation so dense it couldn't be hefted.

He hesitated momentarily, then decided upon the unvarnished truth. "Not this time, Caroline, but I *have* seen her ... several times. In fact, so often that, for me, in some ways, she's still with us."

"Me too, daddy." She spoke almost reverently, all the tension gone from her voice, as if they were now initiates sharing a sacred experience that could at last be spoken of aloud. "I've seen her too, and she's talked with me."

He said nothing and each of them simply listened to the breathing of the other hundreds of miles away.

Caroline spoke first.

"I saw her first the night she died. She just came and stood at the foot of my bed and told me she was all right. Then, since that time, when I feel like my heart is going to explode with missing her, she sometimes comes back again in the night and we talk. Once, she even played with my hair like she used to do when I couldn't sleep."

"Oh, Caroline," was all Jason could manage as tears flushed his eyes and his heart and throat constricted with emotion.

* * *

On a guano-stained railing post, a large gull with two of its three toes missing from one foot cocked its head against the blue of the sky and begged scraps from the table of nearby diners.

Jason sat nervously on the edge of a bench located on the elevated restaurant patio that overlooked the main dock of the Grosse Pointe yacht club. He'd arrived a little early to assure that the kids would not have to wait for him.

His palms were perspiring despite the freshening breeze that tousled his hair. He wiped them anxiously against the blue sailing shorts he wore and scanned the parking area for the arrival of the limousine. When it entered the lot in a lazy wide turn he was already up and bouncing down the steps leading to the unloading zone. He was waiting when it pulled up and stopped.

The rear door nearest him opened and a young muscular man in his mid twenties had just put one foot on the ground when Michael came spilling across the man's lap diving headfirst out the door yelling, "Dad."

Jason rushed to the vehicle and caught his son as the boy tumbled out and into his arms. Two arms squeezed his neck in a frenzied welcome and Jason turned in small circles of joy holding his son to him and repeating simply 'Michael', over and over again.

"Here, let me see you boy," he finally said setting the child down at arm's length and examining him while the boy beamed.

"You've grown another foot since I saw you last!" he exclaimed.

For an instant the boy looked puzzled and glanced down at his feet. "Nope, dad. Still just two, but it was a good joke. I almost believed you."

They both laughed.

The young man was out of the limo and had gone to the other side to open the door for Caroline. Michael grabbed hold of his father's hand and began pulling him around the rear of the automobile.

"C'mon dad, Caroline's over here with Tom."

They arrived at the opposite side of the vehicle just as Caroline stepped out and stood up. She was wearing a spaghetti strap sundress and her bronze tresses fell casually upon bare shoulders. Jason saw she was wearing lipstick, light make-up and an expensive cameo choker which he recognized, with a twinge, must have been chosen from her mother's jewelry that he had given to her as per the specifics of Annette's will.

She was exquisite and he stopped short of sweeping her into his arms, pausing first to appraise her head to foot before emitting a facetious low-pitched 'wolf whistle'.

She blushed violently.

"Oh, daddy, you're still just as big a dork as ever," she said as she held out her arms to him but he could tell she was flattered by his appraisal of her as a full-grown woman.

They hugged each other each in silence for a moment and then he felt her hand rise to the back of his neck and stroke his hair the way she had seen her mother do in so many past embraces.

"Oh, Caroline," he sighed and squeezed her more tightly to emphasis his joy at seeing her.

When they stepped back from each other, he saw her quickly dab at her eye to blot away a tear. She was wearing white gloves. Grandma McLean's touch.

Michael grabbed his father's hand again and began to pull him toward the dock area. "C'mon, dad. All the good jet skis will be gone if we don't hurry up."

"Michael, you're forgetting your manners," upbraided Caroline. "Daddy hasn't even met Tom yet and you're already running off."

"Oh," said Michael, slowing down only momentarily. "Dad, that's Tom. He goes everywhere we go. He says he's not a babysitter but he really is."

The introduction finished, Michael was straining at his father's arm leaning his whole body weight into the task of directing him toward the dock.

Pulling against the boy, Jason addressed the bodyguard over his shoulder. "Tom, nice to meet you."

The bodyguard simply smiled and touched a hand to his forehead in an informal salute.

At the small watercraft dock a dozen jet skis bobbed about on their tethers. Each bore a registration number in blue decals and a red unit number just above it. Michael had already scrambled to the line holding a macho machine boasting 'Turbo' in streamlined lettering on the hood which was painted in a motif of windswept flames licking back toward the driver's seat.

"This one's mine, dad. I saw it racing yesterday on TV. I know I could drive it real good!"

The boy was obviously shooting high, knowing in advance that his ploy wouldn't succeed.

Jason decided to let reality rein in his son's ambition. "Well, just take your driver's license to the registration window over there," he said gesturing to the end of the dock, "and tell the man which machine you've chosen."

Michael looked quizzically at his father then said, "You know I don't have a driver's license yet dad. Can't you rent it, *then* I'll drive it?"

"Mikey, it's a one man machine and I'm afraid either Tom will have to use that one or we'll all four of us go on the two-seaters."

"Two-seaters, dad? They're for little kids and old ladies like grandma!" he protested.

Caroline interjected, "How do you think grandma will feel about you calling her an 'old lady'?"

"Well, she *is* old... and besides she's not here and won't know what I said unless you tattle again," Michael riposted.

"Wrong again," said Caroline, her eyes sparkling mischievously. "Tom tells her everything. Right, Tom? That's how she knows things… Not from me."

Tom shrugged his shoulders non-committally, having already learned the folly of getting caught up in the sibling wrangles of his charges.

Jason interrupted, "Mikey, there are several two-seaters over there. Make your choice from among them."

"Aw, dad," whined the boy as he slouched toward the plainer jet skis without the dashing multicolor motifs.

"Caroline, you can either ride with Tom or drive your own machine. What'll it be?" asked Jason.

Caroline's face flushed crimson and she approached her father, lowered her chin and spoke softly enough that Tom couldn't overhear. "Dad, what'd you say that for? I'd have to hold onto him and everything..." and her voice trailed off in embarrassment.

"Sorry sweetheart, I meant," and he deliberately spoke loud enough for Tom to hear, "Do you want to drive your own machine or ride with me?"

She smiled and took his arm, sliding her free arm around his waist. "I'll ride with you, dad."

"What about me? I don't want to ride with Tom either," protested Michael.

Tom, who had sidled up to the macho machine and was pulling it closer to the dock against the tension of its rear anchor line, spoke up. "Mr. Turner, there's enough room on this model for *two* if one person is small."

Michael dropped the line of one of the tamer machines he'd been pulling in and spurted in a dash toward Tom shouting. "Hey, I'm small enough. I can either sit in the back or the front."

"Your choice, Mikey, ride with me or with Tom," said Jason.

"Tom's ok. I'll ride with him," the boy volunteered brightly.

"Well, then let's choose our wetsuits and get on with things," said Jason heading in the direction of the registration window and a rack of wetsuits hanging along a wall.

Caroline still clung to his arm.

The afternoon was spent in an effervescence of shouts and mad dashes across the water on the jet skis. Michael and Tom literally ran circles around Jason and Caroline who feigned frustration at their own lack of speed in order to heighten Michael's enjoyment.

Towards the end of the afternoon, Jason and Caroline took a leisurely five mile ride alone along the shore which was fronted by luxurious homes with lawns and tennis courts facing the lake.

Michael and Tom had disappeared in a froth of white water accepting a challenge to race with two other machines that had zipped into an informal starting line with them and then tossed down the gauntlet with a series of surging roars that set the jet skis on their tails momentarily.

Caroline had laced her arms under her father's and placed her palms against the front of his shoulders while she lay her face against his back. Without the interference of noisy engines, they spoke freely of their feelings and, protected from having to see her face when he spoke, Jason even talked to her of Amy and how they had met.

She missed nothing and interrupted him in the midst of his enumeration of Amy's qualities. "Do you love this Amy, dad?"

He was taken aback and his hand relaxed on the throttle precipitously. The craft which had been plowing easily through the water, suddenly wallowed for an instant before he regained his composure and edged the throttle forward again.

"Why do you ask that, darling?" he evaded.

"'Cause you talk about her like you do, dad."

Jason winced, even her direct-to-the-point manner was like her mother. However, she still snuggled against his back reassuringly and he decided to venture part of the shocking truth.

"Yes, I think I might love her, Caroline."

There was a long pause during which his anxious thoughts spun frenetically like the flywheel of a clutch disengaged from its gears.

Finally, she spoke, but didn't pull away from his back, "You *think* you *might* love her?"

He laughed uneasily. "I guess I do love her, darling."

"*Guess* you love her?"

"No, I'm not guessing. I *know* I love her."

He felt his daughter move her face away from his back and the cool air that fell into the gap between them suddenly felt like a frigid blast that immediately sent a chill deep into his bones. He almost gasped at the sensation. He shuddered quickly, briefly and knew that she could not have missed feeling or seeing it.

Her voice seemed to come from far away. "And mom?... What about her, daddy?"

He had to clear his throat before he could answer.

"Darling, I love your mother still. There are times when she fills my heart so profusely that I feel my love for her spilling into every corner of my body and mind. She owns my soul and I have wanted literally to die to be with her again."

He paused.

"So what can you give this Amy if you still love mom so much?" she asked.

"I'm not sure. We're still working it out. There're some things about Amy that are so much like your mother that I sometimes get them confused."

"*I* could *never* do that, dad."

"I wouldn't expect you to, Caroline and I'm not sure you could understand what I'm experiencing."

"I know I could never have *two* mothers."

"I can understand that..."

"But *you* could have *two* wives?"

"Not exactly... It's hard to explain."

"Remember what mom used to tell me, 'Just say it like it is, Caroline, and I'll probably figure it out'... That's good advice, dad."

"Yes, it is, sweetheart. So here it is: *I love them both and one is not replacing the other.*"

"But mom is still first, right?"

"Yes, your mother is, and always will be, my first love. That will never change."

"Promise, dad."

"Cross my heart, darling."

He felt her settle herself back against him, and the chill he had been feeling dissipated instantly.

"Then, I guess if this Amy chick is satisfied with second best, that's her business."

Sudden elation exploded in Jason's chest. He sat up in the seat, punched the air and yelled, "Way to go, Caroline!" as he yanked back on the throttle rearing the jet ski upward like a spurred bronco and roared up onto the waves.

As they skimmed the top of the crests pounding out small explosions of foam, he could hear Caroline screaming half in delight, half in fright and her arms pincered themselves around him so tightly that he suddenly knew not even death could separate them.

* * *

Jason and the children had returned to the hotel after the yacht club outing and Jason had been obliged to spend almost an hour playing follow the leader with Michael at the swimming pool. True to his word, he went down the two-story waterslide until finally his son tired of the challenge of finding another novel position in which to negotiate the chute.

They dined quietly in the Marriott's rotating restaurant atop the hotel and, during the whole time, Tom was only a few steps away.Jason had wanted to be alone with the children but, after discussing the situation with Tom, he agreed that if someone were planning to harm the children it might be inviting disaster to leave then without a professional nearby.

It was decided, however, that Tom would not be in the suite of rooms with them that night but in a connecting unit next door.

When they had unpacked their bags and Michael had quietly investigated every nook and cranny of the suite, they gathered in front of the television in the living room where Jason brought out one of the videotapes Annette had made several years ago for the children's sake.

"Kids, you remember the tape Mommy made that we all watched after she died?" he asked somberly.

Both of them nodded but said nothing. Their level of anxiety had sealed their lips.

"This tape is another one which she made to be played if a certain situation developed."

He was also ill at ease and his tension was betrayed by an excessively somber tone of voice.

Just after dinner that evening, Caroline had come to Jason and asked her father if she could speak to Michael privately about Amy and what her father had told her.

The two children had spent at least fifteen minutes alone in the lounge section of the restaurant. Jason and Tom watched from the restaurant doorway as Caroline sat next to her younger brother and spoke earnestly. Uncharacteristically still, Michael listened raptly. At one point, the child had appeared to be crying and Caroline had pulled him next to her so that his head rested on her shoulder while she stroked his hair.

When they'd returned to where their father and bodyguard stood awaiting them, Michael's eyes were bloodshot and Caroline was unusually taciturn. Without comment they'd taken the elevator down to their floor where Tom left them and they went into their suite.

Michael appeared to have been briefed well by his sister and, despite several openings offered by his father to ask questions, he chose no to do so.

In silence, Jason inserted the tape into the video player and adjusted the sound. A grainy screen of gray disappeared without warning and Annette was suddenly walking away from the camera. The video had been shot in the couple's bedroom and Annette was dressed in silk pajamas with heavy brown wool leg warmers pulled incongruously over the fine tissue of the pant legs. She plumped the pillow and settled back into an easy relaxed pose lying on the bed and looking at the camera.

"I wanted to be comfortable for this one kids, because when you watch it, I'm sure you won't be comfortable. Take a hint from me, move around, if there's a pillow handy get it out and snuggle down. What's happening is not as bad as it may seem to you at the moment."

Jason took a throw pillow and handed it to Michael.

"While you're getting comfortable, I want to tell you that I've thought about what I would say to you on this subject for a long, long time. You can take notes if you wish or just replay the tape again and again. It isn't going to be long but it is very important that you understand how I feel about your dad. By the way, he has promised me that he will not have cheated and previewed this or any other of the tapes. You'll all be seeing them for the first time together."

"I'm going to start by going back long ago to before either of you were born, to the time when I met and fell in love with your father."

"Maybe you didn't know it but my dad and I didn't get along. He is or *was*… I'm not sure if he'll still be alive when you watch this tape… a bossy kind of guy and we often argued because he didn't like the way I ran my life. Deep down, I think I always wanted more approval from the 'judge' than I ever got. I even became a lawyer hoping he'd approve of me, but he didn't."

She paused and fluffed her own pillow before continuing.

" Anyway, the lack of closeness with my own dad left me a little bit crippled on the inside where people look at themselves privately. Maybe I was like that beautiful Canadian goose that lived in our pond by the barn. You'll remember... the one who limped. She raised beautiful goslings and had a handsome mate but she always limped just a bit. Well, I was like that because of the problems between me and my dad."

"I didn't *like* bossy men, yet I seemed to be attracted to them. So, all my boyfriends before your father were bossy, powerful guys who tried to tell me what to do and we would fight just like I did with my own dad, who I kind of loved and kind of resented, too. Both things at the same time."

"And then I met your dad. At first, and I know you won't believe it, but I thought he was a wimp because when I met him, he had a very beautiful girlfriend and boy did she try to boss him around! I wanted to tell him, 'Hey, guy! Tell her to get lost and leave you alone,' but, of course, I said nothing."

Michael who had been wiping his eyes every few seconds since the tape began, gave a choked little laugh and half turned his head toward his father whose attention was riveted to the screen.

"We were living in the same community, so I saw your dad several times and every time he was with the same bossy beauty. We knew each other a bit by then and, one evening at a party, I got him alone for a minute and I told him, 'Look, I know it's none of my business but Lacey (that was the girlfriend's name) is always telling you what to do. Why don't you stand up to her and tell her you can do what you want?'"

"Know what he said? He said, 'But I do what I want.' And I said, 'But she's always on your case, you shouldn't let her do that.' And then he says, 'So you think I should do what *you're* telling me to do rather than what *she's* telling me to do? And I'll be better off?'"

"Well kids, I just kind of said 'oops' quietly to myself and thought of an excuse to get me out of there. In one short sentence, your dad had had shown me that *I was just like my father. I wanted to boss people around.* I had never seen that clearly before and it was a revelation to me."

"I started to watch your dad and I soon learned from my watching that he wasn't a wimp. *He did do just what he wanted but he didn't fight with anyone because of it.* I was beginning to like and admire him. After a short time, only may be a couple of months, I told my last bossy boyfriend to get lost and I had my eye on your dad. I was real nervous around him because I wanted him to like me and I was afraid my bossyness would come out. I did everything I could to be close to him. I even followed him to the library and grocery store and I'd arrange to bump into him. Isn't that funny?"

Michael laughed out loud and hugged the pillow closer.

"Well, one day I learned that he had told this super beautiful, super rich, super smart girl who really wanted him that he didn't want to be with her anymore. I was so happy! I remember dancing around in my room singing when my girlfriend told me over the phone that they had broken up."

"It was the summertime and guess what I did? I got the sexiest bathing suit I could find and then I talked my girlfriend into having a small party on a houseboat and inviting your dad along. Without a date of course! And I even paid the $300 for the boat rental!"

She stopped speaking and made a funny face.

This time, both Michael and Caroline laughed.

"When he came to the boat party and found that I was the only female without a date, I think he caught on to my plotting, 'cause he avoided me at first, but that was a real *hot* bikini I was wearing and I just kept walking by him and stretching out on my towel around him. And, well you know your dad... He gave in. He asked me out and the rest is really history."

"I'm telling you all this to let you know how special your father is. He doesn't tell people what to do. He never tried to stop me from doing what I wanted to do all the time we were together. I loved him so much for that and for a million other reasons. If I hadn't met him, I don't know whether I would ever have learned to really love a man because I had been so busy fighting with them all the time. Because of your dad "...

Her voice quavered and, in the room, a stone silence reigned until she spoke again and everyone dared to breathe...

"I learned to love my old curmudgeon of a father, too. So I owe your dad a lot..."

She wiped her nose with the sleeve of her pajama... "And we were *always* happy. We learned a secret: if you are more concerned about your partner's happiness than you are about your own, you'll both be deliriously happy... and we always were."

"If you're watching this video, *and I hope that there is a reason for you to watch it*, it's because your dad has found happiness again and he's got a girlfriend. Even though I am not there, I want to tell both of you that your happiness and your father's happiness are my deepest desires. If some very, very lucky woman..." and Annette picked up a Kleenex from a box on the bed beside her and waved it in the air... "I'm a sucker for happy endings"... and then wiped her eyes with it before continuing.

"If some very, very lucky woman has found even a little tiny bit of the joy I had with your father and he is happy with her, too... I beg you, don't be bossy and tell him what to do. Don't place your own happiness ahead of his and don't try to defend me by fighting off all the women of the world who know a good thing when they see it."

"Your dad's happiness has always been my first priority ever since I met him so long, long ago. Believe me... Please, believe me, I am deeply grateful to the woman who will make your daddy happy again now that I am gone."

She stopped speaking, leaned forward and smiled at them. Tears were spilling from her eyes. Almost a full minute later, after several Kleenex and crooked smiles, she blew them each a kiss.

"I love you all and I'll be with you, *each one of you,* forever."

Suddenly the screen went blank.

Michael was hugging the pillow and crying "Mommy... mommy."

In the same instant, Caroline and Jason dropped to their knees on either side of him and joined their tears with his.

CH037

Jason had said his good-byes to the children at the hotel when the limousine came to collect them. It had been a tearful, draining experience and he was exhausted well before his taxi arrived at the metro airport.

The sky was clear with a limitless ceiling and vapor trails laced the azure vault that hid the stars behind a transcendent sunlight. Kerosene fumes assaulted his nostrils as soon as he opened the taxi door and the roar of jet engines at full throttle caused him to grimace.

He used a curbside Delta check-in service and was about to head to the departure gate when an older portly Italian man whom he recognized as Tony Gallo's companion, Rossi, limped slowly toward him. As he got close he held out a cell phone to Jason.

"Dr. Turner, Tony Gallo would like to have a word with you."

Jason took the phone and put it to his ear. "Jason Turner, here."

"Thanks for taking my call, Dr. Turner. I'm calling to make you aware of new developments in Albany. My man learned that Smith has been replaced. In fact, there may have been two CHC agents there all the time. What I know now is that a guy name of Walter Murphy has been there for about a week now."

"Is he taking up where Smith left off?" asked Jason.

"He seems to be, yes," replied Gallo.

"What can you tell me about him?"

"He's a PI from the west coast. He's done time and he's dangerous. Smith looks like a choirboy compared to him. I advise you strongly to steer clear of him and keep Ms. Davis away as well."

Jason was surprised that Gallo knew about Amy.

"How long have you known about Ms. Davis?"

"That's not important, Dr. Turner. What matters is that she not be allowed to follow him like she did Smith. She's out of her league and in danger. Besides, her ex-husband from Atlanta has someone looking for her as well. We haven't got his name but he's black and turns in different circles than my man down there, so he'll be harder to keep track of."

"Just who all is involved in this?" asked Jason, a little taken aback by the information Gallo had provided.

"Counting my guy, at least three men from out of state and I'm not sure we've got a line on all the locals. You'd know more about them than we do, I suspect."

Jason had been speaking quietly but in a conversational tone. He lowered his voice and turned a few steps away from Rossi. "Gallo, I need to know if your people moved on Smith."

"Why?"

"Well, I'm the one along with Ms. Davis on the front line down there."

"Do you really expect a comment on Smith from me?"

"Yes, I do."

"No disrespect intended, doctor, but I won't discuss what happened to Smith. I *know* nothing about his problems." The Italian's voice was terse.

When Jason said nothing Gallo added, "We're doing our best to cover you and your interests, doctor. We're still digging on the C-4 used in the car bomb that killed your wife, too. It's military. So far we know it was part of a shipment sent to Robbins Air Force base three years ago."

"How will you get in touch with me if you learn more?" asked Jason.

"Don't concern yourself with that. We're handling things and if you need a warning we'll get one to you... By the way, congratulations are in order, aren't they?"

"About what?"

"The upcoming nuptials of course."

"How do you know about that?"

"Who do you think Tommy works for now, doc? Anyway, I'm glad to see you're getting on with your life and frankly, if the kids like her that'll influence any decision the court makes on custody."

"We agreed that those proceeding would be kept in abeyance." Jason's voice had an edge to it.

"Sheesh! Calm down, doc. Nothing's happening. I'm just trying to be pleasant."

"Sorry, I'm sensitive about that. I still intend to keep my kids away from McLean."

"Wouldn't expect it to be different, doc. I'll be in touch. Meanwhile, keep your head down and your fiancée's too. Ciao," and the line went dead.

Jason looked up at the four-faced clock hanging from the ceiling. He had twenty minutes until flight time. Without a word he handed the phone back to Rossi who limped off after snapping it shut.

CH038: CASTRIES, ST LUCIA

Vincent Malik picked up his bottle of Carib beer and slowly rolled it in his blunt fingers across his forehead, exchanging the cool condensed droplets on its surface for the beads of sweat on his brow. His eyes seemed to be studying the pattern of scratches in the varnished tabletop between them as if they contained the secrets of the ages. After a significant pause during which he'd weighed the American's introduction in his mind and found it suspect, he raised his steel gray eyes and locked them onto the man's face.

"You say that some feller name of Jed Haycock in Antigua gave you my name as 'a good man who worked well and who knew how to keep his mouth shut'?"

"That's right," replied the stranger, apparently not in the least intimidated by the short man's piercing gaze, "Said you and him had done a few jobs together in Trinidad several years ago, back during the oil boom."

Malik remembered Haycock but he remembered him as a loose-lipped drunk who had nearly gotten them both buried in shallow jungle graves by the Chinaman they'd been scamming. A recommendation from Haycock was suspect at best and simply raised the squat expatriate Brit's natural wariness to the level of overt suspicion. However, times had been lean in recent months and he couldn't afford to let a good opportunity pass him by.

Vincent Malik had a nose for money and around this American he could virtually smell it. His eyes roved over the stranger's face but he said nothing.

The man was handsome... movie star handsome, with chiseled features that set off hazel-green eyes below expressive brows. A mesh of unruly jet-black hair curled across a forehead that looked dry and cool despite the sweltering heat and humidity. Perfect teeth gleamed white against a country-club tan when he spoke and he exuded the calm self-assured air of someone who is accustomed to the easy use of authority and the ready acceptance of it by those with whom he deals.

His manner was almost nonchalant, although *he* had deliberately sought out Malik in the grimy Castries bar and offered him a beer after a brief conversation with the bartender.

He wanted something and Malik knew it. If he wanted it bad enough he'd pursue it. Malik decided to test the strength of the stranger's interest by rejecting the recommendation.

"Haycock was a fool who almost got us both killed," he said flatly still holding the man's face with his eyes.

The American's expression remained unperturbed as if Malik's message didn't merit comment. He swished his beer in the mug and took a long slow swallow then, cupping the mug between both hands, he leaned back in his chair as if to bring the Englishman more clearly into focus.

"I see you have all the money you need to live off the fat of the land here in paradise", he said. His eyes rambled over Malik and paused just long enough at the threadbare collar of his white guayabera to signal that any pretense at affluence would be pointless. Their relative positions in any bargaining to be undertaken were as obvious as the Rolex versus the Timex watches they respectively wore.

"A chap can always use a bob or two extra, or at least that's what my New York broker's always telling me," replied Malik curling his lips in a sarcastic half-smile that let a gold incisor flash briefly.

"Are you looking to invest in the islands, mate?"

"Could be. I may have a brief job that pays well..." he said as he topped up the beer in his mug from the bottle that sat in front of him, tapping the edge of it against the glass to dislodge a trailer of foam.

"How well is '*well*'?"

"Ten thousand up front and the same when I have proof the job's properly completed."

Malik nodded and let his breath escape in a low-pitched whistle. "Must be important... perhaps *dangerous* work..."

"Important, yes... dangerous?" the American said shaking his head... "Not if you're prepared..."

"Is this the kind of work I'm going to have to leave the island for after it's finished?"

Malik was leaning forward conspiratorially and had dropped his voice almost to a whisper as if every ear in the bar were trained on their conversation. His eyes flickered back and forth from the American to the several patrons seated at the bar.

The handsome man made no effort to participate in the attempt at dissimulation and replied in a normal tone of voice. "I guess it might be a choice, but if you are efficient, no one will be the wiser..."

"So it *is* illegal," Malik said, still whispering.

"How many jobs that pay twenty thousand dollars a day aren't?" said the stranger arching his eyebrows slightly at Malik's apparent naiveté.

"Well, you need to know that I don't take credit cards or checks except for charters..." Malik's eyes narrowed to slits and he had continued to whisper.

The American dropped a hand below the table momentarily and returned it holding a wad of hundred dollar bills in a silver money clip. He snapped one out and waved it at a waitress clearing glasses from a nearby table.

She was a painfully thin young woman with skeletal arms and greasy Rasta braids that swung when she walked. Her manner was careless and lackadaisical as she slapped at some crumbs on the table she was cleaning with a soiled towel.

When he caught her eye and she glimpsed the money, the transformation was electric. She almost dropped her tray and rag in her haste to cover the ten feet between them.

"Yessir," she said following the movement of the bill in his hand with her eyes as if it were a hypnotist's pendulum. "What can I get you?"

"Two more Caribs, please... and keep the change."

With the appearance of the money, Malik's eyes had sprung wide open like a starving man's in front of a feast and now his hand snapped out quicker than a frog's tongue snaring the bill just as the stranger passed it to the girl.

"Elaine, get the beers and put them in a bag. There'll be ten of this for you when it's done."

An edge of menace had been added to his usual adenoidal tone when he spoke.

The girl's face flushed with a mixture of disappointment and intimidation but she only said, "Yessir, Mr. Malik," and turned toward the bar.

Malik snapped the crisp new Franklin between his thumbs and forefingers till it popped audibly. "Haven't seen any of these new bills here yet," he said fingering it greedily then folding it. "Hope you understand that we can't let you corrupt the help here with extravagance. I'm in here often enough... She'll get the hundred in due course, you can be certain of that, mate."

He grinned wickedly as if some agreement had just been concluded between them, then nodded his head toward the door. "Why don't we walk down to the harbor. Shame to miss the local color an' all... I'll show you my boat."

The American had been smiling wryly since the action with the girl and the money had begun. Malik's recruitment hadn't been much of a challenge thus far but he still needed to assure himself the pudgy expatriate Brit was his man.

"Why not?" he shrugged and pushed back his chair.

The 'Hangman's Noose' bar was on Gilbert street at the upper edge of Castries' old section. Above it, loomed the luxurious villas of the privileged jutting out from the verdant mountainside like the roosts of birds of prey overlooking the crowded warrens of the rodents upon which they depended and fed. Below it, wound the maze of narrow streets and alleys of the old town twisting gradually downward toward the harbor that glistened emerald green in the distance.

When the two men had stepped into the bustle of the dirt street Malik began to speak at normal volume again. "Damn sun... near hot enough to fry your brains in your hat."

He fumbled in the square pocket of his guayabera for a pair of greasy sunglasses which he fitted clumsily over his broad flat nose. A sea captain's peaked cap that had hung on a peg by the door of the bar sat perched, almost comically, on his oversized head.

The Brit's face had the blunt flat features of an Olmec stone head. With no neck and his thick trunk and stubby legs bracketed by long simian arms, he had the appearance of a normally proportioned man who had been dropped from a great height onto his feet and compacted in the process.

Well-tanned arms the color of dried tobacco bulged with muscles that flexed with even the slightest movement. He moved with an unusual, almost bulldog-like gait in which he shifted his weight from side to side as if his body had been a heavy fridge being walked on its corners. But beneath his apparent clumsiness, the American could sense the deceptive quickness of an alligator capable of bursts of deadly speed and power.

"Watch yourself in these streets and keep your hands in your pockets or some little black mongoose will swipe your wad and you won't feel it gone till he's down an alley and away... That's why I always carry a switch."

As he spoke, he strode over to the trunk of a towering Banyan tree just across the street from the bar and, with a worn but razor-sharp clasp knife, nipped off one of the slender air roots. He slashed the air with it and was rewarded with a whistling hiss.

Two barefoot black children, shiny with sweat and clad only in ragged shorts, who had fallen in behind them as they left the bar, scampered away out of reach, white eyes wide and staring at the switch. Malik feinted at them with the rod raised and they turned and ran, one howling as if he had already been struck.

The Englishman laughed, a raucous, gargling sound. "He remembers me, that one..."

"How far is the boat?" asked the American, who still looked cool and at ease under the brim of an Aussie bush hat with one side snapped to the crown that he'd slipped on as he left the bar. "I've got a five o'clock flight and would like to be on time."

"Not spending the night with us, guv? There's a bevy of lonely German lasses at the Holiday Inn and they're giving a bash this evening..." he stopped on an expectant note.

"No thanks, I've business that won't wait back home."

"Home?" asked Malik, not really expecting an answer to his probe.

"Yes... home," replied the American flatly, then added abruptly in a chilling non-sequitur. "Have you ever killed a man, Mr. Malik... for money, I mean?"

"Sounds like you're asking me to incriminate myself, mate. And why pray tell, would I do such a silly thing as that?"

"Think of it as a job interview, if you will. I'd never hire a bricklayer whose hands hadn't been in mortar as much as they'd been out of it."

He paused but hadn't dropped the inflection in his voice and Malik knew he wasn't finished. "I know for example, that you spent three years in a Halifax penitentiary for armed robbery and I find the effort, if not the result, commendable but it doesn't qualify you for the work I have in mind." The American continued looking straight ahead while he spoke.

"Well now, I'm impressed, I am," said Malik. "You've done your homework well, mate... And what else do you know about my past?"

"Enough to make it interesting, if I *were* a cop... which of course I'm not."

Malik could see the smile lines tensing into relief on the man's cheek as a fan-shaped wedge of wrinkles tightened almost mischievously at the corner of his eye.

'*The bugger's having himself a laugh at me own expense*,' he thought.

"Then, I suppose you heard about the one-eyed Dutchman in Curacao that fell across my filleting knife, poor soul..." said the Brit inviting a more approving comment.

"Gutting a half blind cripple in an argument over cards, really doesn't impress me, Mr. Malik... Yes, I heard the story from Mr. Haycock".

"That lying wetbrain! …The Dutchman was as big as a house... Blocked the sun, he did... and spry as a cat he was too... *until the accident*."

"Then that makes *one*, Mr. Malik..." The American's voice remained level, unimpressed.

"Very well... but you need to understand that if I tell you my dirty deeds and we don't strike a deal to seal our lips… I'*d have to kill you*."

Malik had intended the threat to banish the humor from their discussion. Thus, he startled visibly when the man roared with gut-felt laughter for a moment.

"You'd have to kill me?' he chortled.

"And what is so damn amusing about that?" asked Malik doing his best to sound indignant.

"It's just the picture that floats across my mind's eye when I try to imagine it, Mr. Malik. Don't be offended, please..."

Malik's lower lip jutted in an aggressive pout, leaving no doubt that he *had* been offended.

"You'd laugh less if you'd been the Chink I strangled in Port of Spain or his Hindu bodyguard who I knackered at the knees with a machete before he could draw down on me." The stubby Brit's voice had become almost petulant... Totally asynchronous with the violent content of his message.

The American said nothing, but nodded his head and murmured, "Uh, huh!"

Malik waited for more but they continued walking in a pregnant silence that kept Malik ill at ease.

'Nosy son of a gun, this Yank... asks about the very guts of my life then lets it drop as if we'd been discussing the time of day,' he thought and then decided to ratchet down the intensity of their conversation in order to control his anger. The American could be testing him.

"I gather you're not much for mere idle chitchat, mate," he said as he turned to look at the stranger beside him whose eyes seemed to be snapping pictures for storage in his brain, taking in every detail of their surroundings.

"As you said, Mr. Malik... It would be a shame to miss the local color."

The unpaved street they were following was flanked by single-story clapboard buildings perched on stubby brick stilts to foil termites. All were in need of paint. Their blistered facades shimmered in the heat of a sun that, like a laser hole burned into the firmament, blazed down white hot from a cloudless sky.

Above paneless windows, square wooden shutters like vertical trapdoors were propped open at the bottom with sticks. Spicy cooking odors wafted out from darkened interiors.

Changing the topic, the American asked without turning to Malik, "I can't see into the houses. Are they all private dwellings?"

"Dwellings, yes. But anything except private, mate... The locals crowd into them eight or ten to a room... Wall to wall snoring it is each night and the rats running over them nibblin' an ear here or a nose there. A few of them have hammocks, but I doubt you'll find a real bed or mattress in this whole street. They crash out on sleeping mats just like their ancestors did back in Africa two hundred years ago... Progress or what?"

"Who owns the houses?"

"Business types, mainly... They rent them out for a few dollars a week to a man who might have a job on the docks or at the tropical oil plant... You and me couldn't live like that, what with the bugs and rats and all, but they're as happy as pigs in muck... Don't know no better and that's not likely to change, no matter what his nibs the Premier promises..."

As they made their way down the street the American fell silent again, attempting to work out the details of how he could gain sufficient control of the situation to guarantee that Malik would keep his end of any deal they struck that day.

For his part, the homely Brit chattered on from time to time when they passed something that struck his fancy. "Check out the utility poles, mate! See how each one's got a rat's nest of wires drooping off the top... You Americans gave the boys at government house an endless spool of telephone line. When one line stops working, they can't follow it through the mess, so they just string up another."

Malik doffed his cap and ran a hairy forearm across his brow to wipe away perspiration before continuing his travelog.

" Every three years or so, we get one of those storms from hell that rattles the town to its foundations. Things get all torn up what with branches, tin roofing sheets an' such swirling around. When it's over they restring the whole bloody network. If you look careful like, you can see the meteorological history of St Lucia recorded in the larger knots of line. Some birds get hung up in the mess and die there, then you might see a rat or two crawling out to gnaw on a feathery sun-baked meal... Did you know there's three rats to every human on this island?"

"Do tell," replied the American, dryly.

Between the dingy clapboard buildings intermittent starbursts of crimson bougainvilleas or hibiscus mercifully perfumed the air subduing the sour smell of poverty and poor hygiene.

Every hundred yards or so the canopy of a stately mango tree threw a merciful circle of shade in which people clustered like fish under a coral outcropping. Vendors, hawking sugarcane juice or flavored shaved ice from fly-covered two-wheeled carts, stood with their backs to the trunks.

Animated knots of men in T-shirts, shorts and flip-flops and women in nondescript dresses congregated around the carts. A dozen pairs of eyes peering out from the shade would follow the two white men striding by, the babble of conversation dimming as they approached and rising as they passed in a reverse Doppler effect.

Having finished the mental elaboration of his plan of action and deciding that both greed and fear would be needed to keep Malik in line, the American allowed himself to begin coversing with the Brit again.

"No one works here?" he asked pointing to the groups of people lounging aimlessly under any blotch of shade.

"Most of them work, but just not all at once or for very long. We've got the ideal job-sharing scheme down here... about one job for every four men and they split them up. As long as a willing face shows up everyday most employers don't quarrel. The jobs aren't anything that requires training just a strong back and a docile spirit."

They were approaching lower town and the hum of traffic and the blaring of horns signaled the start of the pavement. The occasional decrepit taxi like the one that had carried the American to the 'Hangman's Noose' had pushed by them on the side road but otherwise vehicles stayed in the center of the town.

The exertion of the walk had painted circles of sweat under each man's arms and a swatch of dampness down his spine.

"We can get a taxi over there," said Malik indicating the nearest paved intersection where the town's perimeter was marked by two-story buildings whose balconies overhung sidewalks and storefronts.

"It was quicker to walk than to wait for one to pick us up from the `Noose'," he explained.

The American just nodded. He'd put on sunglasses, and with his eyes hidden, the Brit couldn't even guess at his reaction to the fact that they had walked in the torrid heat when they needn't have.

It was now important to Malik that the American remain well disposed toward him because he'd pretty much decided to hire out to the chap if the job looked feasible, even though he instinctively disliked him. He didn't want to piss him off... but he wasn't prepared to kiss ass either.

The Brit waved an arm and the driver of one of two ancient Toyotas parked at the curb got up nonchalantly from a chair propped against a wall.

After climbing into his vehicle in slow motion, he pulled the car over to the pair of white men now standing in the shade of a balcony. They slid into the overheated rear seat slick with seat covers that appeared to be jury-rigged from industrial plastic sheeting by some local entrepreneur. An inadequate trickle of cool air filtered back from the dashboard AC vents.

“To the cove, mate, and step on it,” Malik told the driver, slapping his hand on the back of the front seat for emphasis.

They rode in silence as Malik had apparently decided to cut short the commentary on local color. He appeared to be deep in thought as he traced the outline of his chin back and forth nervously with the end of his blunt index finger. He glanced from time to time at the American who was watching the town slide past through the side window of the Toyota.

The back of the driver’s sweaty black head was cropped so closely it looked like a bowling ball that had been sprayed by a vaporizer in preparation for polishing. It swiveled with the demands of driving while the image of his face on an ID card suspended from the rear view mirror swung to and fro’.

When he wasn’t leaning on the horn or cursing someone impeding their progress through the narrow streets, he hummed a hidden tune from inside his head tapping out its rhythm with his fingers on the edge of the steering wheel.

At one point, when a truck with ‘Culligan’ lettered on its side and loaded with large transparent bottles of water blocked an intersection, he gave a blast on the horn after cursing out his window and then turned around to ask.

“You gentlemen trying to catch the tide to go fishing, Mr. Malik?”

“No, not today, mate,” replied the Brit and then, almost as an afterthought, snapped, “You’d best be minding your own affairs and get us round yonder bloody truck.”

“Ok, mon, ok!” replied the driver raising his arms and shrugging to indicate both comprehension and mild disgust at Malik’s ill manners.

In ten minutes, the Toyota pulled up alongside a three foot high stonewall shaded by the lily pad leaves of a row of Manchenille trees squeezed between a cracked sidewalk and the wall. Several men clad in the T-shirt-shorts uniform of St. Lucian males slouched along the wall, two with their backs against it, one straddling it and a fourth man lying on his back atop the stones.

As he got out of the cab, the American reached across the seat with a twenty dollar bill and told the cabby to wait. The man grinned his thanks and turned off the car.

Beyond and above the fringe of Manchenilles, the outriggers of fishing boats hidden from view by the wall and the trees wavered against the horizon like the silvery antenna of several huge mythic sea creatures lying below the surface of the harbor and sampling the air above.

A tight ring of several gulls, so high up they seemed but white specks, circled against the azure sky. Below them a frigate bird rode the wind currents on motionless ebony wings, its forked tail twisting like a rudder controlling its wheeling patrol over the waters of the tiny cove that sparkled like a billion silver coins in the sunlight.

Malik led the way along the wall to a set of stone steps that descended to an ancient jetty upon which several huge mooring tees, large enough to tie up a cruise ship, bled rust onto crumbling concrete.

Large threadbare truck tires were hung edge to edge along the jetty's front and produced a low-toned gurgle, like a giant swallowing, each time the light chop that swelled up their sides slurped back out of their barnacle-encrusted bellies.

Six charter boats bobbed lazily beyond hand-painted wooden signs on ten foot poles set into the jetty that bore their names and those of their captains. Redundant messages of 'charter boat' or 'fishing charters' were on each of the six. Only one slip lay empty testifying of the low demand for their services which had honed Malik's interest in the American's proposal.

"She'll be at the far end of the slips," he said over his shoulder as he skipped his considerable bulk nimbly down the uneven steps.

The American followed watching several naked young boys taking turns running off the jetty into the water, their laughs and shouts splashing back against the wall. He didn't smile or appear interested beyond the simple noting of their activity.

The 'Saucy Lady' was a thirty-six foot Bertram at least twenty years old but her paint and trim were immaculate and the canvas sunshade suspended over the flying bridge was crisp and white. Her teak rails were smooth and had been recently oiled. Malik grinned noting the American's perusal of her lines as they approached.

"She's a beauty, eh, mate? She's the only woman in my life and I sleep with her every night... A bloke couldn't ask much more than that, could he now?"

By the time they had come opposite the stern, a black man with a salt and pepper brillopad of hair and a withered arm that he carried in a rigid right angle at the elbow like a piece of bent pipe, had appeared out of the boat's cabin. His face was split with a lopsided smile that followed an unnatural crease up his left cheek almost to his ear. Whatever had mangled his left arm had chewed out a groove in his face as well.

Four gleaming white teeth, two in the upper and two in the lower jaw, like he was growing a new set and had not gotten past the infant stage, gave him the appearance of an ugly cartoon rabbit.

"This here's George, me boat boy," said Malik as he gestured to the American to move onto the gangway that George held grinning from the other end.

"He's as thick as a boot sole and doesn't speak much cause he's really only got one lip, but he's handy and can do more with one arm than most locals can with two."

As he got closer to the man, the American could see the smile was a permanent distortion of the fellow's face since the upper left cheek was a mass of scar tissue pulling the top lip so tightly in its stricture that it appeared to be absent, at first glance.

George bobbed his head several times in welcome but didn't speak a word.

"Propeller got him about ten years ago, long before my time. Flayed him open like a Wahoo hit by a shark, it did... Now, the Saucy Lady's the only female in his life, too." He chuckled at his own humor.

"Here, George, take those beers and sling 'em into the icebox and bring us two cold ones," Malik ordered pushing the plastic bag he'd carried from the bar toward the boat-boy who scurried away.

When George had fetched their beer, they sat at a small table just outside the cabin but out of the sun under the protection of a Bimini top.

Their conversation lasted twenty minutes. Most of the time was taken up by questions from the American that Malik answered, his expression gradually moving from flippant levity through sober interest to quiet pondering. Finally, the American wrote something on a paper and pushed it, along with a photograph, across the table to Malik who stared at the two items without speaking for a minute.

"Twenty's not half enough if I'm to do them both, mate... And I'll need the two thousand in cash now to bribe the other boat owners." He watched the American's face for a reaction but saw none except for an ominous hardening of his eyes and a knot of muscle that began working rhythmically in his jaw.

Malik continued. "There'll be no choice for me but to leave, after I've done it. If two tourists disappear from my boat, I'll be obliged to move over to Guadeloupe or St. Barts because the rumors here would do me in."

The American's expression, as he listened, had become wary as if he suspected that the shorter man's resistance was a lame attempt at a shakedown. Perhaps, he was simply a blowhard attempting to weasel out of the job. But the man had already seen the photograph of the victims and the die was cast. When he spoke, his voice was steel on ice.

"Malik, you told me you'd killed before... If that's a lie, I'll find out and *then* you'll have to go further than just St. Barts. You already know too much and you've bragged your way into a corner you can't get out of, you shriveled little worm. If you haven't got the guts to kill them both, then I've made a mistake and *I never leave my mistakes uncorrected*," he growled.

"Yes I've killed before... Just like I said, but never a woman. I've got my own rules, mate, and you're asking me to go against them..." His lip curled as his voice matched the intensity of the American's tone becoming low and menacing. "And, I don't take kindly to being threatened aboard my own boat."

He leaned across the small table to get closer into the American's face. It was a mistake.

So fast that Malik felt nothing before the small blade stung the skin beneath his jaw over his jugular vein, the American had grabbed the Brit's hair with his left hand and pushed his face into the tabletop.

The scalpel must have already been in his right hand, perhaps slipped surreptitiously from a pocket. The tiny blade set in a steel handle didn't even dent the skin as he pressed it carefully inward. The tanned flesh sprang apart as if it were warm rubber under tension and blood dribbled rapidly in dark red blotches onto the table-top.

"I don't *threaten* Mr. Malik, I only *promise...* Now that we are business partners, you'll carry out your end of the deal for thirty thousand and not a penny more... Is that understood?"

Malik could taste the salty tang of his own blood that, pooling quickly on the table, had trickled across to his lips. He felt nauseous and thought he was going to piss himself.

"Ok, ok, ok!" he whispered hoarsely in a throat tight with terror. "I understand... clearly.... Please drop the knife." His voice sounded like it came from deep within a rusty drain.

The American increased the pressure of his left hand on the Brit's oversized head levering himself up to a standing position as he did so. The man groaned and pleaded again. "I've got it …It's ok, I tell you."

"Very well, Mr. Malik. I *promise* you that no one ever crosses me in business... You may sit up now and attend to your little shaving nick." The man's eyes were veiled with a homicidal glaze that Malik took in with the same degree of apprehension as he did the scalpel still glinting in his assailant's right hand.

He clutched at his neck and yelled for George who must have been watching because he appeared immediately with a cloth in his hand. The black man's eyes were wide and the fear in them clashed with his grin. He backed away quickly from the two men groping behind him with his good hand for the cabin wall, then crabbed sideways until he reached the steps and scuttled down them into the cabin again.

Malik had risen as well. He said nothing, his eyes mirroring the obvious sentiments of his boat-boy as he pressed the cloth so tightly to his jaw that his knuckles blanched with the effort.

"In two days you'll have fifteen thousand dollars in an account at Barclays' Bank here in Castries. I'll contact you through the 'Hangman's Noose' once I know the date."

The American's face had relaxed instantly and he spoke almost nonchalantly as if there were suddenly no further need for intimidation. He'd pulled a handkerchief from his pocket as he talked and seemed to be absorbed in wiping the blade of a small scalpel, the steel shaft of which was disguised as a pen. He replaced its cap and put the deadly pen back into his shirt pocket.

When he looked up again at Malik he was smiling and extending his hand. "Do we have a deal, Mr. Malik?"

"We do, sir, yes, we do," stammered the stubby Brit who took the American's hand in a boneless moist grip that spoke volumes on his inner turmoil.

“Very well, have a pleasant day, Mr. Malik,” said the American as he stepped onto the gangplank and began retracing his steps along the jetty to the head of the stairs where the taxi stood waiting.

Malik watched the man’s back going up the stairs before he pulled away the blood-stained cloth, felt the oozing begin again, and re-applied it. He spoke in a mumble.

“I’ve killed three people and when I’ve done with your two, you bloody bugger... I swear on my life that I’ll do you for my own count and pleasure.”

CH039: CASTRIES, ST. LUCIA

The evening of their arrival in St Lucia, Jason and Amy had talked until well past midnight with Brigham Landry. It had been pleasant but light conversation until the doctor become serious.

"When Jason called and told me that you two were planning to be married, I must admit, I had mixed emotions. Hospitals and their ilk are notoriously dangerous places to strike up emotional relationships and I feared that the rule may have held true in your case... but..."

Pausing, he stood up to his full six foot seven inches and extended one huge arm out over each of their heads as they sat at the table grinning sheepishly.

"I pronounce you both whole, fit and competent to enter into the bonds of matrimony here tomorrow morning on our beach!"

"We needed that blessing, Brigham. At least, I needed it," said Jason. "I got badly sleep deprived about two months ago and hallucinated up a storm. I told Amy about it and she's been looking at me a little strangely ever since."

Amy got up from her chair, leaned sideways toward him, took his face in her hands and kissed him gently on the lips. "I'm taking you with all your flaws revealed, darling."

It was his turn to stand up. He turned to her and swept her into his arms and kissed her.

When they persisted in their embrace, Landry coughed, then spoke.

"Too bad you have to sleep in different villas, tonight... It's an old St Lucian law that is written on the back of every marriage license issued here. It's on the one I got for you... I checked."

Jason opened one eye and winked at Landry over Amy's shoulder.

* * *

After leaving Landry they retired to their villa and without exchanging a word, both searched for their swimsuits and changed into them. Words would have been superfluous. Amy waited for him at the door while he went and brought two towels from the bathroom, then they walked, arm in arm, down to the beach.

"Look at the moon, darling..." she said.

"Yes, it's just like the first night I saw you… You know, I can still close my eyes and see you exactly as I did then..."

She looked up at him, an impish smile on her lips, "Really?"

"Absolutely... down to the last detail."

"Are you certain, darling," and planting her toes against his, she took both his hands in hers and leaned back away from him until her long hair almost touched the sand behind her.

"Yes, I'm certain. Why?"

"Because I want to do it, *again*..." She laughed and started to sway from side to side.

"Ok, but why?" he queried.

"Because, Mr. Turner, that first time, *I* didn't know you were watching me until I came back onto the beach after my swim."

"Does it matter all that much?" he asked naively.

"If you were a woman, my darling, you'd understand that it does... A lot of a woman's sexual pleasure comes from *being watched and wanted.* Deep down, we're all just exhibitionists who can't wait to get stared at by someone we *want* to be watched by."

"My face is red. You'll have to stop all this erotic stuff."

She laughed again. "Not hardly... Now, run on down the beach to your boulder. I'll give you a ten minute start... and then," she let go of his hands and posed provocatively... *"I'll show you erotic."*

He laid his towel over his shoulder and started off down the beach at an easy distance-consuming lope.

In a few minutes, he was atop the basalt boulder with the towel folded under him. He tried energetically to will himself into a trance to exactly simulate his previous experience but, knowing that she was coming, he couldn't.

After two minutes, he ceased the charade and shifted his towel so that his line of sight was straight down the beach in the direction from which she would be approaching. He watched expectantly. Looking at his wristwatch, he noted it was exactly one twenty a.m.

The moon was actually higher in the vault of the night then he remembered it. Its image upon the softly undulating surface of the bay was elongated and disjointed.

Jason had been taking a deep breath about every twenty minutes since they had stepped off the plane in St. Lucia. The scent of the tropics was a potent elixir for him and, now, in the freshness of the night air, every extraneous odor having been eradicated by the sun's heat, only a distillation of the most durable and enchanting perfumes remained.

He inhaled deeply, held his breath until his pulse slowed perceptibly, then let it escape slowly from flaring nostrils. The soft susurration of the sea washing against the sand beckoned like a siren's lullaby. He closed his eyes and, despite his yearning for Amy, the magic of the place tugged at him, seducing him to a level of profound relaxation.

He was teetering at the edge of the slope to oblivion and peace when he abruptly caught himself with a startle of awareness and opened his eyes. He looked at his watch, fifteen minutes had passed since he scaled the boulder and begun his vigil. He strained to see if she were approaching far down the beach but he saw nothing except nature's canvas upon which Amy had promised to paint herself.

Aware now of the passage of time as he watched for her appearance, each second became a sensual stroke whetting the edge of his desire, honing it to razor sharpness. Anticipation danced on every nerve ending and, once again, he leaned forward, squinting his eyes to sharpen the images of the night. Nothing... then, much closer along the beach than he had expected, a fluttering whisper of white flashed in the moonlight. But before it could drift down to the sand, it evaporated into the shadows.

He was wondering if his eyes were deceiving him when suddenly it reappeared, a ghostly puff of gossamer floating briefly on the air. This time, it wafted slowly downward until it landed upon the sand.

As he stared transfixed, scarcely breathing, a spectral white figure began to arise as if issuing from the very sands of the beach. It emerged gradually from the shadows, drifting toward the water's edge. At first, the consistency of what he assumed to be white silk seemed no more substantial than shadow. However, when the moonlight fell fully upon her, he could see the profile of outstretched arms, the reflection of copper highlights in a swath of hair cascading over the upper border of the silk.

Below her hair, he could barely make out the exquisite substance of her whole body. As she continued to glide further onto the beach, her back and legs were profiled more clearly against the silk. In the moon glow, her hair alone hung on the near side of the shimmering veil.

Then, abruptly, she drew in her arms and the silk spun into a whirling shaft of copper and white, the moonlight glinting on hair and drape as she twirled toward the water's edge. Reaching it, she suddenly collapsed upon the sand into an alabaster pose from which first one, then slowly, two arms began to stretch skyward.

Over the next few moments, she slowly drew herself fully erect and stood facing him. Her face remained swathed in shadow but her breasts, as if seducing the moonlight to caress their voluptuous curves, appeared strangely luminescent. Her arms, which had remained above her head, drifted down to horizontal and the diaphanous cloth now became the background against which she stood clothed only in moonlight.

As he watched, she approached rapidly with running strides until he thought she intended to come right up to the boulder. However, a mere five yards from him, she veered right, took two splashing long-legged leaps that sprayed water like a silver fan around her, then executed a perfect dive disappearing virtually without a splash, leaving the white silk floating in undulating folds upon the lazy swells.

He watched impatiently for her to reappear in the direction that he estimated she would be swimming beneath the surface. A full thirty feet ahead of where she dove, he caught a flash of moonlight on ivory skin beneath the surface, and as he continued to watch, she drifted up along the liquid plane, gliding easily through the last few feet before rising from the water to stand in silent profile nearly opposite where he sat. She stood still as a marble statue except for her heaving chest.

Her beauty was breathtaking.

He wanted to call out but he was afraid the sound of his voice might shatter the spell. He ached physically to hold her, so that when she turned to face him and beckoned with her hand, he leapt directly from the summit of the boulder to the edge of the water stumbling forward with his momentum before falling into its freshness.

Scrambling to his feet, he ran through the shallows and, when he couldn't run any longer, he dove and swam to her stopping just in front of where she stood. He raised himself from the water almost reverently, never taking his eyes from her. Slowly, she opened her arms in invitation. He approached and enfolded her against him surprised at the ardor of her kiss which crushed his lips beneath hers.

After their embrace, they swam together for a time, then sat quietly cuddling on the sand until the moon had settled low on the horizon. Jason wanted to make love on the beach but Amy, teasingly, refused, saying the marriage would be invalidated according to the terms written on the back of the license. His kisses and caresses could not dissuade her.

As they wandered back along the ebony stand, he asked, "Where did you find the silk?"

She laughed brightly.

"Jason, it wasn't silk, just one of those inadequately thin shower curtains from the room. Necessity being the mother of invention and all that, I ran back to get it from the villa."

Having been refused the physical consummation of his desire he sought at least to satisfy the demands of his curiosity. "What about your breasts. I could see them so clearly..."

"That, my darling, is called *viewing me through the lens of lust,"* and she laughed again.

"No, really?" he persisted.

"Icing sugar from the kitchen... I'd let you taste some to prove it but..."

"I know," he interrupted, "*it would invalidate the marriage.*"

"Exactly," she chided, and then, placing one hand under each breast, she stopped walking and turned to face him holding them up to the waning moonlight, "See, there are traces of it still visible."

He lunged after her and she spurted away from his grasp.

The short sprint immediately became a full-fledged race. He was utterly determined to catch her, but she outdistanced him again, precisely as she had done before. He was three yards behind her when they reached the patio but he had the satisfaction of seeing that she seemed ready to collapse from the exertion.

She literally fell into his arms.

"Sir knight, if you will simply carry this poor swooning maiden to your bed in yon castle, you may have your way with her, for she is beyond the point of further resistance."

He scooped her up into his arms and ran every step to the villa.

Three hours later, in a mutual embrace, they slept soundly.

* * *

At ten the next morning, there came an urgent tapping at the villa door.

"Mistress Amy, Pastor Antonio is here... It is time. Please awaken from your repose."

Amy was stretching languorously, sitting up in the bed while Jason fumbled for an adequate covering to drape his nudity in order to answer Mohammed's appeal. Amy smiled and blew him a kiss as he stumbled toward the door with his feet still only part way into his pant legs.

Outside the door, Mohammed and his mother bowed respectfully and Jason reciprocated stiffly.

"Mr. Jason Turner, sir," sputtered Mohammed with obvious consternation, "It is already much beyond the hour for the ceremony and you, sir, are not yet dressed! Dr. Landry is needing a fan against the heat because he has been sitting, waiting for so long ...and my sainted mother," he nodded toward the waif-like woman beside him who held a snow-white sari draped across her outstretched arms, "awaits to prepare the bride."

The reproach in his words was unmistakable. Jason's face tingled, betraying his blush to himself. He thought of explaining that the *'ceremony'* would be a simple unpretentious exchanging of vows on the sand at the water's edge, but a quick assessment of the consternation on Mohammed's face and he knew he would never understand.

"We're very sorry, Mohammed. We overslept."

"Yes, Mr. Jason Turner, sir... *and on the day of your nuptials*."

Jason realized that further words would do nothing to mollify Mohammed.

"Give me one minute more and your mother may enter."

Running back into the bedroom, he approached Amy, who still sat on the bed hugging the sheet to her and began to admonish her in a lilting parody of East Indian speech.

"Mistress Amy, do you not know that your honored guests are abiding patiently under the trees expecting your *retarded arrival.*"

"*Retarded arrival*!" snapped Amy, her eyes wide in mock annoyance, as she heaved a pillow at Jason who was cowering in an exaggerated crouch, positioning his hands to protect his head from her imaginary blows, and dancing on the spot with little stuttering steps.

"Oh, Mistress Amy, do not beat me, I pray you. I am full of apologies and regrets for my multiple inadequacies."

Amy, who had been smiling in amusement despite herself, looked momentarily past Jason and her face became suddenly somber.

"Oh, welcome Mohammed..." she said, an apologetic tone in her voice.

Hearing her, Jason stood bolt upright in an instant, his back to the doorway, stifling one of his sarcastic protestations in mid-word. He blushed vividly to his bellybutton and looked at her with a startled disbelieving expression on his face that said, '*This can't be happening*!' Then he turned slowly and saw that no one was there.

He spun back to the bed where Amy had burrowed under the sheet and was wheedling, "Oh, please, Mr. Jason Turner, sir, do not chastise me overly much..."

He leapt directly upon her and began to tickle her mercilessly as they both erupted in laughter, then simultaneously thought of the effect it might have upon the two kind, caring people standing outside their door, and they scurried about busily collecting their clothing.

"I sure hope you can fit into the sari that Mohammed's mother has for you. She's so petite, I wonder if it might be too small."

"Jason," she reminded him kindly, "it's customary for the husband to hold off on the derogatory remarks about his wife's changing body *until after* the wedding ceremony."

"What...?" he stuttered.

"Never mind, darling. If the sari is too small, I'll just mince down the aisle wearing nothing but a smile and a veil and provide the entertainment for our guests myself..."

"It's already been done, sweetheart... back in the sixties... Yoko Ono comes to mind... So just suck it in and try to squeeze *all* of you into the sari. It looked lovely."

Her scowl followed him out the door as Mohammed's mother entered.

Jason was ready long before his bride and, clad in a pair of light dress pants, a white embroidered guayabera and sandals, he made quite an acceptable groom. While he waited for Amy, he and Mohammed engaged the reverend Antonio Wilson in quiet banter.

If anyone was overdressed for the occasion it had to be the very short, very rotund black pastor whose bald pate and cannonball head were dappled and glistening with beads of perspiration.

He wore a heavy weave black suit that sopped up the photons. A worn white shirt collar was buttoned snugly around his neck. The force of the fit had produced a pleat in the fat of his neck which was trapped behind a tie, knotted so that the narrow end hung well below the thicker front portion upon which was emblazoned the word 'holiness' in cracked fluorescent lettering.

His feet however, appeared completely at ease in sandals that stuck out from beneath wide trousers that had been shortened to the point in the legs where a tall man's knees would have been.

He was courteous and chatty, his speech punctuated with expressions of religiosity that left Jason a little uneasy and wondering if he shouldn't request explicitly that no '*hallelujahs*' or '*praise the Lord's* be included in the ceremony.

Under the shade of the nearest flamboyant, Brigham Landry, his wife and the enormous cook sat on rattan chairs fanning themselves with dried palmetto leaf fans. Behind them, two yard boys fumbled ineptly with an electric fan on a tall stand and a knotted orange extension cord that they were tugging on for some needed slack.

Just beyond where Jason and the pastor were standing, two strands of scarlet flamboyant and hibiscus blossoms laid upon the sand marked a narrow corridor, leading to the water's edge. A few of the blossoms had been liberated by the sea from their final task and glinted like drops of angel's blood upon the water.

Suddenly, the cook gasped and exclaimed loudly, "Lordy, lordy... She be beautiful like dee rising moon!" and everyone turned to look.

Mohammed's mother was approaching with small nibbling steps, an air of beatific serenity on her features. From a small basket in her hand she scattered handfuls of white flower petals high in the air before the bride who walked serenely behind her.

A long trailing white veil, of such insubstantial material that it floated out behind Amy on the evanescent sea breeze, partially masked her features but Jason could see the joy resplendent in her eyes. In the middle of her forehead, was a ruby red dot the size of a small finger smudge that Mohammed's mother must have insisted upon to ward off evil spirits.

The sari had been modified to fit her impeccably and its flowing lines hugged the contour of her legs and thighs more snugly than the classic cut of such apparel. Her right shoulder was bare and a graceful swath of tissue lay across her bosom, then rose and disappeared over her left shoulder.

Jason's breath caught in his throat at her radiance and he and the two men with him stepped aside while the guests under the trees stood up.

Behind Landry, the two yard boys, in a veritable panic, were indiscreetly thumping on an old ghetto blaster that must have been supplied to provide taped music. Perhaps the wedding march. Landry silenced their whispers and commotion with a harsh hand signal that they obviously recognized and obeyed.

When Amy came to Jason's level, he stepped into the midst of a puff of petals which floated down upon them both and held out his right arm for her to take.

With undignified haste, the little pastor squirted in front of them and scurried down the corridor of blossoms to turn and wait for their approach. As they progressed toward him, the guests fell in behind stopping at a short distance from the place on the sand where the ceremony would be performed.

Pastor Antonio showed enormous restraint and read from only two classical marital scriptures, one from the Old and the other from the New Testaments. Then, diluting his natural fervor considerably by refraining from any expressions of evangelical enthusiasm, he spoke quietly of the responsibilities of the state of matrimony that they were entering. He asked for no objections from the guests and finished his words of admonition with a blessing.

Finally, he turned and, extending a hand to the sea, he prayed, "May your union be as peaceful and blessed as this endless expanse of sea, unblemished from here to the horizon of eternity, and may the eyes of Almighty God watch over you."

Jason and Amy, who had been gazing at each other throughout the ceremony, were both overcome with emotion and when he pronounced them man and wife and invited them to kiss they clung to each other blissfully.

There was silence for a moment and then the cook began to applaud and shouted, "God bless you bot', me children."

Amy and Jason smiled. For another moment, he leaned toward his new wife's ear and whispered a few words that had an electric animating effect upon her. She turned her face to his to kiss him passionately again and, at the same time, flung her arms around his neck, hanging with her feet off the ground.

When she stood up on her own again, she whispered in his ear, obviously a question, because he nodded his head affirmatively.

She stepped forward holding his hand and pulling him after her, closer to their guests.

"Dear friends," she gushed in hushed enthusiasm, "as the finest wedding gift I could ever receive, my husband, Dr. Turner, who is a marvelously talented pianist, has agreed to play for us all."

Ten pairs of hands clapped heartily.

Brigham Landry hailed one of the yard boys and said, "Joseph, bring us a variety of drinks to the reception hall." Then turning to Jason, he asked with exaggerated politeness, "May I kiss your bride, if she doesn't object."

Jason looked at Amy who stepped toward the huge man, leapt lightly into his arms and planted a genuine kiss of affection on his hairy cheek.

Following a few more expressions of congratulations and best wishes, during which Jason failed in an attempt to get his arms around Eulie, the cook, everyone retired to the reception hall and found a place to sit.

Jason and Amy stood whispering beside the magnificent grand piano and she was apparently attempting to convince him of something. Finally, he shrugged his shoulders, put an arm around her waist, and turned to address their guests.

"I am a private person and do not speak either easily or articulately about my emotions, as Brigham can attest. However, Amy has convinced me to share the story behind my piano playing… or rather, I should say, my lack of it."

Amy was hugging his arm fiercely and seemed as excited as a schoolgirl receiving an award.

He continued, "In a strange way which I hope you may understand, my talent as a pianist doesn't really belong to me. With the exception of one magnificent composition which I played only infrequently for my late beloved wife Annette, I have essentially not touched a keyboard since the death of my dear mother fourteen years ago."

He paused and seemed to be studying the floor in front of him for a few moments before he looked up again at the group.

"Her name was Olivia Jensen Turner, and the reason why you do not recognize her name as a household word is that she withdrew from the concert stage, in the prime of her professional career, as one of the world's foremost female concert pianists..." His voice began to quaver with emotion but he caught himself and continued, "in order to raise her only child. She taught me to play but it was always her within me, the mother inside the child, who loved her art and thrilled to play. When she died,…" and again, he paused for several beats, "I could no longer play alone."

There was a hushed silence in the room.

He resumed, "Annette Annelise McLean, was my first wife, my first love and the mother of my children. She died tragically some time ago. She has been the only person since my mother..." and, turning to Amy, smiling, "and now, my new wife, who has inspired me enough to place my fingers back on the keys."

He paused once more, as if collecting his thoughts.

"I believe in eternal life," and Jason glanced over at Pastor Antonio who was beaming with pleasure, "and no argument premised upon the logic of men can convince me that the bonds of love are not as eternal as the immortal spirits of those who belong to one another. The veil which separates us from our loved ones who have preceded us in death is thin and, I am firmly convinced, that there are special occasions when our merciful God permits the fleeting reunion of the living and the dead. And so, at Amy's request, I dedicate this rendition of Rachmaninoff's piano concerto in C minor to my dead wife, Annette."

He stopped speaking, seated himself formally on the piano bench and bent his head as if in prayer, his hands poised above the keyboard. A minute or more of absolute silence followed, and then suddenly, his hands touched the keys and the music was born.

Amy had quietly moved to the side of the room and sat upon the floor, her back to the window glass, exactly as she had positioned herself when she had first stolen into the hall to hear him play during that night months ago. Her eyes were closed and her visage serene.

Around her, the music soared as Jason's fingers flew over the keys. His eyes were often closed and he was, almost always, positioned either prayerfully bent over the keyboard or head flung back, his face raised to the arching ceiling above.

The intensity of his efforts, despite the air conditioning of the reception hall, had daubed the back of his shirt between his shoulders with a swatch of perspiration. A dew of the same moistened his temples and upper lip.

With the exception of Eulie, the cook, everyone present had closed their eyes, although pastor Antonio, used to years of peeking during prayers to check on the pious attitude of his flock members, occasionally and furtively, would steal a glance around the circle of listeners before quickly closing his eyes again.

Others stirred between the concerto's three movements but Amy remained enthralled, to the point of trance.

At last, the final crescendo boomed and then silence, sudden and total... yet still filled with the spiritual echoes of the music... fell upon the room. Jason slumped forward on the bench. No one applauded but, one by one, they arose quietly and, taking their cue from Brigham Landry, passed by and touched the pianist's shoulder while he sat overcome with emotion.

Then they left the hall.

It was at least ten minutes before Jason lifted his head and looked around. He saw his wife in her beautiful sari sitting on the floor as if in a deep sleep and, as he had done on that first night, he gathered her gently in his arms and carried her tenderly to their bed.

CH040

Amy awoke well before dawn.

It was a gentle awakening, a soft progressive awareness of the metronomic swish of the waves upon the beach drifting in through the open curtains of the balcony. Outside the villa, the moon must still have been high, for a muted fluorescence lit the balcony and fell halo-like upon the foot of the bed.

She sighed and stretched cat-like in contentment, her calf brushing up against her sleeping husband's leg.

Her husband. The alchemy of the phrase and its implications, even as she thought it, filled her with a fuzzy tingle. No longer alone. No longer hidden away. She belonged to him and, as she rolled up onto her elbow to look at his sleeping profile, she realized that he was the *first* male she had ever really loved. Even the simple contemplation of sharing the rest of her life with him caused a surge of such elemental emotion that her eyes began to fill with tears of joy.

Her childhood had been stark and barren, bereft of the attachments to powerful adults that allow children to grow up unafraid in a world full of peril. Even as an adult, she had survived by fleeing attachments with others... and now, she was attached. She belonged to someone other than herself. And he belonged to her.

She didn't want to disturb him, but she was overcome by the physical need to touch him. Cautiously, as he lay with his back to her, she began to toy with a lock of hair that fell haphazardly upon the nape of his neck. She rolled the hair between her fingers, repeatedly picked it up and then let it fall back upon his neck. With a finger she traced the profile of the rest of his hair along the side of his neck up to the crown of his head, almost mesmerized by the process of touching him. Silently, she marveled at the transformation she felt stirring within her from being connected to another person after a lifetime of solitude.

Eventually, her arm began to tire and she allowed herself to rest it on his arm while she continued her stroking. When he didn't awake, she became bolder and slid carefully across the space in the bed that separated them until she felt her breasts compressing comfortably against his back.

Like a child sneaking incrementally nearer some object of powerful attraction, she continued to snuggle closer to him, until the warmth from his skin seeped into her, his scent filled her nostrils, and she brushed her lips against his neck flicking her tongue out to taste him.

When he moved slightly and murmured something, as if he had been summoned from the realm of dreams by her attentions, she froze. She wouldn't have been able to explain *why* she was touching him while he slept and the experience would still be too novel for him to dismiss without explanation. So, she lay very quietly against him until he was still and silent again. Then she, too, slipped back into her dreams.

When he woke her with gentle kisses that wandered around her face and neck, the green of the clock radio dial glowed 7:10 and the sun was already perched on the balcony railing.

"Wake up sweetheart. We're already late."

"Late for what, Jason?" she said, squinting against the light.

"Diving... You've forgotten, haven't you?"

“Oh,” she smiled sheepishly, “yes, I did. I’m sorry.”

“No need to apologize but we need to get going. Mohammed was just here at the balcony, gawking in at us. He told me that the van was ready and waiting for us.”

“Oh, Jason,” she purred, reaching up to pull him down to her in the bed, “let’s just stay here in bed *all day*... In fact, let’s stay in bed for the whole week. We can go diving in our next lives.”

“Amy,” he pleaded trying to extricate himself from her grasp, “Brigham has made all the arrangements. The boat’s chartered. The fish have sent messages that they’re waiting for us... You’ve got to get up.”

Unable to escape from her, he abruptly changed tactics and burrowed his face into her abdomen, locked his arms under her shoulders and waist, and began bulldozing her across the bed toward the far edge. She panicked, coming fully awake in a flash at the prospect of crashing onto the floor off the bed with him on top of her.

“Let go, Jason... Stop it or we’ll fall and be killed on the rocks below,” she joked, but when he continued pushing she dug her fingers deep into his hair and pulled ferociously. “Stop it now!”

“Ouch, okay... But do you promise to get up,” he whined.

“I’m not letting go until *you* promise to stop pushing,” she said through clenched teeth.

He nudged her again playfully, and she pulled even harder on his hair.

“I mean it, Jason... I’ll pull it all out... *let me go*.”

“Alright,” he proposed, “cease-fire on three… one... two... *three*...”

Then, just as she loosened her grip on his hair he gave a huge shove, and with her screaming all the way, they slid off the bed and into a jumbled heap on the floor.

“Oh, Jason... you liar... I’ll get you,” she hissed playfully, snatching at him as he stumbled up off her and scrambled on all fours toward the bathroom door.

She pursued him into the bathroom running and tumbled headlong into the Jacuzzi where he had jumped. He'd already filled it before she awoke. She broke the surface grabbing for him, finally catching his face between her hands.

"Jason, listen to me," she said, her face screwed up in mock irritation, "I'm not... *absolutely not*, going diving until you make love to me right here and now in this Jacuzzi. Do you understand?"

* * *

When the van pulled up beside the fishing pier in Castries, Malik and his boat-boy were waiting with a wobbly-wheeled cart to load their diving equipment and food coolers. The Brit roughly pushed the black man toward the back of the van where Mohammed had headed when he got out of the driver's seat. Then he walked toward the clients.

"Good day to you, missus," he said, obsequiously doffing his cap to Amy.

Turning to Jason, he extended a gigantic hand, "My name's Tony Malik and I'm your captain for today's excursion."

His grip was vice-like and Jason winced as the bones in his hand were ceremoniously kneaded to the point of real pain.

"Careful, Tony or I won't be able to hold my spear gun," he quipped, pulling back his hand.

"Beg your pardon, sir, but I'm so used to hauling lines that I forget my own strength. The locals aren't much for handshakes and I'm out of practice," he smiled thinly and a gold incisor glinted.

As Jason and Malik talked about the details of the reef where they would be diving, Amy sized up their captain.

He was a curiously misshapen creature with a normal, even larger than normal torso, but truncated legs and an absent neck. His overall appearance was that of a dwarf whose major genetic errors had stopped at his pelvis. His arms, which were also of normal length, almost reached his ankles. They were thick as bowling pins and corded with muscle under a fleece of curling sun-bleached arm hair. When she noted his outsized hands, she shivered involuntarily remembering Smith's attack and his palm which had covered her whole face.

She took an immediate dislike to Malik as a result of his association in her mind with Smith.

At the rear of the van, the clinking and clunking sounds of loading had stopped and a door slammed just as the boat-boy rounded the corner of the vehicle straining to push the cart loaded high with supplies.

"George," Malik called out, pointing to the far end of the sidewalk above the dock, "push it down to the end of the walkway and then pass the items on down to me."

To the clients, "S'cuse me folks, but I'll just help with the loading. Join us when you're ready," and he left them in order to help with the cart.

"Which boat is it, Jason?" Amy asked.

Jason pointed to the last boat at the dock. "See the big blue and white one with the flying bridge? That's it. She's called the 'Saucy Lady'."

"Looks big enough," she commented.

"In fact, it looks to be about the nicest of all the boats. Brigham did a good job of picking her. Captain's a bit of a weirdo, but if he knows the fishing grounds and reefs, we should do well. He looks prosperous enough with all those gold chains and bracelets hanging off him, so I guess he's good enough to satisfy his customers."

"If you ask me, he looks thoroughly dishonest and I'll bet he makes his money smuggling or something equally disreputable," countered Amy.

"Well, aren't you melodramatic this morning... Remind me never to make love to you before breakfast," he joked, "It makes you paranoid."

"Shush, Jason, he'll hear you," and she playfully reached up a hand to cover his mouth.

"I'm not the one impugning his character," replied Jason dancing away sideways from her attempt to muzzle him.

"You're impossible sometimes, you know," she pouted, then sidled up to him and kissed him on the shoulder.

"C'mon, let's go down and check out the boat," he suggested.

Jason took her by the hand and moved off toward the stone steps leading down to the dock.

Two young boys about eight or ten years old were laying on their bellies looking down into the water between a pair of large truck tires fastened to the edge of the dock as bumpers. One had a piece of fishing line in his hand and he jerked on it every few seconds. Amy let go of Jason's hand and went over to kneel beside them.

"Watcha catching, guys?"

Both children turned up shiny black faces full of bright white teeth to see the speaker.

"Stripers, missus. But they ain't bitin'. We don't got no bait," and he pulled up the line to show a rusty hook far too large for the small wrasses she could see patrolling lazily around the submerged portions of the tires.

"Can I try," asked Amy, reaching for the line.

"Yes'm," said the boy obediently passing it to her and then sliding sideways to make a space for her between them.

Amy got down on her belly and Jason watched while she emitted dramatic little shouts and comments each time she jerked up on the line. The two boys laughed in amusement.

After several minutes.

"They're too smart for me. No dinner tonight," she frowned.

The boys sat up and laughed even louder, exchanging knowing glances about the strange white woman.

"Missus, does you eat stripers?" queried one of the boys incredulously.

"Haven't yet and I guess I never will... unless," she paused, now sitting up with them, "I have you boys catch some for me."

The two scrambled nimbly to their feet.

"We kin do it, missus. We kin catch a whole bag full, if you likes!"

Their eyes were shining with excitement at their good luck.

"Then it's a deal, boys. A bag full of stripers for, let's say, ten dollars."

"Ten dollahs," echoed the second boy, his eyes wide in amazement.

"That be too much, missus. We be Christian boys and the honest cost be jist two dollahs," said the first, crestfallen that his conscience and training were forcing him to pass up such an opportunity.

"Back in the U.S. where I came from, the price would be *ten* dollars and I insist on paying that much."

She winked at Jason who was getting out his wallet.

"Besides, you boys need new hooks and lines or I won't have any stripers. Is that okay?"

The boy stared at his feet obviously arguing with himself and silence hung between them.

Amy spoke, "Ok, *two* bags for ten dollars. That's a deal for you and for me."

The larger boy looked up and his face brightened at the solution.

"Yes, missus. Two bags for ten dollahs is ok."

Jason passed a ten-dollar bill to Amy who shook hands with the older boy and gave him the bill.

"What time you come back fer the fishes, missus?" asked the lad.

Amy glanced at Jason.

"What time, darling?"

"Just before sundown," said Jason.

"We be here," said the boy, almost over his shoulder as he started off down the dock toward the stairs.

The smaller boy, who had the piece of old line with the oversize hook, tossed it unceremoniously into the water and scampered off after his partner. She could hear them chattering excitedly. She smiled as she took Jason's hand. "Well, if we get nothing spear fishing, at least we'll have stripers," he quipped.

She took his arm, snuggling close to him. "I'm a great shot with a spear gun. I promise you I'll get you something so big, you won't be able to lift it."

"And if you don't?" he teased.

"Then," she winked and squeezed his arm a bit tighter, "I'll be your slave girl to command as you wish for the rest of the honeymoon."

"Deal!" he said emphatically and turned her toward him to seal the bargain with a quick kiss.

By the time they reached the Saucy Lady, the gear had all been stowed and Malik was waiting for them at the end of the gangplank.

"We've a ways to go, folks. You ready to put off?"

"We are, captain," said Jason, as he held the rope which formed the side of the gangway for Amy to cross.

When they were settled on an upholstered bench at the stern of the boat, Malik climbed to the cockpit and the twin diesels rumbled smoothly to life. George cast off the lines and then leapt, almost gracefully, from pier side onto the gunnels of the boat as it moved away from the dock and turned out into the bay.

A gull plummeted from the sky braking sharply at the edge of the boat's creamy wake. Its head snapped to the side at the nadir of its plunge as it snatched up some morsel and wheeled away toward a distant beach.

"I'm always jealous of such grace and maneuverability," said Jason, noting that Amy had been watching the gull with him.

"Me too. My second favorite dream is when I can soar like a bird and look down at the world from enormous heights."

"*Second* favorite dream?" he echoed.

"Yes... and my favorite dream is none of your business," she answered.

"A fantasy... You have fantasies, Amy? You can tell me. I'm your husband, after all."

She was suddenly blushing, as if he'd been able to look inside her head and steal a glimpse of her private world. "*Everyone* has fantasies, Jason. Nothing wrong with that," she said defensively.

"Then, why are you blushing?" he teased.

"I'm not... It's the sun. Dig into that beach bag for me and give me the sunscreen."

Although he complied and searched in the bag at his feet for the sunscreen, he kept talking. "It's not the sun, Amy. You've got erotic fantasies hidden in your head. I know you do."

He'd found the suntan lotion and handed the bottle to her.

She took it and slid closer to him on the bench and whispered in his ear. "Well, darling, unless I have to do the slave girl thing, you'll never know, will you?"

"Oh, I'll know alright because *you talk in your sleep," he retorted.*

"I don't, do I?" she blurted, truly mortified.

"Yes, darling, you do... A steady stream of secrets." He was smiling.

"Then, I'll sleep alone from now on," she pouted.

"Ok, I lied. You sleep like a stone, silent and solid."

"What do you mean by 'solid'?" and she pulled back from him squinting to look at his eyes carefully.

"It's just a word, darling... Seemed to go well with silent. You're not *solid* at all."

"So, what's the opposite of solid... flabby?"

Jason looked at her in mock disbelief. "You truly love to tussle don't you? I'm going to get a drink. Care for one?"

"Seven-up, please."

The play of the sun on the water brought out an almost emerald hue when it pierced the swells that rose and fell behind the boat. Amy's exposure to the ocean had been limited to two vacations to Mexico and Antigua and yet, she felt such a profound attraction to its power and vitality that it seemed as if there were some profound link binding her to it.

She recalled the awe she'd felt in Antigua when she'd been exposed to the beauty of the undersea realm during her scuba training. She'd literally spent her every waking moment either with tanks on or snorkeling among the reefs. Yet, no matter how many schools of fish, coral gardens or solitary sea creatures she saw, each encounter was an adventure experienced anew.

Despite her teasing with Jason this morning about staying in bed, she could feel her excitement growing at the imminent prospect of once again plunging beneath the waves.

Their diving equipment had been lashed to the side of the boat with bungee cords and she proceeded carefully across the tilting deck to examine it. It belonged to Brigham Landry and she and Jason had never borrowed it before.

A short inspection allowed her to identify the US diver's logo on both tanks and jackets. It was identical to the gear with which she had trained and the familiarity was comforting. Beside the scuba equipment sat a shallow wooden box with slots in the bottom that held the spear guns.

The thick tubular barrels of the guns themselves told her they were pneumatic CO2 weapons. 'Sporasub' in fluorescent yellow lettering along the side of the guns revealed their French origin. She'd need to examine them more closely never having used anything but Champion rubber sling guns in the past.

She hefted one and was surprised by the lack of weight and the comfortable balance and fit of the handle even when it was out of the water. In contrast to the rubber sling guns, there seemed to be no cord attached to the spears which were no more that two feet long. An empty set of clips on either side of the barrel evidently could hold some of the additional spears that now were standing upright in holes drilled in the box's floor. As she fingered the razor sharp spear tips, she heard a lisping voice behind her.

"Missus would like her soft drink?"

Swiveling toward the speaker without standing up, she gave a perceptible startle and saw a flash of anxiety in the black man's eyes. It was the badly disfigured boat-boy proffering a sweaty Sprite bottle, almost timidly. Instinctively aware that her surprise had been generated by the horrific scarring on his face, he turned himself obliquely away from her as he continued to hold out the bottle and it seemed as if he were preparing to flee as soon as she took it from him.

Recognizing his distress, Amy attempted to put him at ease, demonstrating her acceptance of his disfigurement by not abbreviating the encounter.

She stood up and, when she reached out to him, it was to place a reassuring hand on the fellow's shoulder.

"Thank you, George... It is George isn't it?" she asked, looking him squarely in the face and flashing a friendly smile.

"Yes, missus. Me name be George," he answered nervously, again turning his face away seeking to avert his scars from her examining eyes.

"May I please see your face, George?" she asked, gently reaching out with her other hand to take his chin. "I'm a nurse."

The boat-boy said nothing, doubtless being unable to refuse the client's request, but also obviously taken aback by such an unaccustomed reaction to his disfigurement. He passively allowed her to study him with her face no more than ten inches from his own.

"George, come over and sit with me on the bench, if you please," she said, and she turned his shoulder with her hand toward the bench where she and Jason had been sitting.

He complied with only a moment's hesitation. In the years since his accident, no woman had ever taken a second look at him with anything but disgust or fear in her gaze. Now, this white woman was looking at him with a mixture of compassion and interest that he found quite astonishing. They reached the bench and he sat down turned toward her, still holding the Sprite, while she took his face in both hands. She continued to examine him for a moment. Then, using her forefinger, she traced the scar which ran from his sagging lower eyelid to the mutilated upper lip which had been hemmed up by the strictures of his wound into a perpetual sneer leaving half the teeth of his upper jaw exposed.

"An accident?" she asked kindly, still touching his face.

"Yes, missus... a boat, she hit me when I were swimmin'. Many years past."

The scar below his eye was thick and braided, as if a mesh of white twine had been tucked under the skin and sewn unevenly in place. The lack of black pigment and the almost serrated pattern along the scar's edge gave it the appearance of a miniature lighting bolt frozen into flesh. The propeller had also obviously sliced off almost all the flesh of the right half of his upper lip. Where the normal plump convex curvature of the lip should have been, a concave welt of pink tissue glistened, stretched tight as saran wrap across a bowl.

"Can you open your mouth, George?" Amy queried.

In response, the man complied. Amy saw how the scar tissue, where the lip should have been, tethered half of his mouth so that he could open the left side of his mouth fully twice as wide as the right side. As a result, his teeth had been worn down crookedly by years of uneven biting and chewing.

His mouth still open, she palpated the tension of the scar, slipping her index finger into his mouth behind the lesion and between his skin and teeth, to judge its thickness.

"Thank you, George," she said, smiling again as she dropped her hand to her lap.

He made a move to rise from his seat and she placed a restraining hand upon his shoulder.

"No, wait here, please."

Jason had climbed to the cockpit beside the captain. When he heard Amy call him, he came carefully down the ladder and crossed to where she and George sat.

"Take a look at his scar, Jason, and tell me if you agree that a graft should be possible for the lip and one could also do a release of his stricture up here," and she touched the corded scar tethering the lower edge of George's eyelid.

As she slid over to make a space for him on the bench, Jason slipped into the spot she'd vacated and began an examination of the old wound. After a minute of palpation, he spoke to her while still looking at George.

"A flap from the lower jaw could be pulled up to form a new lip and, since he doesn't seem to form keloids, we should be able to ablate the scar under the eye easily. It would take time and work but it wouldn't be too difficult at all. It could even be done under local anesthetic at the clinic. Trang could tell me how to do it if we had good pictures from which to work."

Amy looked into George's eyes which were brimming with emotion. She wondered if his feelings arose from the awareness that someone, seeing his plight, had done something more than simply avert their eyes and mutter some inaudible comment or, worse yet, snicker audibly.

Wanting to help with his confusion, she reached over her husband's shoulder to touch the man's arm in a gesture of reassurance. "George, Jason is a doctor and we think we can help you with a small operation to fix your scar."

She expected an expression of agreement or gratitude, but instead, the man's eyes scampered anxiously between her face and the cockpit of the boat before he bobbed his head twice in an amorphous gesture, thrust the bottle of Sprite into her hand and left them, almost running.

He crossed the distance between their bench and the cabin and disappeared inside without a word.

"Maybe he's afraid of needles," quipped Jason, in an attempt to dispel the whiff of uneasiness the patient's abrupt departure had left hanging in the air.

Amy continued to watch the passageway into which the boat-boy had fled.

"He's afraid of something, that's for sure," she said, shifting her gaze to the captain of the boat who had been staring down at the threesome and who now turned back to his business of steering a course.

To the right of the boat, no more than a half mile distant, long sleek beaches had replaced the cluttered tin shantytowns which surrounded Castries. An occasional black figurine could be seen on the beach but no boats were anywhere near the numerous azure swatches of sea that marked the shallows overlying reefs.

"I'm surprised that no fishermen are on the reefs," said Jason, shading his eyes with a hand as he surveyed the length of sea visible both ahead and behind the boat.

"You spent too much time in the Jacuzzi, darling," replied Amy, giving him a playful poke in the back.

"They got their fishing done early and are already at home having siestas."

He acknowledged her comment with a wry smile and then pointed slightly ahead of the boat to a large light area of sea that must have been almost a half mile in length. "Look at that reef, shallow enough to have curlers breaking over the inside edge and deep blue water on this side. It looks like it might be a wall."

He turned to face her, excitement in his eyes, "Wanna go explore it?"

"Are we near the places you talked about with the captain?"

"No. He told me we'd go north to some place called 'Anse des Anges' then head thirty miles out to where there is a wreck lying in about seventy feet of water off a shallow reef that ripped out the bottom of the ship. But I'm anxious to get in the sea, aren't you?"

"Yes, but what if this place has been fished out. It's pretty close in and the local fishermen must surely work it on a daily basis," she commented.

"So we just take a look, darling. We've got three tanks apiece," he said, pointing to the equipment stash, "and the whole day in front of us. Besides, even if the reef has been picked clean, it fronts onto deep blue and there's gotta be a few sharks and some king mackerel or carvallos cruising by."

She smiled at his almost childlike enthusiasm, unable to delay his gratification for even a two hour boat ride. "Ok, I'm game. I'd like to try out the gun first anyway. I'm not used to pneumatics."

Jason's face split into a wide grin and he headed for the ladder to the bridge of the boat. When he reached the bridge, Amy could see him talking to the captain who took his hand off the helm to stab a finger at his watch then gesture emphatically several times toward the seaward horizon. Jason was shaking his head and pointing to the nearby reef he'd just shown her. There was an obvious disagreement. It persisted for several minutes before Jason come back down the ladder with an irritated expression on his face.

"This guy is unbelievable! First, he told me that this area was a local fish sanctuary and when I said, 'Great we'll get to see things undisturbed by fishing', he contradicts himself by telling me that these inshore reefs have a lot of fish with ciguatera and we'll be in danger of poisoning."

"How would he know about ciguatera being here? You can only get the disease by *eating contaminated fish* and you don't catch fish in a sanctuary?" Amy asked.

"I know. He's lying for some reason and the runty little fart is stubborn. I finally had to pull rank and order him to go to the reef. Even now, he insists we don't use more than one tank here. He kept talking about the monster groupers waiting for us at the wreck."

"Did you make some deal with him about the catch? Maybe he wants to sell it and is worried we will waste air here and get fewer fish."

"That's just it, I *did* make a deal about the catch. He has two fee schedules for the trip, one if he takes the catch and another if we keep it. I thought we'd bring a few good groupers back to Renaissance and then give away the jacks and other stuff we might get to the clinic staff. I told him I'd pay him the higher rate. It was only thirty bucks more."

"So what's the problem? It's no skin off his nose even if we never fire a gun."

"I know," replied Jason, putting his index finger to his temple and spinning it in the universal sign for mental debility, "he's goofy."

"Careful, Jason," said Amy as she reached for his hand, "he'll see you and we need this guy to show us where the big ones are… We've got a wager, remember?"

His eyes lit up. "You bet I do. *'Something so big I won't be able to lift it'*, you said. Right?"

She nodded. " Or I'm your slave girl for two hours."

" Two hours! No way, you said *'till the end of the honeymoon,"* he exclaimed in mock annoyance.

"Alright, *two days,*" she conceded, leaning over to kiss him on the cheek.

He pulled her toward him, nibbled on her earlobe and whispered, "*Two hundred years*".

She laughed, pushed him upright and said, "We're getting close to the reef. Let's get on our equipment."

Within ten minutes, the boat had slowed and begun maneuvering with the clunk of gears and the rumble of its complaining diesels unaccustomed to brief shifting movements as the captain expertly nosed the Bertram's bow into a wedge of deep water between two arms of coral reef only ten feet below the surface. Amy and Jason had had sufficient time to put everything on but their swim fins. They had tested the regulators and Jason was explaining the Sporasub guns to Amy.

"The cord is on a reel hidden inside the barrel. It self-retracts and brings the spear back after a missed shot. This snap-swivel here," and he tugged on a stainless steel piece hidden under the far end of the gun's barrel, "clips over the ring on the end of the spear shaft."

Amy was watching the demonstration attentively.

"How do you reload?" she asked. "I mean, I know how to set the spear in the barrel but how do you get another charge of CO2."

He turned the gun sideways. "See this button here behind the trigger guard. It's recessed so you won't hit it by accident," and he pointed the gun at the deck and depressed the button.

Amy heard a brief hiss and a sharp snap inside the handle. "There, it's charged and ready. The safety lock is in the trigger itself. You have to squeeze once to disengage it, then squeeze again and it fires."

The engines had stopped and the captain yelled to George, who had clambered out of the cabin through a hatch on the fore deck, to let go the anchor. They heard it splash a moment later.

"Want to fire it over the side into the water and see how it feels?" Jason asked, looking at Amy who was examining her gun.

"No, they probably kick like hell if you fire them out of the water," she said.

"Surprisingly they don't. The kick isn't anything like the sling guns."

"No. I'll wait `till I'm in the water," she replied.

Malik was down from the bridge and crossing the afterdeck coming toward them. "Only little fish here, ma'm. You won't need the gun. Just have a look and when we get to the outer reef, there'll be big fish aplenty... S'cuse me an' I'll get the gate for you."

He squeezed past them and unlatched the gate through the stern allowing easy access to the swim platform from which they would enter the water.

The sea was calm and the gentle swells which nudged the Bertram didn't even reach the swim platform on which they now stood checking their dive calculators.

"How deep is it here, Mr. Malik?" asked Jason.

"I read about one hundred and sixty feet before we moved up over the wall which is where you see the water color changing," he replied pointing to starboard.

"Are you ready, darling?" Amy asked.

Jason had already placed the mouthpiece of his regulator between his teeth and nodded vigorously giving the thumb's up signal.

Amy took a hissing breath in through her own regulator, held up three fingers which she dropped in succession three… two... one, and they both toppled backward off the platform hitting the water simultaneously.

Her inner ear blipped in alarm for only a second until her momentum carried her through a summersault and to an upright position just under the surface. She blinked and lifted a hand to adjust her mask and saw Jason doing the same thing. An effervescent cascade of bubbles was wobbling up toward the surface all around him as if he'd just plunged into champagne. She breathed and heard the reassuring sizzle of her air delivery.

Jason was turned her way and tapped his spear gun with his left hand. She shook her head negatively. She'd wait until she had something to shoot at before trying out the gun.

He pointed down and seaward away from the boat's dark shadow which seemed to be lazily scratching itself against a craggy coral head like a bear against a tree trunk. She turned and followed him down the gentle slope of the coral-strewn bottom.

A duo of very large multicolored parrot fish looped hesitantly just outside gun range watching the divers closely. They were territorial, only reluctantly abandoning their turf, and the cautionary distance they kept confirmed that spear fishermen were a known and dangerous quantity on this reef.

Below them several small striped wrasses swirled around an enormous lump of brain coral with convoluted patterns so starkly reminiscent of real cerebral cortices as to suggest that the cranium of some Goliath had been split open and its content dropped in the sea.

Sea fans, glinting either a muted purple or a blue-gray in the ripple-rinsed columns of sunlight wavering down from the surface, seemed to beckon the visitors onward.

As he swam, Jason checked his depth-gauge and read just over thirty feet. Visibility was excellent and he could almost read the date stamp on Amy's tank as she passed ten feet below him skimming the sea bed and pausing momentarily to glance under any collection of coral large enough to hide a lobster. Her mesh specimen bag alternately billowed and collapsed at her waist with her movements and her exhaled air bubbles blossomed from her regulator like silver bursts of paradoxically buoyant liquid mercury.

They were now past the depth at which the snorkeling St. Lucian fishermen, who couldn't afford tanks, could dive and hunt and, almost as if cued by that fact, the number of fish around the coral outcroppings multiplied perceptibly.

A school of glistening fry hung like an undulating ten-foot curtain of silver cloth across his passage twenty feet away. Abruptly, a squadron of about six yellow-tailed jacks burst into his peripheral vision heading straight toward the school of tiny fish which, as if in response to some shouted alarm from a sentry, yanked itself surgically in half opening a fruitlessly empty corridor of attack for the jacks which sped through and then wheeled in a broad arc beyond their prey to charge back. Their course took them above Amy who had been swimming more rapidly that he had.

She had stopped swimming and her outstretched arm holding the spear gun pivoted to follow the group of onrushing jacks which seemed oblivious to her presence.

Just as the fry bunched once more for evasive action, Jason heard a high-pitched snap like a glass rod breaking and the largest of the jacks was driven sideways transfixed on Amy's spear. In his experience, speared fish, even the size of the twenty inch jack, inevitably struggled and bucked when hit. However, Amy's jack gave only one desultory lunge and then began to quiver as it was pulled downward by the weight of the spear. He swam down for a closer look as she retrieved the line and drifted slowly downward.

The spear had struck the fish just behind the pectoral fin, the only place except a headshot that would bring about near instant death. A trickle of dark blood wafted up from the fish's wound like a streamer of cigarette smoke gradually dispersing to invisibility.

He tried to discern the expression in Amy's eyes but he was still a little above her and the sunlight had turned her mask into a mirror. Efficiently, she retrieved the fish and, by the time she'd worked the shaft of the spear back through its body, he had removed the stringer from his waist and handed her the end to thread through the jack's gills.

An empty plastic coke bottle, into which he'd allowed some air from his regulator to escape, was attached to the other end of the tether and would keep it and the fish floating safely above them avoiding both entanglement of the line in the coral or the danger of shark attack if the catch were kept too close to them.

She reloaded the gun and came up to hang in the water opposite him. Now he could see her eyes and they were sparkling with pleasure. He hoped she could see the admiration in his for not only had she hit the rapidly swimming jack but she hit it *exactly* where she had aimed.

He turned again and this time, she followed him.

The bottom had leveled off at forty-five feet and, although the coral heads were scarce and the bottom mostly sandy, there was a profusion of fish ranging from clusters of silvery jack and gray carvallos patrolling between the corral heads, to much larger groupers parked like sentinels outside their coral caves watching the divers with pectoral fins and tails barely moving enough to hold them in position.

Off to their left, Jason saw a fair-sized eagle ray rooting like a miniature dredge for crustaceans in the sand but, when they approached, it bulleted away into the distance suddenly diving and vanishing from view. *The wall.* It was just ahead.

With his pulse ratcheting up in excitement, Jason pumped his legs vigorously traveling along the same line the ray had followed. Amy was almost directly behind him.

The wall itself, so named because of the sheer vertical drop of the seabed where such formations exist, was impressive. Jason was swimming rapidly when he shot over the edge and the effect of suddenly being suspended over a precipice plunging hundreds of feet was tantamount to the sensation of being flung off the top of a tall building during the brief instant before you plummet to your death. He involuntarily caught his breath, froze in surprise for a fraction of a second as he peered into the depths, then briefly flailed his arms and legs to assure himself that he was safely suspended in water and not air. Behind him, Amy was reliving the same experience.

When the shock dissipated, wonderment and awe flooded into the vacuum left.

Below them, the water transitioned from clear to turquoise, then finally to a dark and murky emerald beyond the range of sight.

The same sea fans, corals and marine formations that decorated the seabed behind them now dotted the wall, as if the earth had suddenly been tipped at right angles to its original position. However, despite the similarities, the sheer majestic expanse of the panorama sweeping away on both sides imposed the impression of being thrust into a very different realm where life in a myriad of novel forms flitted and pulsed around you.

Amy signaled her intent to descend the wall but Jason knew that expending time at greater depths here would make it impossible to dive the wreck later that afternoon because of decompression precautions. He shook his head and tapped at the face of the dive computer on his wrist. She held up one hand with fingers spread pleading silently for five minutes only. He returned the signal shaking his own hand to emphasize *five* minutes as he conceded to her supplications.

As she sprinted down the section of wall directly below her she was literally herding a gradually increasing multitude of small brightly colored fish before her as they abandoned their corals in alarm.

Jason remained at the upper edge of the wall watching dozens of butterfly fish negotiate the angle from wall to seabed and back, flitting in zigzagging choreography among the corals upon which they fed. They reminded him of bees in a meadow of blossoms.

Above him about three feet under the surface of the water, the coke bottle float and the trailing jack had found an easy equilibrium of weight and buoyancy. However each time he moved, the tethering line, now tied to his waist, tugged and this action was transmitted upward to the dead jack causing it to intermittently jerk as if badly wounded.

This action had attracted the attention of a patrolling barracuda which now circled the jack high above him.

Intrigued by the interplay, he decided to attempt to provoke an attack by the barracuda since the jack was a poor eating fish and the entertainment would pass the time while he waited for Amy. Carefully he jerked the line teasing the predator which flashed forward jaws agape to stop with abruptness only a foot from the jack. Staring and studying its potential prey, it remained motionless for a few moments and then, its curiosity satisfied, it sped forward again shearing the jack into two neat pieces and sectioning the line as well with its shear-like bite.

The barracuda raced away with half the jack and Jason watched the second half drifting lazily downward trailing a new blood trail. The stringer cord fell even more rapidly and he began retrieving it hand over hand.

From nowhere a small school of razor-toothed Spanish mackerel appeared and began savaging the remains of the jack with darting attacks that in less than a minute left the water clear of even the tiniest particles.

Having enjoyed his interlude, Jason turned again to survey the wall.

Far down to his left a blunt shadow was climbing steadily upward from the depths moving into sharper focus as it rose. It was large, and at first, he thought it was a huge grouper patrolling the wall face but, as it approached, he could make out the half-moon profile of an enormous sea turtle rowing its way up the wall with long lazy strokes of its powerful fins.

Evidently possessing remarkable visual acuity, the beast seemed to spy him from a distance. It abruptly changed course angling out away from the wall so as to preserve all spatial options for escape should it become necessary to flee. Tethered however, by its curiosity, it continued to approach inspecting him now from no more than forty feet away.

Jason pivoted slowly without any sudden movement and continued to watch silently as the terrapin drifted nearer cocking its head a little sideways like a bird does when staring at some object of interest. No more than fifteen feet away, it paused and hung motionless with only the occasional quiver of its fins.

The silent mutual inspection between man and beast persisted with neither moving as Jason imagined that the turtle was staring at his mask trying to process the image of this one-eyed monster through its data banks and finding no match. For his part, he studied the turtle closely, somewhat amazed that its carapace was dotted with barnacles and even had a streamer of green moss trailing from the rear.

Suddenly, the turtle broke gaze dropping its head first, then tilting its whole body downward for an instant before exploding into action and bolting hastily seaward. Below him Jason saw Amy swimming obliquely upward toward him, a large rock lobster hanging motionless in each hand. Her gun had been clipped crossways to her weight belt.

When she was next to him, she held up her arms displaying the lobsters. He reached out to carefully grasp one of the clawless but spiny crustaceans with his free hand and take it from her. Amy pointed in the direction of the boat and, when he nodded his agreement, they began swimming in tandem toward the Saucy Lady.

No more than ten minutes later, the shadow of the hull hung above them, the anchor rope trailing into the depths and a border of lacey fluorescence outlining the bottom of the boat against the silvery ceiling of the surface. Their ascent had been gradual and the limited bottom time meant that no decompression was required.

Amy preceded him to the swim ladder hanging from the platform at the stern of the boat. He saw her lift her spear gun and then the lobster before she reached down to remove her fins and climb from the water. He stood off from the boat about ten feet and surfaced continuing to watch her scramble lithely onto the platform and drop both gun and lobster over the stern of the boat.

He had expected that the boat-boy would be present to help them aboard but he was nowhere in sight. Amy turned and signaled him in with a wave of her hand.

When he got to the ladder she'd already divested herself of the tank and her mask and her face was creased with a smile below the ring of redness around her eyes and nose where the mask seal had pressed against her skin.

"Isn't this great, Jason," she enthused not waiting for a response.

"I got both of those sweethearts from the same crevice. There were several of them in just about every crack in the wall."

He had passed up the lobster to her and she held it up as it flipped its tail vainly in the air.

"What a beauty!"

She reached down with her other hand to take his spear gun and turned to pass both lobster and gun off to the boat-boy who had belatedly appeared at the stern rail.

When he was aboard and had removed his equipment, she passed him the towel she had used to dry herself while George rinsed the gear with freshwater from a short green hose.

"George, give me that hose for a minute," he asked. "I want to wash off the saltwater before I towel down. I hate the stickiness it leaves."

The water was tepid and pleasant and when he'd rinsed his body he took in a mouthful and gargled before spitting it overboard.

Amy hadn't waited for him to towel off before she snuggled close to him, her face sideways upon his chest.

"I'm so happy, Jason. You wouldn't believe it," she purred.

"You're getting all wet again, darling," he said, tousling her hair playfully.

"Don't care a bit. I didn't rinse off so all my salt will stick me to you and you'll never be free of me."

He leaned forward to kiss the top of her head.

"I never want to be apart from you," he whispered before bending to scoop her up in his arms and carry her to the stern bench where he put her down, "except for the thirty seconds it takes me to dry off."

She stretched and yawned, arching her back and pointing her toes as she raised her arms high above her head on the bench.

A moment later he sat down beside her.

"I'm hungry. Think George could boil those lobsters?" he asked.

"They've got a galley but I don't think they can boil water while we're moving."

"I'll ask Malik. He must be up at the anchor," said Jason as he got up and moved toward the bow of the boat.

"George," called Amy, "can you cook us both of those lobsters?"

The boat-boy continued to work at straightening up the diving equipment. He had his back to her and didn't answer. She asked again.

"George, could you come here, please for just a minute."

At that, the fellow got up from a squat and turned slowly to face her. As he did, she saw that his right eye was puffy and contused and his ear on the same side of his head was also swollen.

“What happened George?” she asked sitting up and motioning for him to approach which he did slowly and reluctantly, glancing nervously over his shoulder toward the bow of the boat several times.

When he was close enough for her to touch she reached solicitously toward his face. He put up his own hands to fend her off and whispered in a harsh frightened voice.

“Missus, no go in dee water any more... danger.”

She looked puzzled, then suspecting he was concerned about underwater perils she responded.

“George, I’m an experienced diver and I’m also very careful. Nothing will happen to me... Now, let me see your eye.”

Again the boat-boy avoided her touch, this time by stepping back. He repeated his warning again, “No go in dee water... no go at all!”

Then he pivoted on his heel and hurried toward the cabin just as Jason and Malik came round the cabin from the bow.

“Captain says George can use a small pressure cooker they have to steam the lobster tails for us, darling,” said Jason as he came across the deck toward where she sat.

“We have two hours more sailing to reach the outside reef which gives us plenty of time to eat before we dive again.”

Malik was in the gangway barking orders down to George about the lobsters.

When she felt certain they wouldn’t be overheard Amy beckoned Jason to sit down.

“Something weird just happened, Jason.”

“What?” he asked.

“Well, George is swollen up on his face and ear. Looks like he’s been punched.”

"By Malik?"

"Who else?"

"Well, I don't like to butt in on private business but I'll say something to Malik, if you want."

"No. I don't think that would do poor old George much good."

She lowered her voice. "Remember how I told you he was afraid of Malik?"

Jason nodded and Amy continued.

"He wouldn't let me touch him when I tried to examine his face and twice he asked me not to go back in the water."

"Not to go back in the water?" he repeated.

"Yes, he said it twice."

"What do you think he's afraid of?"

"I thought he just meant I might be in danger diving... but now I'm not so sure." She was still whispering.

Malik's voice rang out from ahead of them. "We best be getting underway now. George is about preparing your lunch."

"Fine Captain," called back Jason.

The Brit climbed to the cockpit and a moment later the diesels rumbled to life.

CH041

Amy took the last scrap of lobster shell and held it above her head teasing the pair of terns that had been wheeling over the wake of the boat deftly catching every morsel she'd thrown to them before it hit the churning water.

"You're being cruel, sweetheart. They can't eat that."

"No, I'm not. Look at them trembling with anticipation so overpowering that it almost drives them to approach my hands."

"And how's that not cruel?" he said poking her with his finger in her belly button as she stretched upward to coax the birds even closer.

She flipped the shell skyward and both birds nearly collided attempting to snatch it away.

"Finished torturing the birds?" quipped Jason.

In response, Amy slid silently away from him across the bench and struck a provocative pose with eyes half-closed and seduction written on her face.

"Have you forgotten already how heady a brew anticipation can be, darling," she cooed.

He began to slide toward her but she raised one bare foot and planted a pointed toe squarely in his chest. "Look, but don't touch... Keep your distance like the birds and concentrate on the prize."

She reached one finger under the strap of her bikini top and slid it tantalizingly down her shoulder allowing the suntanned orb of one breast to peek out from the cloth.

Jason took her foot in his hand and kissed a toe, then wheedled, "Just a little closer, darling."

"No," she pouted emphatically and placed her second foot in the center of his abdomen effectively blocking his efforts to slither past her other foot.

"Use your imagination …Savor what you haven't yet tasted," and she dropped the bra a little lower until the edge of her nipple, like a beckoning eyebrow, winked out for a moment to his view before she slid the bra back up.

"C'mon Amy," he pleaded.

"What are you feeling now, darling? Anticipation?... Want to go back to watching me feed the birds?"

"You know what I want."

She laughed a quick spirited laugh then leapt to her feet and skipped past him to stand at the far rail of the boat, arms outstretched above her, her back turned to him.

Just as quickly, he found his own feet and closed behind her sliding his arms around her, one hand cupping her breast as he kissed her neck.

She dropped a hand backward to tousle his hair.

"Still think the birds were being tortured?" she quipped and gave a little yank on his hair for emphasis.

The onshore breeze that had been present earlier, riffling the water when they had explored the wall, had disappeared now that no land was in sight. The azure expanse of the sea stretched to the horizon as calm as the doldrums and the shadows of mountainous cumulus clouds stacked in towering ranges against the blue of the firmament wandered across the surface like slow moving herds of gossamer pachyderms.

"Does it get any more beautiful than this?" breathed Jason into her hair.

Recognizing that no response was necessary, she lowered her lips and kissed his hand where it lay on her breast.

They studied the scene before them, lulled by the baritone purring of the twin diesels which needed only three quarter throttle to skim the Saucy Lady effortlessly across the slick surface at optimum speed.

"We should be there real soon at this clip," volunteered Jason swinging his gaze from starboard to the endless vista before the boat.

Amy slid around to face him, slipped her arms behind his shoulders and leaned backwards studying his face while squinting against the sun. Then, moving quickly forward, she stopped just short of his face and flashed her tongue out, lizard-quick, to touch the edge of his lower lip before leaning back again. She made a small chewing notion.

"Notice how good that lobster was, just boiled in its own juices? In a restaurant we would have had to have butter sauce, a bit of garlic etc?" she asked.

"Is that what you were after?... A crumb of lobster I had on my lip?" he asked quizzically.

"Just protecting you from the birds, my love."

She smiled as she pecked him full on the lips again.

He smiled wryly in return.

"Sometimes, you really surprise me," he said.

Leaning closer, she kissed him first on the cheek, then above one eye, and whispered in his ear. "If that's true, I hope it never changes."

As she finished speaking the engines suddenly decrescendoed and the Saucy Lady slowed perceptively.

On the bridge, Malik was sweeping the horizon ahead with binoculars, then looking down he consulted the GPS readings and nudged the helm slightly to starboard.

"Are we almost there, captain?" called out Jason.

The Brit looked down and seemed to study them briefly before answering. "Yessir, coming up on the wreck in a minute or two. I'll be setting us off her stern just over the edge of the reef that gutted her."

"We'll get suited up then," replied Jason

"As you wish... About ten more minutes `till we're over her grave."

"`Over her grave'... how cheery," quipped Amy as she headed for the scuba equipment stowed on the opposite side of the deck.

Malik had overestimated and, in much less than ten minutes, he'd reversed the engines and was squinting into the fish finder undoubtedly lining up his position over the wreck of the Brazilian cargo ship that had gone down ten years ago on her maiden voyage, full of frozen beef bound for Antigua.

Malik had told Jason that salvage ships had quickly picked over the ship's carcass and left all the refrigerated lockers open which lead to a two month feeding frenzy of sharks gorging themselves on the beef. That initial effervescence of marine life had been a favorable omen for sport fishing and, after the trolling for the sharks had dropped off, the fact of the ship's cavernous holds all being open had produced a natural fish haven long before the shrouding sea growth had transformed it into an artificial reef.

Too far from St. Lucia for locals to reach and in an area of dangerous reefs that kept trawlers away, it had become a spear fishing paradise.

As Jason was dressing he'd been filling Amy in on the details the captain had confided to him about the wreck's history.

Malik had finally given George the order to release the anchor rope and now had come down to join his two passengers. He wore a wide grin exposing all his gold-capped teeth and, with one ham-sized hand, he was tipping back his seaman's cap and scratching his sweaty forehead.

Amy shuddered inwardly looking at the hand.

"Well, we're here mates. St. Lucia's best spot for spearing trophies. I promised you a treat and here she is, the Maria Esmeralda *sleeping with the fishes*, so to speak," and he grinned again before digging in a pocket of his shorts for a tattered sketch which he knelt on the deck and spread out, smoothing away a multitude of wrinkles. It was an ink drawing of the ship as she lay on the bottom.

Pointing to the bow with a frankfurter-sized finger, he noted, "She lies bow down at about a thirty-five degree angle. Stern's only at about thirty feet and most of the cargo holds being this end, most of the fish are also in shallow water."

He looked up from under his cap at Jason. "However, the giant groupers like a little more depth and the bridge and bow are cluttered with the biggest damn Jewfish you'll ever see."

He poked the frankfurter at the image of the ship's bridge and superstructure. "She's on her side so access to her bow is simple, just follow the deck down. My best advice to ye would be to go down the ship to the bow first while there's air a plenty. Then later, if you're out of air, you can always snorkel down to the stern and still spear enough fish to fill the boat."

Jason, who had been finished his preparations first, was looking over Amy's shoulder at the sketch as her helped her on with her tank and vest.

"Isn't spearing Jewfish illegal?" he asked.

Malik smiled conspiratorially. "We're outside territorial waters here... Anything goes, doctor, and before we tie up at the wharf, George will have everything in steaks and unrecognizable. Your pictures will be private proof of your take. No game wardens here."

As Amy buckled on her weight belt and tested its fast release, Jason was preparing the two spear guns.

"Here, darling, your gun was lucky earlier so I'll take it and you can try the old clunker I had," he joked handing her the weapon.

"You'll need the advantage," she smiled, then winked, "if you're to beat me and don't forget the prize."

"Fat chance," he answered as he shouldered his fins and made his way to the gate leading onto the dive platform at the rear of the boat.

Malik followed him and Amy picked up her fins and was about to follow in his footsteps when she felt a tentative tap on her arm.

Turning, she saw George, his red-veined eyes wide in obvious fright and with a finger to his mouth enjoining her silence. He darted close to her and spoke softly but with urgency.

"No go in dee water, missus!"

He looked as if he wanted to say more but suddenly fear flared higher in his eyes and Amy heard Malik bellow from behind her.

"George, get your skinny black arse below and prepare for the fish."

And the boatboy squirted away like a frightened mongrel menaced by a mastiff.

Amy glanced in Jason's direction but he had already fitted his mask and was settling himself in a seated position on the swim platform.

Suddenly uneasy, she glanced around and met Malik's eyes which seemed to bore into her and she wondered if he'd heard or understood the boat-boy's warning. "Just looking for the message slates... George didn't know where they were," she lied to protect the boy.

Malik pointed a blunt finger at a vinyl pouch at the side of the wooden box where the guns had been stored. "They're in that pouch, miss."

Amy retrieved the two slates and the underwater pencils used to write messages.

She was fumbling to fit the elastic of one slate over her wrist as she made her way onto the swim platform.

Holding one set out to Jason she pointed, "Put this on, dear."

When her own mask was set, regulator tested and a check of the dive calculator completed, she gave Jason a thumb's up sign and slid off the platform into the water, her heart beating rapidly to the adrenaline of apprehension and wondrous excitement.

She righted herself, evacuated a bit of water that the mask had allowed in on her entry to the sea and, still adjusting her mask, took two strong sweeps forward to where Jason was waiting for her six feet below.

She wanted to catch his eye but knew that he could see no more of her face through the Cyclops mirror of her mask then she could of his so, she fell in behind him as he pointed at the stern of the wreck only forty feet away.

Below them on the wreck, the water was clear enough to see a dozen different varieties of very large fish patrolling the stern area of the Maria Esmeralda. Nearer them, and seeking the proximity of the reef, was a truly impressive shoal of sardines that stretched as far to the right as Amy could see and which hung like a glittering undulating curtain from the surface of the sea to the reef thirty feet below. She had never seen such a large school before and she almost gasped in admiration, momentarily forgetting George's warning.

Jason had also stopped and was hanging motionless just taking in the scene. This offered her the opening she needed and she swam up beside him signaling to him to read her slate even while she fumbled with the grease pen on its tether.

She wrote: '*Stay near the stern*'.

'*Why*??' he wrote back with two question marks after the single word.

She swiped the slate clean with the side of her hand and wrote '*must do something*', then looked up at Jason who shrugged and wagged his head from side to side.

Amy turned to look back at the boat then began swimming toward its bow where the anchor rope disappeared behind the curtain of sardines halfway down its length. As she approached, the sardines parted creating a small shimmering cavern around the rope to allow her passage. Jason followed her as she traced the course of the rope to the bottom.

The anchor was a standard two flange design that weighed almost too much for a single man to haul aboard. The Saucy Lady had a power winch to retrieve its bulk. The rope itself ended about six feet from the anchor where it was braided through a coupling attached the anchor chain.

As they got closer to the anchor, the rope made contact with a coral head about twenty feet in diameter and ran along its top before disappearing over one side. Spread across the top of the coral head like large warts on a giant's pate were several bulbous brain corals at least two feet across and set upon sturdy stocks.

Below the coral head, Amy saw the anchor laying sideways on a bed of crushed white coral, its chain coiled across it. The sea being calm, the movement of the Saucy Lady was slight and, although the sardines hid the boat from sight, the rope alternately tightened enough to pick up a foot or so of anchor chain and then slackened allowing the rope itself to touch the seabed.

Amy turned to find Jason right behind her. She signaled for him to take her spear gun for a moment and then, standing on the coral head itself, she picked up a length of anchor rope. As the boat above moved and the rope slackened she deftly flipped a loop into it, which she dropped over the top of the largest brain coral. With the next cycle of the rope's waxing and waning, she slipped a second loop after the first then watched as the coral firmly held the boat.

Jason handed her the gun, stuck his own between his knees to free both hands and wrote *'paranoid'* on the slate. It was Amy's turn to shrug.

Jason retook the lead and went down the side of the coral head to where the sea floor sloped down toward the stern of the wreck. To their right, two large propeller shafts protruded from the ship. The huge brass propellers which had once turned on them had been removed by the salvage teams and now they held only a collection of new coral.

A black grouper about three feet long lay motionless in the water directly under one of the shafts. Amy pointed at the large fish. Her heart was pounding. She wanted to go after it. Jason shook his head and extended his arms fully signaling that the impressive specimen was still 'too small'. He then waved his arm and started down heading away from the shafts to where the edge of the deck loomed in shadow to their left.

They approached the shadowy gallery, guns at the ready knowing that the truly large denizens of the area had already picked up on their presence and would be hiding to assess the threat. You didn't sneak up on a fish whose lateral lines could sense substantial motion a hundred feet away. You shot them either when they underestimated your threat or mistakenly felt they were safely hidden from you.

Jason went first peering intently into the heavy shadow of a passageway along the side of the deck. The gloom extended out about four feet from a metal bulkhead that, because the ship was lying on its side, now formed a ceiling to the corridor which was bounded on the other limit by a railing.

Hanging cautiously with just his head and shoulders into the shadow, he searched for any movement or forms which would betray large fish. Seeing nothing, he gestured with his free hand motioning Amy to follow him in as he glided into the penumbra ahead.

Ascertaining that her weapon pointed downward, posing no threat, she gave two easy strokes of her fins to follow him.

Ahead and above her, she could hear the tinkling of Jason's expelled air bubbles clinking along the bulkhead above them. She watched as several of them shimmered flatly against the metal but most rolled lazily along the bulkhead before slipping out of sight over the slightly tilted edge.

The noise of their breathing apparatus was the spear fisherman's greatest handicap and why so many of the world's best spear fishing enthusiasts had learned to dive to depths of eighty feet or more without tanks and their telltale exhaust bubbles. Amy began to skip breath to reduce her own air noise.

They had proceeded down the passageway about twenty feet when they came upon an open bulkhead door hanging vertically downward. Jason swam easily under it. Amy had passed half her body length under it as well when Jason suddenly lurched sideways ahead of her and a large tubular shadow slammed heavily into Amy's leading shoulder with such force that she was pushed downward roughly into the barnacle encrusted railing below her and felt the neoprene of her wet suit snag, then snap free of the sharp shells.

The large fish, which had struck her, caromed off the door above her before it frantically hammered the water in the passageway with several desperate tail thrusts generating shock waves which struck her in the chest like padded karate kicks.

Although all the action took place in less than three seconds, Amy experienced it as if it were slow motion and, even in the dim light, she identified the fish as a huge grouper about five feet long.

After jolting the door, it had fled into the companionway behind it.

She spun around drawing her legs from under the door then pushed off cautiously to peer into the inky blackness of the corridor.

Jason, who must surely have been struck by the panicked fish, was almost immediately at her left side. He squeezed her arm in excitement then outstretched his own arms to their full extent. Hastily he collected his slate and scribbled '*want to go after him*?'

Amy nodded her head emphatically, then wrote on her own slate '*Flashlights*?'

In the velcroed side pocket of their vests each had a small but powerful underwater flashlight which they quickly disengaged. She reached out to Jason and caught his hand in a gesture signaling him to leave his light off. Then tugging on his arm to follow her, she backed off from the passageway moving away from the ship to the edge of the shadow where the sunlight streamed down from the surface in wavering green columns.

'*How*?' he wrote on his slate realizing that she had already formulated a plan.

She wrote quickly in cramped characters on her small slate. '*Both us in passageway opposite door. Two headshots point-blank.*'

He looked at her and shrugged pointing at his previous message, '*How?*'.

'*Noise. Single spear companionway blind shot*,' then, when he nodded his comprehension she wiped quickly and wrote 'T*hey hate vibration. Use spear line irritation. Shoot when runs.*'

Jason looked puzzled but shrugged his agreement.

Cautiously, she checked her gun and he did the same. She tugged off the detachable tip to check it and then refitted it to the shaft. Finished with her preparation, she stroked carefully back to the passageway.

They positioned themselves, one above the other to the left of the door. Jason was in the lower position. She took off the slate from her wrist and put it with her flashlight stuffing both items in the pocket of her vest. Jason followed suit with the slate but kept his flashlight out.

Amy nervously checked her gun a second time. A five-foot Jewfish could weigh upwards of three hundred pounds. Their shots would have to be accurately placed or their equipment would simply be ripped from their grasps and lost when the fish bolted out of the companionway.

Pointing to her own neck she signaled Jason where he needed to shoot the fish. He nodded.

Holding onto the upper edge of the open doorway with her left hand she pulled herself forward enough to peer down the darkened companionway. She would only have a moment to get off a shot and then another moment to wrap the line from the spear around the large butterfly nut at the edge of the doorway that had apparently served as a latch. She ran her hand over it, then pulled out her knife from her leg scabbard and scraped heavily around the latch shaft removing sharp barnacle edges that might slice through a cord under tension.

Satisfied that all was ready, she replaced her knife, extended her right arm into the doorway and positioned herself for the initial shot. Jason looked up and, on her nod, switched on the flashlight. Its probing beam, like a Star Wars' light saber, sliced narrowly into the gloom.

At first, all they saw was a set of stairs coming up from below deck. The passageway was no more than fifteen feet deep. Jason's heart sank as he imagined that the beast had fled down the stairwell but, as the beam probed higher, a huge pectoral fin broader than a grown man's face quivered in the darkness.

He was there, resting at the top of the short hallway just below the ceiling.

Cautiously, Jason slid the beam from left to right about a foot and a second fin came into sight. He knew that a head shot with these guns would be useless against the bony plates of the grouper's skull. Amy needed a shot well placed into soft tissue that wouldn't tear loose.

She let herself slide carefully downward to increase the angle of her spear's trajectory into the monster's belly behind the bony brace of the pectorals. In position, she gave a nod of her head and Jason directed the beam behind the center area between the fins and the pale cream colored expanse of the belly was spotlighted.

Amy's heart was pounding. If the grouper simply recoiled from the flesh wound and didn't bolt for the doorway, she'd have time to tie off the spear and reload her weapon. Her finger depressed the trigger and she felt the safety click off, then focusing upon a palm-size area on the belly, she pulled the trigger and felt the gun thud back comfortably into her palm. She heard a brittle snap at the same time the spear leapt forward to bury itself haft deep into its prey.

There was a flash of white then black in the light's beam and Amy was buffeted against her face mask by the shock wave of the fish's violent movement. The line sang out from the gun with an audible whir then suddenly stopped. As she'd expected, the fish had retreated only a few feet further back into the darkness.

Jason swung the light onto the door latch and Amy deftly wrapped the cord five or six times around the latch shaft before cutting it with knife and taking two half hitches firmly around the portion of it that disappeared into the darkness. Then, just as dexterously, she pulled out the rest of the cord until it stopped at about six feet in length, all that was left on the internal spool of the gun.

From her belt she extracted a second spear, also with a detached head, and threaded the cord through the ring at its blunt end. Once the gun was reloaded, she tapped Jason excitedly on the shoulder requesting his flashlight.

Taking her own slate out of the pocket she wrote '*Neck shot, darling, don't miss!*' then using the elastic of the slate wrist harness, she moved out to a two inch round metal post that ran from the railing up to the side of the ship and lashed the flashlight in place adjusting its beam to illuminate an area of the metal door just outside the cavern of the doorway. Jason nodded his approval.

They took up new positions now, side by side just opposite the door and midway between the ceiling and floor to permit a shot either slightly above or below them if the grouper burst out in either position.

Once in place, she pointed to Jason's leg scabbard requesting his knife. Holding the knife in her left hand she reached into the doorway and began to rub the backside of the blade along the taut spear cord. Blunt, it posed no risk to the cord's integrity, but it would set up a vibration in the cord that would pass down to the embedded spear causing the grouper to believe it was being attacked again in the same place. In less than thirty seconds of rubbing, the cord tightened even more and Amy would feel the mild turbulence tumbling out of the door as the fish tried to free itself of the tethering spear and line.

Abruptly, the cord was yanked sharply downward and then went slack. Amy repositioned herself two feet lower and Jason also floated down. The cord jerked twice more and then the huge head of the grouper with bulging eyes, gaping mouth and nostrils the size of silver dollars burst into view. The beast hesitated only momentarily and then bolted straight into the beam of light.

Jason saw the head pass Amy and heard her shoot. He held his own shot only a split-second longer until the fish reeled upward under the impact of Amy's spear and when he fired he saw with excitement and satisfaction that his spear had disappeared into the soft tissue just back of the gills.

Blood gushed from the two lethal wounds, which proved to be within four inches of each other, and both ideally placed to enter the grouper's heart.

In a desperate death lunge the enormous fish slashed at the water with its powerful tail which slammed against the passageway door raising a cloud of shattered barnacles and ocean debris and snapping lose the one hundred pound test cord wrapped around the door latch.

Amy, holding fast to her gun, was immediately jerked by her shortened cord after the fish and over the railing. Jason's line had more slack, giving him time to reach for his knife which he had replaced in its scabbard before he too was forced to follow Amy over the railing.

The grouper's desperate flight had carried it away from the shadows into the light and, as Amy trailed behind its momentum, she quickly saw that the spears had found their marks and the fish was no longer swimming forward but was actually falling slowly sideways to the seafloor only twenty feet below.

As it lay, gasping its last, she released the gun and stretched and re-stretched her arm which had taken a beating from the fish while she was trying to get around the door as well as during its death throes. Her gun, under the effect of its buoyancy packet, floated up to hang impotently over the cord tethering it to the spear which had all but disappeared into the side of the fish.

Jason joined her and she reached for his slate. '*A beaut! Good work*!' He shook his head in excited agreement.

After a moment's admiration, they set about with their knives to retrieve the two spears from the fish's side. The minor butchery produced a cloud of blood and, already, dozens of fish were spinning about the bleeding carcass nibbling here and there like sparrows attacking a crippled crow.

As she was refitting her spear tip and returning the tether cord to the gun, Amy heard a sustained clinking noise of metal upon metal. At first, she couldn't locate its origin but after a moment or two of turning her head and holding her breath to extinguish air sounds, she knew it came from the anchor of the dive boat.

What she had feared was happening.

She poked Jason who was still trying to force his spear from the grouper. When she looked up and back to the dive boat and yanked urgently on his arm, he nodded that he understood.

Without waiting for him she swam rapidly upward toward the coral head and the anchor.

From a distance she could see the dust rising from the coral bed around the anchor which was standing on end, the chain pulled taut above it. She thrust upward as fast as possible passing the anchor and could hear the whining vibration of the Saucy Lady's winch struggling to free it. Reaching the top of the coral head, she quickly saw that the largest of the brain corals around which she had looped the rope had been sheared off by the winch's power and only one more coral stalk still held the boat to the bottom.

She swam desperately toward the shadow of the boat's hull, etched on the ceiling of the sea, heading for its stern and shedding her bulky tank and safety vest as she went.

When she was a mere five feet below the twin props, she heard the engines gargle to life and saw the water churn suddenly white as the screws spun into motion and the Saucy Lady moved slowly forward.

Her glottis had started to snap spasmodically against her larynx as the need to breathe jerked at her lungs.

When she broke the surface just behind the boat, the diesel-laden steam of the exhaust bubbled around her. Despite the fumes, she took in a deep breath and, with three sharp arm strokes which pulled her forward, she grabbed onto the last rung of the swim ladder trailing behind the dive boat.

Still gasping from her efforts to reach the Saucy Lady she felt herself pulled forward by the boat. Then, abruptly, the engine hiccupped momentarily before sliding into reverse. Effortlessly, she swung herself up onto the swim platform using her forward momentum as the boat surged backward toward her.

'*He's trying to use the boat to break the anchor free… That's what George meant, Malik was planning to abandon us out here*!' she thought.

A surge of icy realization washed over her and she flattened herself against the platform to avoid being seen over the transom. Malik would be on the flying bridge and if he took his eyes off the anchor rope and glanced backward, as he reversed his engines, he'd see her.

She slipped off the swim fins and peeked over the transom. Malik was at the helm yelling at George whom she assumed was operating the winch at the bow.

"Cut the bloody rope an' do it *now!*"

Amy heard the engines shift again and felt the boat advance once more. She knew she needed to act fast.

Quickly scanning the rear deck, she saw a third spear gun with three spears beside it still standing in the storage box. Glancing up and noting that Malik remained preoccupied with the anchor, she slipped over the transom and across the stern bench to drop silently on her knees beside the spear gun.

The metal of the gun was hot to the touch having been exposed to the sunlight but she ignored the unpleasant sensation and snatched up both gun and spears before scuttling unobtrusively across the open deck to flatten herself against the outer wall of the cabin directly below Malik.

She had to squint to bring the bridge into focus as her eyes had not fully adjusted to the glittering brilliance of the sunlight. Without looking down, she fumbled the spear into the barrel of the gun then tested the trigger to see that there was a CO2 charge in the chamber.

Above her, Malik's tree-trunk leg was all she could see from her sequestered position. Her was cursing at George who apparently finally sawed successfully through the anchor rope as the boat surged suddenly forward unrestrained.

Amy's breathing was fast and shallow and her gun hand trembled perceptively. Her thoughts were racing. Jason was behind and still in the water and she would have to tackle Malik alone. She really had no plan but knew that every second she hesitated the boat was moving faster away from Jason.

She sprang out from her position against the wall and stepped backward to where Malik's full bulk came into view above her. She trained the spear gun on his back and mustered enough courage to yell out, "Malik! Don't move", in the most intimidating tone of which she was capable.

The Brit swiveled his neckless head toward her and looked down with the expression of someone who has just heard the click of a land mine's trigger depressing under their foot.

"Get your hands off the helm and hold them above your head!" she barked.

Malik's left hand slowly opened palm toward her and the surprise drained from his features as he realized what had happened.

"Both hands! High above your head..." Amy repeated, jerking the spear gun upward to emphasize the direction of her command.

The Brit's eyes flickered momentarily, quickly scanning the aft deck before his face softened into a grin.

"Miss Amy, what do you mean? I was just repositioning the boat... The current's turning"...

"I know what you were doing Malik. Now get your hands up and cut the engines or I'll staple you to the control panel with this spear."

Malik's face expanded into a full smile. "And how am I to cut the engines with both of my hands in the air?" he asked as he slowly raised only one hand.

In his surprise, he had pushed the helm to starboard and Amy could see that the Saucy Lady was following a lazy curve to the left at low throttle in the direction of the sun.

She assessed her situation and shuffled back a couple of steps, her feet spread wide for better balance. If they continued to curve they'd move back past where Jason should be by now.

"Lock the wheel. I know you can do it!"

“As you wish, Miss” and Malik did something with his other hand that she couldn’t see and then slowly raised it as well above his head.

The Saucy Lady held her circular course.

“Now, climb down to the deck. Slowly. With your hands where I can see them. Face the ladder and keep your back to me.”

She didn’t want him leaping at her from part way up the ladder.

Although she had an obvious advantage in the confrontation, the Brit kept smiling as if he knew some secret that was tipping the balance of their mutual predicament in his favor. Amy found it unnerving and licked at her dry lips nervously as the captain turned and began his descent.

She was glancing about the deck hoping to find something with which to bind her prisoner but could see nothing useful. Her eyes fell upon the large fish box and she was mentally gauging its capacity when suddenly the boat leapt forward with such explosive force that she lost her footing and was slammed full length to the deck on her back.

The spear gun discharged as she landed and she saw the spear strike the side of the boat at too sharp an angle to imbed itself before it skittered across the deck and ricocheted off the cabin bulkhead below the ladder holding Malik.

Her momentum backward combined with the boat’s forward thrust, sent her skidding rapidly toward the stern, the slick deck as slippery as an ice rink.

Something blistering white detonated in a starburst of incandescent streaks in front of her eyes. She blinked rapidly and the white flash receded into red before settling into a distorted view of the deck that wobbled drunkenly. She’d struck her head with damaging force against the bench that lay across the stern. Nausea tapped at her throat and she panicked at the sensation of fainting which was threatening to overwhelm her.

Lose consciousness and die.

She screwed her eyes shut in an effort to squeeze away the visual distortions and swore loudly as she ground her teeth and grimaced in pain.

When she opened her eyes she found herself lying on her side crumpled against the bench. Malik had somehow managed to climb back to the flying bridge and was staring over his shoulder at her with a maniacal expression, half-grin, half-madness as the boat was now racing forward with both diesels howling like demons under the decking below her.

She fought against the nausea and the boat's force thrusting her backwards into the bench until she got her feet under her and pushed herself up into a crouch. Ahead of her across the deck, the cabin door had come unlatched and swung open. She pushed off with her legs and scrambled awkwardly on all fours toward it, moving with surprising speed.

Almost at the door, she reached a hand out to grab at the passageway sill and, as she did, she felt a scorching pain rip through her upper arm as if she had been stabbed by a red hot ice pick. She cried out but nonetheless drew herself into the passageway just as the second slug from Malik's .38 splintered a jagged hole in the deck from where she'd scrambled one instant before.

'*He has a gun!*'

She began to reach up to grab the swinging door with her right hand but pain clamped like the jaws of a pit-bull on her arm. Looking down she could see a heavy dark red stains against the blue of her wet suit and a small flap of ragged neoprene at the underside of her upper arm bent open under the weight of large dollop of blood, then snapped closed again when it fell noiselessly upon the deck.

'*He's shot me!*'

She used her left hand to catch the latch on the door and hurriedly pulled it closed. Two sturdy-looking deadbolts in steel hasps were located at the top and bottom of the door and she slipped them shut with trembling fingers.

Her thoughts caromed violently about inside her head like dice being shaken in a cup by an obsessed loser desperately willing order over randomness.

Why would he want to kill them?

What did he have to gain?

How could she save herself?

And Jason?

In desperation, she glanced about the starkly furnished cabin. Above her head a dozen rods and reels hung from the ceiling in brackets. On one of two bunks lay a long handled net.

Of no use to her.

The boat lurched to starboard and she slammed into a closet door. Searing pain erupted from her wounded arm and boiled into her shoulder so that she screamed and grabbed at the wounded limb despite herself. Yellow ponchos swung momentarily out of the cupboard door which had sprung open when she struck it. A black rubber boot fell incongruously into the passageway.

Still nothing useful.

He had to be coming. Just outside the door. She winced as she imagined another bullet smashing through the door to bury itself in her chest. She shuffled backwards several steps and a flash of silver in her periphery caught her attention. Above the small galley stove, a wooden rack held two knives, a thick-bladed carving knife and a blunt serrated blade used for sawing. She reached for the pointed knife but her hand was shaking and she hesitated involuntarily.

Knives, as weapons, were too intimately vicious. The wielder had to be prepared to resolutely slash through firm intact flesh to reach the soft organs below and then twist and hack at the victim's vitals if the attack were to be effective. Instinctively, she knew she couldn't do that. She might be capable of plunging the weapon in but, when the warm blood gushed out sticky and pungent over her hands, she'd yank herself away from the gore. It was a mistake she couldn't afford to make with Malik.

She was still staring at the knife, her breath coming in terrified gasps that rasped in an arid throat scorched by fear, when Malik's fist crashed against the door.

She snapped her head back in the direction of the sound fully expecting to see his huge hand tearing through the thin wood of the door panel.

"Open up, miss. You can't escape. Save yourself the pain."

Then to George. "Ease up on the throttle, you black ape, or I'll gut you from chin to brisket."

The boat precipitously lost power and almost immediately stabilized, the howl of the engines dropping to a mere grumble.

A second blow shook the substance of the door rattling the deadbolts. Amy's breath caught in her throat as the screws of one lock hasp sprang out of the doorframe under the force and remained akimbo.

Another thump and he'll be in upon me.

Unarmed.

Paralyzed with fear.

Without thinking, she scampered sideways upon a bunk wishing it were a bed under which she could cower as she'd done successfully several times when a child.

Her barefoot slid into the space between the mattress and the wall and came to rest upon cold steel. She turned and dug her hand into the crevice wrapping fingers around a rod which she tried to tear loose. Four feet of an aluminum handle came free but the far end seemed snagged in the mattress which jumped as she tugged. She let fall the handle and dug frantically at the entangled end. It came loose.

A gaff!

Razor sharp.

And with a handle sufficiently long to render ripping someone in the chest or neck a remote enough action that she knew she could do it.

She glanced about the cabin, then slid the gaff back into place making certain that the point was against the bulkhead and free of the entangling mattress.

Calling out in a voice that surprised her with its calmness, she answered Malik.

"If you promise not to harm me any further, Mr. Malik, I'll open the door."

There was a pause and he yelled something she couldn't understand, presumably to the boat-boy.

Then.

"You've my word on it, miss. Just open the hatch and we'll talk this out."

Amy began stripping off her neoprene wetsuit.

"Just a minute. You shot me and I'm bleeding. I've got to stop up the wound."

Then, picking up the knife, she added as an afterthought, "I'm armed Malik, so don't try anything."

Reaching to the ceiling, she used the knife to strip off a length of nylon line from an overhead fishing rod. Attaching one end of it to the inside door handle of the open closet, she threaded the other end through the crack between the hinged side of the door and the wall and then ran it along to the wall side of the bunk hiding it in a fold of bed covers.

Malik's voice rang out. "I'm sorry I shot you but you had that spear gun on me and I had no choice... Now open the door or I'll break it down and bargaining will be at an end."

Amy approached the door and just before reaching for the remaining viable deadbolt, she pulled down her bikini top on the side of her injured arm, ripping off the strap. With her left breast fully exposed she flipped open the lock, grabbed up the knife and retreated back down the passageway to assume an aggressive crouch beside the bunk with the knife raised. She wanted her face to show desperation and terror which required no artificial effort on her part.

The passageway door clicked open and the Brit's huge head peaked cautiously in. The brightness of the backlight from outside haloed him momentarily in a brilliance that hid his features from her.

He blinked in an effort to accommodate his vision to the shadowy interior. As he saw her at the furthest reach of the cabin armed with only a kitchen knife, he came cautiously down the four steep stairs.

"Stay back," she said… "Stay back," and raised the knife menacingly.

Malik had his .38 in his hand pointing it directly at her belly. As he took in the blood on her arm and the terror in her eyes, a leering smile twisted his lips which he exaggeratedly licked as he studied her nakedness.

"Well, nothing vital damaged, I see."

His glistening agate eyes were lit with lust and Amy could feel them greedily probing at her breast.

"Stay back, I'm warning you," she said again but, this time, she deliberately let her voice vibrate with fear. "You leave me alone."

"Your wound needs tending," he replied never taking his eyes from her breast.

"I mean you no harm. It was an accident. I swear it."

He was advancing slowly, the pistol now drooping and no longer trained on her.

Amy began to cry, a whimpering despairing sound intended to enhance her vulnerability in his eyes.

It worked.

He tucked the revolver into his belt and continued coming. Slowly. Relentlessly. Becoming larger as he approached.

Amy allowed her knife arm to wilt slowly lower as if she were preparing to abandon all pretense of defense. Her knees, however, would not cooperate in the ruse as they *truly* felt rubbery and unreliable. She slid laterally to rest her right buttock on the edge of the bunk in order to steady herself and prayed that he would leave the cupboard door ajar when he passed it.

In Malik's face, she could see the lecherous resolution forming. Rape, then murder.

She recoiled even further sliding her right leg up onto the bunk deliberately retreating from her enemy until she was tucked up into the corner.

She was staring intently at Malik, fixing on his eyes as he came slowly forward when her vision began to blur and his blunt features wavered slowly out of focus. She blinked repeatedly. This was no time to lose control but the more she blinked, the more distorted his features became... and, she realized with surprise… T*he closer he came, the less apprehension she felt!*

From deep within her gut a new churning began. It was no longer the disordered turmoil born of terror but rather a deliberate uncoiling of something animate and powerful that caused her abdominal muscles to tighten and a perceptible flush of energizing warmth to infuse her limbs.

The pain, which had been throbbing in her wounded arm, suddenly ceased and, in the same instant, *Malik's face became her father's face.* His yellow eyes and teeth were the same as she remembered from those nights so long ago. His mouth held slightly open in predatory anticipation.

Amy felt her eyes narrow to menacing slits and her free hand began to viciously knead the cloth beneath it. She drew herself slowly up, sitting straight, her eyes locked on her tormentor.

"You want me, you slime?... Then come and get me." Her voice was flinty with no quaver, no hesitation. Deliberately, almost contemptuously, she tossed the knife to the floor and then reached behind her back and ripped loose the rest of her bikini top. Holding the garment out before the rapist, she challenged, "Come on if you're man enough to take me."

Her attacker, hesitating only for a moment, snatched the cloth from her hand flinging it in one motion behind him as he knelt upon the bunk which creaked under his added weight.

Amy slid her legs down the bed and felt the skin of her back slip along the surface of the bulkhead and down onto the bedclothes. She never allowed her eyes to waver from his.

He bent closer and she could now smell his fetid breath. Resisting a sudden impulse to gouge out his eyes, she instead raised a deceitfully welcoming left arm as her right hand ranged into the crack between mattress and wall, her finger tips brushing the shaft of the gaff.

He was breathing hard now, fumbling with both hands to loosen his belt. The revolver fell from his waistband upon the bed and he swept it impatiently from under him and onto the floor.

Amy waited, the tension in her muscles building almost to the point of discomfort.

He eased his bulk down upon her. One huge hand wrapped itself into the hair at the back of her head and his mouth went greedily to her breast.

She wanted to claw at him, to rip open his skin with her nails and punish his genitals with her knee as he blindly probed between her thighs but again she held back.

Her right hand let go of the gaff and groped for the end of the fishing line hidden in the bedclothes until she found it. She wrapped the line around her hand once and waited until she was sure that his lust had overcome any caution. She yanked viciously on the line and the cupboard door, which had been five inches ajar, slammed shut with a resounding bang.

He startled up raising his trunk off her and swiveling his head to peer down the passageway.

Amy grasped the gaff sliding her hand as far down the handle as possible and lifted it free of the covers and mattress. It hung poised above the thick calf of his leg.

With all her force she pulled down and forward and the four inch hook buried itself in his flesh.

He screamed in pain and pulled his leg sharply to the left which simply imbedded the gaff more deeply. Amy twisted as hard as possible, at the same time levering the handle against the side of his thigh thereby exerting pressure upward on the hooked flesh.

He continued screaming and reached down to clutch at the wound as he rolled off her in an attempt to escape. With her left hand freed from under him, she placed it as well on the gaff handle and yanked upward as she rose to a sitting position. The force she exerted twisted his leg into an unnatural contortion above him where he lay now on the deck. She watched as the buried hook of the gaff tunneled through the muscle and emerged gleaming through the skin of his thigh.

She tasted blood and realized that she had bitten into her lip as she exerted herself.

Retaining a controlling grasp on the gaff handle, she shifted down the bunk and dropped to the deck, taking care to stay well away from the huge hands which grasped vainly at the hook of the gaff where it remained buried in his flesh.

She wanted to get at the revolver but it was hidden under him and unavailable.

Amy suddenly released the gaff and he instantly drew up his mangled leg. When he did, she delivered two kicks in rapid succession into his groin doubling her toes downward to protect them from injury.

He jerked himself into a sitting position on the floor, his eyes wide in pain and his mouth open in a scream. She leaned forward and spat in his face just as his chest bucked convulsively and vomit fountained from his throat choking off his scream.

She turned and ran to the hatchway scrambling up the stairs. As she burst into the blinding sunlight, she involuntarily jerked her uninjured arm protectively across her eyes, squinting as she searched for the spear gun she had dropped earlier. The blast of light searing her retinas was like standing behind a flaming jet engine but, despite the handicap, she glimpsed the gun laying against the stern bench.

Remembering her earlier fall, she scrabbled across the deck on all fours and seized the weapon, pulling frantically upon the cord to retrieve the spear she couldn't see. After two pulls, the cord went taut and refused to release. The spear was jammed somewhere. She yanked in desperation but the cord remained fast.

From the cabin she could hear the bellows of pain and anger becoming louder as Malik struggled toward the hatch.

She considered running to the hatchway and waiting for him to get close enough to kick in the face but he would probably have the gun again. Casting about, her eyes fell on the extra air tanks but they were too heavy to wield effectively even as a bludgeon while hiding at the side of the hatchway. Then she spied the two extra spears standing in their slots. Her heart leapt and she ran the three steps necessary to retrieve one.

Even as she worked efficiently at fitting the spear into the gun she marveled at the energy and resolve she possessed.

She was going to kill him.

She knew it.

And she relished the thought.

No warning this time.

As soon as he appeared he was a dead man.

She knew that the spear risked not penetrating his chest deeply enough to kill him, and yet, a gut shot might not be sufficiently disabling to protect her. A head shot in order to be lethal would have to pass through the thin facial bones of the eye sockets and nose to assure that the spear didn't graze off the rounded surfaces of the thicker cranium.

She'd go for his throat.

The boat had slowed even further and was relatively stable. From close range, it would be a high percentage shot and if she struck him squarely in the throat, the spear would likely shatter the fragile vertebra of the neck and sever his spinal cord high enough up to paralyze him immediately.

She could hear him at the stairs as he hobbled on his savaged leg. One bloody hand appeared on the sill of the hatchway amid a storm of curses and groans.

She quickly crossed the deck playing out the cord from the gun to permit her unhampered movement and took up a position to the left side of the door.

Malik heaved himself up to stand at the bottom of the stairs. His leg, where he had extracted the gaff, burned like the fires of hell and the blood that still pumped from the wound made his deck shoes slide dangerously with every movement.

The revolver in his right hand still held three rounds, enough to do away with the bitch if he could see her.

As he stared at the brilliance beyond the hatch, he knew he'd be blinded when he stepped out. He paused, blinking and squinting. His heart was pounding thunderously in his ears and he felt unsteady, not solely because of the leg wound, but also from the substantial blood loss gushing from his severed leg artery. He didn't have much time.

His mouth was cinder dry and sour even as the perspiration poured off him stinging his eyes. He cursed the lack of caution that had allowed her to ambush him. She'd pay dearly.

What if she were hiding just outside the hatch waiting to strike again as soon as he emerged?

He licked his lips and calculated. Two of his three shots would be needed to guarantee his safety before he climbed to the deck. The wood from which the bulkhead was fashioned was thin. Even a .38 caliber slug would tear through with enough force to mortally wound anyone beyond it if it struck them. Cautiously, he identified two sites on either side of the hatch where a well placed shot would have the greatest probability of striking a hidden attacker. He rapidly fired off two shots, one on either side of the exit, and was rewarded with a cry of pain from the right.

Ignoring the pain in his leg, he pushed off firmly from the bottom step and, at the same time, pulled with his left arm and heaved himself clumsily but effectively through the hatchway and onto the deck. He lost his balance, fell to one knee and, as he did, saw her standing in front and above him.

Face contorted in rage. Eyes green and reptilian.

He swung his gun hand up just as she fired the spear gun.

Abruptly, the world shifted to slow motion. As his arm moved slowly upward, the spear gun bucked and the spear left the muzzle traveling toward his throat. He didn't feel it enter his neck but he was tossed backward, folding at the waist upon his wounded leg. He marveled that there was no pain and exulted that she had missed him... but when he willed his finger to squeeze the trigger, it didn't move... When he tried to turn his head to see his assailant, it didn't turn... When his brain screamed for oxygen, his lungs refused to expand... When he crumpled to lay face up on the deck, eyes to the blazing sun, it plummeted from the sky burying him in a blazing brilliance.

Amy looked at Malik, the spear protruding from his throat. His spinal cord sectioned. His brain firing at seizure speed vainly attempting to animate a body already dead. His life winking out in a frantic fluttering of eyelids.

As abruptly as her anger had exploded, the rage was extinguished and relief and fatigue flooded into the vacuum within her.

Her arm began to throb again and she felt a burning in her left side. Looking down, she saw she was covered in blood from mid-flank to her foot. Numbly, she placed a hand over the wound, watched the blood well up and spill over her constraining fingers, then feeling suddenly nauseous and light-headed, she slumped to her knees and fainted.

CH042

Amy's eyes opened slowly. She'd been ordering them to open for several seconds ever since she'd become aware of voices around her, but the lids were so heavy that it seemed she was attempting to lever up the edge of the world with those feeblest of muscles.

She stared blankly in disorientation at the shadows of two faceless heads hovering over her. Behind them, the tropical sun blazed viciously causing her to squint instinctively.

"It's me, darling… It's Jason," and, even as he spoke, she felt his fingers caressing her cheek.

Jason was in the water. Could they both be dead?

"We're on the Saucy Lady," he said answering the unspoken question she was attempting to form with dry lips. Her mouth seemed filled with sand and she couldn't speak but, driven by the urge to dispel the unreality of the moment, her hand rose and she touched his face. Unless spirits possessed flesh and bones, he was real and *neither of them were dead.*

She closed her eyes in relief and drew in a shuddering breath which she held for several moments then released in a long sibilant sigh.

"Malik's dead but he hurt you. You've been shot in the left arm and a second bullet grazed your side. Neither wound is dangerous and I've dressed them both. The bleeding has been controlled."

She rolled her head toward his voice and forced her eyes and lips to open. "Are you alright?" she slurred with effort.

"Yes, I had a nasty moment or two when the boat left the wreck site but George knew the co-ordinates and returned to pick me up. Said he didn't know what to do with you and had to come after me."

Amy turned to the other shadow which now had a glistening mouthful of teeth and touched George's face as well. He drew back but proffered a green glass bottle through which the sun's rays shattered into a dozen glistening facets.

"Missus must try and drink, please," he said directing a bent straw to her lips as Jason placed a gentle hand under her head and raised it slightly.

The cool Sprite stung where she had bitten her own lower lip but it soothed her parched mouth and trickled, welcomely, down her throat. She swallowed several times and felt immediately better.

"I can sit up now, Jason."

"Not yet, darling. You need to drink more than that."

She smiled at his solicitude. "Jason, I'm lying in a pool of blood that may not all be mine. I *need* to move."

His face, which was visible now that her eyes had adjusted to the sunlight, filled with sudden concern.

"Oh, I'm sorry... I never thought..." and he slid an arm under her shoulders and knees lifting her from the sticky deck. "George, get the hose please and spray the blood off madam's back and legs while I'm holding her.

As he waited for the boat-boy to comply, he shifted position so that Amy's own shadow fell across her face banishing the glare of direct sunlight. He leaned down and kissed her forehead.

"Oh, how I love you... When the boat left and I thought I'd never see you again, I just wanted to give up and drown."

She felt him begin to sway slightly from side to side, rhythmically like a parent might rock a frightened child. There were tears rolling down his cheeks. She sensed a little humor might be in order to reassure him she was rapidly returning to normal.

"Are you certain you still want me now that I'm full of holes and have a blemished boob?" and she glanced down meaningfully at her right breast which was still bare and bore the linear pink scar from St. Lucia.

He smiled through his tears. "You lovable goof," was all he said.

The water from the hose was pleasantly warm and as he shifted her in his arms so George could remove all the blood, she could see the dilute effluent roll in pink sheets across the deck and part around the inert mound of Malik's body. She saw the spear protruding from his throat but, strangely, she felt no connection with the events she knew had led her to dispatch the man.

The dissociation was puzzling.

"George, hose down the body too, then cover it up with a tarp or sheet or something," ordered Jason as he noted her studying the cadaver.

"I'm going to put you down to rest in the cabin, young lady."

A gush of anxiety rose in her chest at the suggestion. She spoke firmly. "No, Jason. Not down there! Put me on the bench and get me some towels so I can cover up from the sun. I think I'm getting badly sunburned, particularly my breasts."

He sat her down on the bench, kissed her again on the cheek and disappeared into the bloody hatchway returning a moment later with a clean bed sheet and two towels.

"I've got some Loracet in my kit. Finish your drink and then I'll get you another. You need lots of fluids."

George was hovering nearby. "A coke, missus?" he asked shuffling his feet nervously.

“A coke would be great, George. Thank you, and not just for the drink. You saved both our lives and we’re deeply indebted to you.”

The praise was obviously disconcerting to the boatboy who had continued to shuffle anxiously and whose hands also began to open and close in a sign of increased discomfort. “Your drink, missus... you need your drink,” he stammered and then hurried away.

She had draped herself in the sheet, covering everything except her face.

Jason was standing beside her with two white tablets in his hand when she finished her task of covering up.

“Let’s get back to Castries as quickly as possible, Jason. There’ll probably be problems with the police.”

She saw Jason’s expression darken.

“Malik wasn’t working alone. I hope no one else is waiting,” he said with foreboding.

* * *

In fact, there were no problems with the police. Jason had radioed ahead asking to have the police meet them at the sport fishing dock. A young Caucasian sergeant, on loan from Scotland Yard to train the local constabulary in detective work, was in charge of a team of three officers. He appeared to be quite competent and within an hour photos and statements had been taken and crime scene evidence collected.

It was no small relief to Amy and Jason that George had not only been able to testify to the events as they had recounted them but also told the officers about the funds Malik had recently received at Barclay’s bank. As well, he told the story of an American visitor, not a tourist, who had discussed business with Malik before they had an argument and the stranger slashed the captain’s hand with “one of ‘em little knives what doctors use fer cuttin' folks..."

It appeared that Malik's local reputation for shady deals and his record of imprisonment for assault with a deadly weapon in Canada, had tipped the balances of justice in favor of a simple self-defense explanation for his violent demise. He had gotten his just desserts in everyone's opinion.

* * *

It was a somber overcast evening with lowering clouds that smothered the stars. The flash and rumble of electrical arguments in the heavens punctuated the soprano chorus of tree frogs that waxed and waned to no discernable tempo. The oppressively humid air was laden with the heavy scent of tropical blossoms unleavened by even the slightest breeze.

"We're in for it tonight," groaned Brigham Landry wiping his brow and neck with a damp cloth as he looked up from his patio chair and scanned the darkness above. Sometimes, I'm surprised that we don't grow moss or mold on our legs down here with all this humidity during the rainy season."

A large cockroach scuttled over the top of Amy's bare foot under the patio table and she instinctively jerked her leg away then winced in pain as the flank wound rebelled against the movement.

"Are you alright, darling?" Jason asked, noticing her discomfort.

She managed a wan smile and touched his hand. He could see the swatches of weariness painted under her eyes. They'd been discussing the events of the day with Landry for the past two hours. Much of their discussion had been pure speculation since the facts were scarce but they all agreed that Malik had no motive to act on his own in plotting their murders.

From George's testimony, it was obvious he'd been paid to kill them and the likely candidate for his accomplice was the unknown American the boat-boy had mentioned.

Tomorrow, the police would search the immigration records for the past two months looking for the names Amy and Jason had supplied to them but it was a low probability activity. Passport control was lax for tourists and Jason knew, from personal experience, that an American twenty dollar bill could become the equivalent of photo ID at the airport.

Otherwise, the money trail from the wire transfer to Barclay's bank (they'd learned that same afternoon that Malik had received fifteen thousand dollars three weeks earlier *and* he'd already spent the bulk of it) was the firmest and *only* other lead.

"I know you are busy with clients, Brigham," said Jason, "but any influence you could exert with the locals at the bank in tracing the origins of Malik's funds, would be a big help. We'll be gone by this time tomorrow."

"I'll keep the pressure on, Jason. The local police tend to follow an 'out of sight, out of mind' policy with crimes involving foreigners but your case is high profile because of the attempted murder and Malik's death. They don't want unfavorable press. And besides, that young British sergeant was impressive. I think he'd like to use your case to teach from and he's got all the resources of Scotland Yard at his disposal to track the money."

"We don't want anything in the press either. It would tip off the American. We only have a few days as a window of opportunity within which to do our own digging back home before he learns of Malik's failure."

Amy broke in, "I'm sorry guys but not even your charming company can keep me awake anymore. I hurt everywhere so I'm going to take a Xanax and limp off to bed before I fall off this chair."

The two men stood simultaneously and Jason took her arm.

"C'mon, darling. It's time to check your wound anyway."

"I apologize, Amy. Didn't realize how badly off you were," explained Landry as he moved a chair from her path to facilitate the short walk to the bungalow.

*   *   *

"The stitches in your side aren't leaking and the oozing from the arm wound has apparently stopped. Are you nauseous?... You look very pale."

"It's not the pain. I don't think the erythromycin agrees with my stomach."

"Maybe you should eat something."

"I couldn't. I'd vomit for sure."

"Just a mouthful... half a banana maybe?"

"Stop talking about food, please. I'm going to upchuck if you don't," she pleaded.

"A cool cloth then for your forehead?"

"That would be nice, thank you."

She'd been sitting naked on the side of the bed while he examined her wounds and now she stood while he dropped a light nightdress over her head. She lay back on the bed with a sigh and he could see her staring vacantly at the slowly turning blades of the ceiling fan.

He shut off the lights and turned up the fan until he felt the air from it stirring the hair on his forehead. He was about to lie down beside her when he realized he'd forgotten the cool cloth.

"Oops! Forgot your cloth."

She reached up and took his hand. "The cloth doesn't matter, darling. Please lie down. I need to talk."

"You need to sleep. Besides, you've taken the Xanax," he countered.

"No. I need to talk, Jason... I killed a man today."

"He was a monster, Amy. It was him or us. You saved our lives."

She pulled on his hand. "Lie down, please, and just listen."

He complied and joined her in watching the shadowy blades whirl above them.

A puff of breeze tossed the flimsy curtains of the open balcony inward and the smell of imminent rain went swirling about the room mixed by the fan.

"I never told you, Jason but you deserve to know. My stepfather molested me when I was a child. It went on for years until I could escape."

Her voice quavered with emotion and, although she stopped speaking, she was listening acutely for any telltale reaction from him. A sudden intake of breath. A comment... She heard nothing.

She was about to put her hand upon her belly in a gesture of self-soothing but, as she lifted her hand, he took it gently in both of his and placed it palm down on his own bare chest.

Thus encouraged, she began again. "I learned to hate him. I wanted him gone. Dead. I finished by wanting to kill him myself and then, several months ago, *I almost did kill him.*"

She paused, but he said nothing and only pressed her hand more tightly against his chest. She could feel the steady, regular beat of his heart and wondered if perhaps he'd placed it there so she could monitor his reaction to her confession.

"If my mother hadn't stopped me, I'd have blown his head off... and I'm not sure where I'd be now. Probably in prison."

Suddenly a hissing crack of lightning lit the room for several nanoseconds and a deafening clap of thunder followed almost immediately. Amy startled so sharply that she cried out and sat bolt upright.

Jason put his arm around her shoulders and lowered her back down to the bed.

"It's alright, darling. Just a lightening strike. Struck very close, but nothing more," he soothed.

Then he took her hand to place it again on his chest.

A violent gust of wind, strong enough to invade the room and smother the ceiling fan's efforts, blew a vase off the small table near the window and it crashed to the floor.

Immediately, the sky opened and the din of a million driven drops reverberated like a timpani roll across the tin roof.

Jason began to sit up.

"I'll close the shutters."

"No, please. I love storms. The lightning startled me but I'm ok now. Nature's turmoil fits right in when I'm talking about my childhood." She raised her voice to be heard over the noise of the storm.

A tree limb cracked in the distance with the sound of a rifle shot.

"When I attacked my father, Jason, I really lost it. It's hard to describe but I became like a savage animal. If I could have torn out his throat with my teeth, I think I might have tried. At the time, it was all happening, doing something as bizarre as that seemed ok to me... As if it were supposed to be like that. But afterward, when I thought about it, I was terrified."

"It wasn't so much what I actually did to him because that was just assault.... minor payback... But what scared me was what happened *inside me, what I became when I was enraged*. Can you understand that?"

She waited again for a reaction but he still said nothing. His heart rate under her hand remained steady and unchanged.

Lifting her head from the pillow, she saw that he was still staring at the fan. While she was still studying him, he turned to face her and peered deeply into her eyes for several heartbeats before leaning over and pulling her face down to kiss her.

She sank back onto the pillow and began again.

"Today, when Malik was trying to smash his way into the cabin, I had a kitchen knife and the gaff. I also had a rational plan. I was terrified but

I knew, that with my breasts in full view, I would be able to distract his attention and then attack. But when he started coming at me something snapped inside me again and suddenly I was filled with the same crazy blind rage. It was instantaneous."

And she snapped her fingers to illustrate.

"Just as quick as that and I had no more fear... In fact, I wanted to go right at him tooth and nail. I even threw away the knife! I had to really hold myself back. It was exactly like it had been with my step-father."

She paused and Jason spoke. "I can understand all that, Amy. The reasons for what happened aren't all that hard to decipher."

"But that's not all Jason. There's something even more unbelievable."

"Tell me. Please."

Amy hesitated.

"You'll think I'm crazy, Jason. I know you will because I think it myself when I remember what I saw."

"I promise you, no judgments. I just want to hear and try to understand."

She could feel her face flushing with something akin to, but more potent than, embarrassment. She blurted out, "Malik became my step-father."

"He what?" asked Jason raising up on one elbow.

"Malik's face... it became my father's face. And it stayed that way all the time we struggled in the cabin. Even afterwards."

She stopped speaking and her eyes began to fill with tears.

"When I shot him with the spear, *I was killing my father, not Malik*. And when I did it, I was *absolutely insane*."

Suddenly, her voice broke and she began to sob uncontrollably, hiding her face in her hands.

Jason slid an arm under her shoulders taking care to avoid her wounds and pulled her close to him while she continued to cry. After several minutes, the violence of her emotions began to subside.

Outside the balcony, the air had been washed clean and freshened by the storm which had passed quickly offshore and was now rumbling away into the distance over the bay. The tree frogs seemed unsure that it was over however, and only a few scattered peeps and the dripping of water falling from leaves punctuated an eerie silence.

Jason began to speak. "Amy, now I have something that I should tell you."

He continued to hold her but now she could feel the tension in his body increase. "It's about *my* father."

Amy stopped sniffling and did her best to make out his features in the semidarkness.

"He was an abusive alcoholic. He beat my mother and he also beat me, regularly. I hated him and I wanted him dead. In fact, I guess we both felt pretty much the same about our fathers except I don't remember wanting to kill mine. Oh, I wanted him dead alright and hoped he'd be killed by a mugger or die in an accident but for some reason, I've always been terrified by the idea that I might kill someone."

Amy shuddered and Jason held her tighter.

"I still have a dream... more a nightmare than a dream, really. It's about me having killed a man. I never see his face but I always end up burying him in the garden of the house where I was raised. It's horrifying and, every time I have the dream, I have to tell myself during the whole next day that it was just a dream, that I am not a murderer."

He stopped suddenly and she could feel the rhythm of his heart against her cheek accelerate sharply. He began to nervously drum the fingers of one hand on her back, as he held her.

When he started to speak again, his voice too quavered with emotion. "*But maybe I am... maybe I really am a murderer.*"

The tree frogs had begun their chorus again and he paused speaking but continued to hold his wife in his arms. Tears rolled silently down his face.

"My father died while I was still very young. He fell down a fight of stairs in our home. Broken neck. My mother always told me he was drunk and stumbled. But someplace buried in my brain, deep down in there with my dreams and such, I think I remember that he was beating my mother and that I pushed him down those stairs."

"*I think I killed my own father.*"

"I think that's why I never see the face of the man I bury over and over again."

Amy pushed herself away from him and took his face in her hands. He seemed to be staring through her at some scene of horror recorded in the past and being played out in the darkness beyond her.

"Jason, you don't really know that that's what happened. Children tend to cover themselves in guilt when they're truly innocent. I know that for a fact."

His eyes refocused and he locked them on hers. Speaking slowly and deliberately he said, "I may not know it here," and he touched his index finger to his temple, "but in here," touching his finger to his chest, "In there, there's *no doubt at all.*"

And he looked through her again, his gaze drifting slowly back into the past and its attendant horrors.

There were several minutes of silence and immobility where nothing but the fan moved in the room. Jason spoke up first emitting a deep profound sigh before he re-imposed a measure of reality on everything by clicking on the bedside lamp and smiling genuinely at his wife. His voice had returned to normal.

"And there we have it. *Our lives uncovered at last.* Not pretty, I admit, but they are *our* lives and no one else can live them for us."

Amy wanted to believe he was right, wanted to believe a light could just be snapped on and everything would return to normal but she needed reassurance.

"What about my psychotic breaks, Jason. I really was insane. You're a doctor. What do I do about them?"

He took her by the shoulders with both hands, stared for a moment into her eyes as if to emphasize the importance of what he was about to say, then raised his lips and kissed her on the forehead.

"Thank God you had those episodes, darling. They're the absolute proof of your sanity just like my disturbing nightmares are evidence that I'm quite sane, too."

Amy looked puzzled. "I don't understand."

"I guess a lot of people would call my logic simplistic but I can't help that. I need some way to deal with stuff like this and, after all the thinking, this is what I'm left with. It's really quite simple. Sane people don't kill others. They can't by definition. But there are times when evil people need to die, or rather, they need to be *killed.* If they're allowed to live, they will kill good people. So sane people, on rare occasions only, are permitted moments of insanity during which they do what needs to be done and what could not be done if they remained sane... and that's it. Understand?"

The bewilderment drained slowly from her face, was replaced for a moment by pure blankness which soon gave way to a smile.

"I sure hope your explanation is right, darling."

"I'm sure psychiatrists would disagree with me. They seem to thrive on dissecting human suffering and, paradoxically, they make it all harder to bear. I've done it their way for most of my life and that kind of agony is completely disabling. I've just decided to see things differently. *I am who I am. I've done what I've done and the past can't be changed* but my attitude toward it sure can."

Amy smiled at him. "How long do you think you can maintain this new healthy attitude?"

It was his turn to smile wryly. "Well, at least for a week... Now, if you'll share one of your Xanax with me, we both could use some sleep."

CH043: ALBANY, GEORGIA

No more *time to screw around. Someone is trying to kill us.'*

Jason was back in Albany. Amy slept quietly beside him and he was sleepless... *again.*

He needed an immediate plan of action and, as he'd worked through recent events, his thoughts had become a confusing mélange of possibilities. Normally, he liked to be certain of his options and carefully select only those that withstood intense and prolonged scrutiny but there was no longer enough time for that.

If West were behind the attempt on their lives, and he seemed to be the logical choice, he was desperate enough to try again soon.

Amy stirred and Jason, who'd been sitting with his back against the headboard of the bed, turned to look at her. His heart filled with softness as he realized again what she had come to mean to him. The possibility of losing her was unthinkable and the depth of his attachment to her was the precise measure of his vulnerability. West wouldn't miss that. Kill her and Jason was finished.

He was going to have to deal definitively with West. It wasn't a choice any longer and, if he had to kill him, he would.

* * *

Apparently West was unavailable. Jason had done some calling around before he ended up later that morning at the anesthetist's office. Roger Atkins thought he'd gone to Chicago but he wasn't certain and West's secretary, Sheila Clark, wasn't letting on if she knew his whereabouts. She remembered the Fish Factory incident.

Roger briefed Jason on the events that had transpired during his absence. It seemed that West had called a partners' meeting for Thursday, still two days off, and Roger thought he intended to test the waters about the CHC takeover again. If there was a substantial division of opinion among the partners, he believed that West was ready to propose the dissolution of TurnerWest.

"What would he gain from that, Rog?"

"Brinkmanship. He ups the ante and changes the alternatives. It's no longer CHC or continue business as usual, but it becomes 'join CHC or accept a striking decline in the status quo as TurnerWest disappears and we all lose what we've worked for years to create.'"

Atkins paused. "It may work in his favor, Jason. It would be about the only argument that could push me toward the merger."

"Do you think he could convince enough partners to split and leave with him?" asked Jason.

"CHC money again. He's got a pile of shekels to spend on new equipment, new building etc... and that's not counting the hidden inducements he'd be offering."

Jason swore and Roger raised his eyebrows.

"First time I've heard you sound off like that, Jason."

"I apologize, Rog, but this place has been a big part of my life and that prick seems determined to trash everything of importance to me."

Shaking his head and kneading a right-handed fist with the fingers of his left, he was walking in a small circle staring at the carpet in Roger's office.

"What are you going to do?" asked Roger, obviously concerned.

Jason didn't answer immediately but kept pacing round his circle. When he did raise his eyes, he stopped walking and pursed his lips, still shaking his head. "Rog, you don't need to know. I mean, I trust you implicitly but you need deniability."

"Deniability?" Atkins looked puzzled.

"Uhuh."

"That doesn't sound good, Jason."

"The time for pussyfooting around is past, Roger... Look, you're a good friend and we've come a long way together but, for the moment, you can't help me anymore. I appreciate what you've done... Thanks," said Turner, extending his hand and the two men shook before parting.

Atkins looked taken aback by what was happening but seeing determination in Jason's face, he knew better than to try and argue.

* * *

The sun was high and strong, bleaching the color out of the grass and foliage. As he stepped out the door to the parking lot, Jason was ambushed by a blast of torrid air that fell over him like a suffocating shroud. Its assault irritated him and he swore in retaliation as he walked, then uncharacteristically, he spat on the sidewalk in front of him.

Two lab techs in tired blues smocks were chatting while they ate at one of the lunch tables under the protective boughs of a nurturing pecan. He'd been speaking loudly and they heard him curse. Looking up, they stopped talking to watch him pass by as if he were a mumbling psychotic caught up in some private hell they could only guess at. One of them hunched her shoulders and raised her eyebrows in a gesture of incredulity at seeing their CEO indulge his passions so crudely. Jason saw them, recognized both, but didn't acknowledge their presence.

Getting into his BMW where the oppressive heat renewed its attack on him, he struck the steering wheel hard with the heel of his hand when the engine didn't fire up immediately. The revolver in his ankle holster had been chaffing and he impatiently ripped open the Velcro fastenings and bounced it onto the seat beside him.

Glancing at the side view mirror, he floored the vehicle in reverse causing the front tires to squeal as the car shot out of the parking slot like a thoroughbred from the starting gate, then slewed around in a vicious arc. He hit the parking lot exit at twenty-five miles per hour causing a UPS van to do a nose plant behind him as he careened onto Jackson Street headed nowhere. In his haste and agitation, he didn't notice the blue Astro minivan slip from the parking lot into the traffic behind the truck he'd just cut off.

Jason had often experienced short bursts of anger. Like summer storms, they could be fierce but they'd always been mercifully brief and, afterwards, level mood had been quickly re-established. He'd been forced, at times, to shore up relations with people he'd offended but he was sincere in his apologies and damage control had been a relatively simple matter.

However, this swing in mood was very different. The corrosive sentiments that had been sloshing around inside of him like acid in a beaker had been eating away at his restraint for three days now. The angry irritability that gnawed at him never subsided for more than an hour at a time and the baseline level of his rage was rapidly rising like storm waters in a sewer. It was as if some gruesome imp from hell had infiltrated his psyche during an unprotected moment and was stoking a conflagration in the nether regions of his mind that threatened to destroy him and anyone who became the target of his wrath.

Jason pounded his fist into the empty seat beside him for no particular reason and his .38 bounced onto the floor. With Mark West unavailable, Jason's aggression had no clear outlet.

A default solution occurred to him. He'd go to the old quarry west of town. It was an unofficial shooting range and maybe he could siphon off a measure of the poison brewing inside him by blasting away at tin cans. There was a box of ammo in the trunk.

The light changed and he floored the car through the intersection with screeching tires headed west.

CH044

The abandoned stone quarry was about five miles out of Albany off old Georgia number 3, the two lane blacktop which meandered through pecan groves and irrigated fields with the occasional farmhouse set back from the road. The quarry itself was at the end of an abandoned dirt track a half-mile within the old Riverside Plantation, a four thousand acre tract owned by northern interests.

Unlike many working or restored plantations that survived on agriculture or by staging bird, deer or wild boar hunts, the Riverside land was untended and largely unvisited except for a few folks who regularly poached bass, brim and catfish from its ponds or shot cans at the quarry. No one would bother him there.

Jason had opened the sunroof and rear windows of the BMW. The air that boiled into the vehicle as it bore south at ten miles per hour over the speed limit was heavy with the scent of pecan and pine. He was absorbed in thought.

Flashing headlights sparkled in the rearview mirror and he could see a blue van obviously wanting to pass. "Idiot, I'm already doing sixty-five," he muttered but he slowed down, pulling slightly right as he rolled down his window and waved the guy forward.

The van had overtaken about one third of the BMW when a horn behind him began blowing with a sustained blast. Jason could see a dark green Explorer with tinted windows and blowing its horn coming like a bat out of hell up behind the van.

"*Two* idiots!" he said to himself and, feeling a surge of increased irritation, he stomped down on the accelerator intending to keep the other two vehicles behind him.

Just as he accelerated, the van slammed into the rear section of the side of his vehicle and the glass of the rear window exploded as a shotgun roared out the open side door of the Astro.

Instinctively, Jason ducked and the BMW's right front tire hooked the gravel shoulder yanking the vehicle crazily to the right and down into a grassy swale that ran the length of an extensive pecan orchard beside the road. The van surged past above him as he rode the bucking steering wheel which lashed first right then left as he slalomed along the slopes of the swale, his front bumper mowing down scrub bushes and wild flowers.

If he rode up over the right embankment, it would be impossible to avoid hitting one of the three foot diameter pecan trunks. Certain sudden death.

On the other hand, braking on the grass would simply flip him into an equally deadly spin in which his vehicle would likely roll multiple times churning him into hamburger at this speed. He had no choice but to ride out the madness until he could regain control, get back on the hardtop and *put a bullet in the brain of the shooter in the van.*

Clods of dirt gouged from the swale's sides and tufts of decapitated shrubs caromed off the windshield as he spun the wheel but, with each crazy gyration to left and right, the vehicle was rapidly slowing.

The Explorer too had flashed past him on the highway.

It seemed like long minutes but, in less than sixty seconds, he had regained control of his vehicle and now he was accelerating carefully along the curving bottom of the swale. Every hundred yards or so there were well-worn tracks that crossed the swale at right angles made by farm vehicles servicing the orchard.

'My tires would grip on the dirt'.

At the next crossing, he pulled the BMW steering wheel left and gunned the engine. The rear tires shot plumes of grass and dirt from under them as he climbed the bank then hit the asphalt with twin puffs of tire smoke and two hearty chirps.

Back on the road, he accelerated after the two vehicles now racing side by side a half mile ahead of him.

The Explorer had claimed the left side of the roadway and, as the heavier vehicle, was taking the offensive in a slamming match obviously intended to drive the van off the road.

Jason had his foot to the floorboard and the BMW was gaining on the dueling pair. When he was only a hundred yards back, the van's tires hit the gravel shoulder just as the explorer struck it broadside. It left the road and shot forward above the swale, momentarily airborne. Tilting perceptibly rightward, the front corner drove into the earth on the swale's side and, immediately, the Astro was launched into the air end over end. It cartwheeled twice before the body of a man was flung like a piece of debris out the side door.

The victim began a deadly high-speed ballet in which he careened across the stage of the orchard, slamming and bouncing off the earth, a doomed puppet in the hands of a crazed puppeteer. With each vicious pirouette his limbs became increasingly disjointed, mocking anatomy and nature as he transitioned from human being to limp rag doll.

The van he'd left continued a violent series of sideway rolls until it came to an abrupt halt as the roof slammed into a pecan trunk just behind the driver's seat and the body of the van pivoted partially around the tree. A very large limb fell in slow motion onto the vehicle's side, as if the tree were retaliating in rage against its mechanical assailant, pinning it to the ground.

Ahead, the Explorer's wheels locked in perfect synchrony in a smoking screech that carried it down the road leaving two lengthy black traces indelibly etched in the asphalt.

Jason had braked even earlier and stopped fifty feet behind the smoldering wreck and opposite the grotesquely distorted body that now lay unceremoniously at rest in the ditch. The man was bent perfectly double with his back in a fatally unnatural extension.

He leapt from his car after grabbing up his revolver and raced down the side of the swale knowing in advance what he would find.

The skin had been flayed from the right side of the man's face by the friction of repeatedly striking the ground. Small twigs and pebbles lay embedded in the exposed muscle like some macabre garnish on a sacrificial victim. An ivory shard of mandible protruded from the ruptured flesh and the upper plate of a set of dentures stuck out of the mouth as if he'd been trying to swallow them when his life had been rudely snuffed out.

The man's heart had stopped beating and blood was only oozing, without pressure, onto the remnants of a white T-shirt which lay under the head of the corpse and stretched out behind it like a ludicrous miniature Superman's cape. The victim's eyes were ratcheted open in the astonished stare of those who meet death unexpectedly.

Jason knelt, fingered the pulseless carotid and lifted the T-shirt over the man's shattered features. No bullet would be necessary to exact revenge against this assailant.

Ahead and above him on the road, the driver of the Explorer had left his vehicle and was standing behind it.

Jason yelled, "Hey, you!" and the man ducked and ran back around his vehicle which then roared away down the highway, the gears changing audibly as the engine surged. Jason had been able to see only that, like the victim in the ditch, he was Caucasian, of medium build and appeared to be balding.

Jason ran forward to the crumpled van which sizzled as if there were a pancake griddle working away in the mangled machinery where the engine had been. He could smell burning oil, gasoline fumes and the acrid heavy scent of warm blood and freshly punctured viscera that only a physician would recognize.

The van had come to rest on its side and the driver's position was now at the top where a human arm clad in a suit coat sleeve could be seen hanging over the edge. Blood dribbled vigorously down the hand dropping almost in a stream from the fingertips. His heart was still pumping.

Jason approached cautiously going first to the back of the van where the rear doors had been. The doors themselves lay scattered in the bottom of the swale behind him along with the rear bumper and a front wheel with the rack and pinion apparatus still attached. He didn't know how many men had been in the vehicle and they had tried to kill him. He'd take his time.

Remnants of seats lay helter-skelter in the rear compartment but the man slumped in the driver's seat appeared to be the only other occupant. He could hear him moaning. As he crawled in through the back of the vehicle shoving debris aside to get to the driver, he heard him cough throatily twice then call out feebly,

"Help me, please."

The man was black and large. He must have stood six feet four inches before his back had been broken and his legs bent grotesquely under the seat where he'd been sitting. He was fat as well and, as he got closer, Jason could see the fish-egg globules of yellow adipose tissue bulging from a gash in his cheek.

"Help me please."

Jason was surprised at the anger he still felt.

"Only if you help me, you prick. You deserve to die."

The man's head, which had been lolling to the side against the still intact shoulder belt, turned slowly toward Jason. One eyeball appeared sunken and had surely been punctured but the other eye blinked and the lips parted.

"Help me, please, mister... I'm only the driver."

"You still need to pay for almost killing me."

Jason's voice was hard and he now extended his arm with the .38 in his hand. Placing the muzzle against the man's temple, he drew back the hammer.

As if he hadn't recognized the weapon until it was cocked, the man reacted with obvious alarm. His remaining eye sprang wide open and he began to plead with a bloody froth bubbling from between his lips.

"I'll put you out of your misery quickly unless you tell me who sent you to kill me." Jason was yelling

The man stammered, "The doctor... it was the doctor..."

"Dr. West?" asked Jason pushing the barrel hard against the man's head.

"Yes… the tall doctor… Mark West."

"Good. Now tell me where he is and I'll call an ambulance."

"He's at the lodge where he hunts... Somebody tried to kill him yesterday... He's hiding at the lodge."

Jason knew where he meant.

"He's alone?"

"Yessir… alone… the ambulance now… please, mista."

“Alright. I’ll call the ambulance but you say nothing about me. Understand?”

And he jammed the gun against the man’s head even more forcibly.

“Yessir... yessir. Nuttin’ ‘bout you.”

Jason crawled back out of the van and up to his car. No vehicles in sight on the little traveled road. ‘*Good*.’

He was gritting his teeth so viciously, as he sped away, that his voice sounded deformed when he placed the 911 call.... It was a formality. The driver’s guts had been heaped like a steaming pile of sausage in his lap. He’d be dead long before help arrived.

CH045

Amy came out of the bathroom still toweling her hair. Showering had been a difficult process and, despite covering her dressings with Saran wrap, they both had become wet. As she headed for the kitchen where Jason kept the gauze and tape, the phone on the counter rang.

"Hello, Turner residence."

"Amy, its Brigham… Everything ok?"

"Not really but I don't expect things to be otherwise. You sound as if you're in an echo chamber."

"These phones do that sometimes. It's irritating."

He paused, then added, "I have news about the money transfer. We got lucky."

"Well?" she asked almost annoyed by the laconic delivery style Landry had developed as a therapist who listened more than he talked.

"The British police sergeant came by late this morning. Seems the unknown American may have counted too much on Malik succeeding. The money he sent was a direct transfer from the central office of the Planters and Citizens Bank in Atlanta. The moneyman apparently didn't even try to disguise it by routing the transfer through a third party or weaving it through the Bahamas or Caymans."

"And who sent it?" pressed Amy, anxiously.

"Don't know that yet. Confidentiality issues are slowing down his identification. The police here have to liaise with the FBI before that information can be released. The sergeant thinks it could take up to forty-eight hours more but I thought you and Jason should know what's pending. By the way, how's he doing?"

"He didn't sleep much last night and this morning he left early to find Mark West. He took his gun and ordered me to stay here at the house. Doesn't want anyone to know where I am. Besides, I'm still pretty much of a cripple and the antibiotics have given me the runs."

"What's he up to?"

"I'm really not sure, but after what's happened, I didn't even try to dissuade him from taking his revolver. Frankly, I'm scared, Brigham."

"Do you think he'd go after West by himself?"

"He's not reckless and he knows enough to evaluate risks but he's really in a state and he could do something foolish."

"Have you considered calling the Albany police in on this?" asked Landry.

"Of course, but I know he doesn't want that. I'm afraid I might damage our relationship irreparably if I did. I just have to trust that his good sense will prevail."

There was a pause at the other end of the line as Landry pondered. "Maybe I could get the police here to call their Albany counterparts," he suggested.

"Are you going to be at Renaissance all day, Brigham?"

"Yes. I've got nothing planned except my regular sessions."

"Then let's do this. I'll wait to hear from him. I think if he cools off he'll either come home or at least call. If he doesn't, then I'll call you and you can have the police make the connection."

"So, you'd be out of it that way?"

"Not really," she replied, "but, at least, I'm not going off half-cocked."

"Works for me. Even if he comes back, Amy, please call me tomorrow. I may have news."

"Is the sergeant going to contact you or is he expecting you to call in?" asked Amy.

No response.

"Brigham, are you still there?"

Nothing, and the echoing quality to the connection was gone from the line. She clicked the flash button. Nothing. Then the disconnect. No dial tone. Puzzled, she hung up the receiver, shrugged her shoulders and reached up for the bandages in the cupboard.

The arm was across her throat effectively cutting off any protest before she could turn around. The roll of bandages fell to the floor as her assailant grabbed her wounded arm and bent it cruelly behind her.

CH046

Mark West's daddy had been an inveterate hunter as had his father before him. As a result, the men of the family, including Mark, had been raised with a rifle or shotgun in their hands. Much of their time away from WestWinds had been spent at a luxurious log chalet sequestered in the center of an eight hundred acre tract of piney woods, river bottom and bird meadows.

Until recent years, an elderly dog handler who kept the kennels at the chalet for the Wests had lived there all year round. He'd died and Mark had never replaced him.

In the long years of friendship between Mark and Jason, Jason had been a frequent visitor to the chalet. He knew the grounds, the outbuildings and the hunting areas well. He wasn't surprised that Mark would retreat there if there had truly been an attempt on his life as the van driver had said. He'd be safer there than anywhere else.

Ironically, the hunting preserve was only ten miles south of the accident site, just off of the old Georgia number 3 inside the Mitchell county line. It would take him less than fifteen minutes to get there.

About a mile from the main entry road to the chalet, a series of ponds, dug to raise catfish, were set a hundred yards off the highway. A smaller track intended for four-wheelers and tractors ran back up and along a low ridge above the ponds to the chalet. Jason would approach from that direction as he was certain Mark would be watching the primary laneway.

Jason glanced down the highway in both directions. He didn't want to be seen leaving the road. No one was coming.

He negotiated a rough track down over an ancient culvert and past a dilapidated wooden gate that hung drunkenly to the side of the track that paralleled the ponds. Beer and soft drinks can littering the path crunched under the tires of the BMW. The preserve obviously had its poachers as well and they apparently made no efforts to cover their tracks.

After he almost high-centered the car twice on hummocks of scrub willows growing in the middle of the track, he pulled into the trees where the BMW would be hidden both from the road and from anyone further up the track on the ridge top.

The noonday air was redolent with the scent of pine gum and the wild flowers that dotted the meadows around the ponds. Catfish swirled leaving small eddies at the surface of the ponds and swallows swooped low over the glassy surface preying on the same hatch of flies that caused the catfish to rise.

Jason took the revolver from its holster which he tossed into the trunk next to the open box of shells from which he's taken a handful that now pressed against his thigh in his pocket. He spun the cylinder and replaced one tarnished cartridge with a new round before snapping it shut.

Unfortunately, he was wearing a light yellow golf shirt which would stand out like a beacon in the brush. He took it off, laid it on the warm hood of the car and proceeded to stain it as effectively as possible with crushed vegetation and a handful of earth. It was a poor camouflage job but still an improvement on its visibility.

After a last careful look around to make sure no illicit fisherman had hidden in any bushes and seen him drive up, he took off on foot up the track which began immediately to climb the ridge. As he walked, he reflected on the past occasions, in more pleasant moments, that he had made the same trip. Whatever the outcome of today's encounter, he knew that this would be his last visit to those woods.

The track left the ridge and open ground to bury itself in piney woods where mature jack pines grew so closely together that their tops formed a quasi-canopy with only the occasional shaft of sunlight penetrating to fall like a spotlight upon the needle-covered forest floor. Red squirrels chirped in alarm at his approach and scampered partway up trunks where they took up sentinel positions, head down and tails bobbing, as they watched him.

A much larger fox squirrel sauntered nonchalantly into the path ahead of him obviously unaware of his presence. When it turned and saw him, it stood on its hind legs like a prairie dog to appraise the intruder before bouncing off into the safety of the trees.

Jason had been on the path for fifteen minutes and was rapidly approaching the clearing where the chalet stood. He slowed his pace and moved closer to the pine trunks hoping no dogs were on the premises to raise the alarm.

' *So far, so good*'.

The trees were thinning and the shadow of the chalet could be seen no more than a hundred yards ahead. The last twenty yards he'd need to cross would be over open ground where the brush had been bush-hogged down.

Taking up a position from which to reconnoiter the buildings, Jason could see the back of one vehicle, an SUV. He didn't recognize it as Mark's . Although he couldn't see the front of the building from where he was, the kennels were visible and mercifully no dogs could be seen in the cemented runs and all the gates appeared to be open.

Surveying the area in front of him, he noted that it was littered with a profusion of dry sticks and brush which meant he had to risk picking his way through it slowly and be completely exposed for almost a minute, or he could dash across and risk the noise he'd make. There were numerous feral pigs in the area which constantly rooted through the underbrush and the noise might go unnoticed, but that was unlikely.

He quietly stole along the fringe of the trees seeking a better view of the house through its windows and searching for a relatively unencumbered pathway to the back porch. About six trees down, he found an area where it looked like someone had tried to rake up the debris and a small path, free of clutter, fully half the distance to the chalet, had been created.

He presumed that Mark would be inside the building and he intended to gain access to the second story by getting to a stairway that ran up from the left end of the back porch to a small balcony outside the master bedroom. He knew the locks here. They were all spring loaded deadbolts that could be opened in a few seconds with a simple penknife. Both he and Mark had done it many times as kids.

He waited a full five minutes motionless behind his pine. At one point, a large woodpecker came flitting to his tree and perched above him with its tail braced against the trunk while it prospected for larvae beneath the bark. Pieces of bark fell in a sylvan shower onto his hair and shoulders and, finally, he waved at the bird startling it away into silent flight. He saw no one inside the house. In fact, the place looked deserted.

He was ready.

Gun in hand and taking care to avoid stepping on debris, he made his way to the path then quickly gained the porch and bent down to hide himself from view behind it.

Two minutes later, he crept silently up the stairs placing his feet on the portion of the risers closest to the edge to avoid any creaking. He skirted the edge of the porch and made it to the second set of stairs without incident.

From a secluded vantage point at the lower corner of a window, he surveyed the interior of the main reception area of the chalet. He could see the huge stone fireplace at the far end and the bar with all its stools empty and perfectly aligned. The couches and dining table were also empty. In fact, no lights or fans were on and he began to wonder if the dying man had lied concerning West's whereabouts.

Going up the stairs, he inadvertently knocked a pine twig from a step and it bounced onto the porch below. The sound was minimal but, to Jason, it seemed like a loud thud.

He froze in position for several seconds, and hearing nothing, he continued on up to the small balcony. The curtains at the small window of the door and an adjacent picture window were drawn and his entry would have to be blind.

For all he knew, Mark West could be stretched out on the king-size bed with a gun in hand waiting for him. He dismissed the image from his mind because entertaining it would bring paralysis and fear which he couldn't afford at this juncture.

He slipped the revolver into his waistband and opened his penknife. It was a simple operation to prize back the deadbolt. The door opened noiselessly inward. The room was in shadows with the sun directly overhead and Jason peeked in. '*No one*'. He pushed through the small opening and closed the door silently. He left the deadbolt unlocked as a precaution.

The house was silent except for the hum of the central air conditioning. '*Someone was here after all*'. His heart surged in anticipation as he thought of Mark and what he'd done to them. The bitter gall of anger had seeped onto the back of his tongue. He drew it along his upper teeth as if he could scrape off the taint and spat silently onto the maroon carpet.

The revolver was back in his hand and he cocked it. He'd do better to risk the click here in an empty bedroom than to have it betray him if he got the drop on West later.

Jason didn't know what he would do to West. He'd considered getting him into the hands of the authorities with a confession but, if that proved impractical, he was quite prepared to kill the man who had murdered his wife. In fact, *he'd clearly prefer to kill him* and it was only the practicalities of being caught and imprisoned that deterred him. In case he did have to kill him, he'd wiped off his fingerprints from the door hardware with his filthy shirt.

He was now at the open door to the bedroom which gave onto a long loft that overhung fully one half of the ground floor. A sturdy balcony railing made of three inch diameter poles ran the full length of the loft with a stairway at the far end. Luckily, it was all carpeted and shouldn't betray him with any creaks as he traversed to gain the stairs.

He slid out the bedroom door, hugging the wall with his gun held against his chest in both hands. Sidling carefully along, he watched as the main room opened incrementally to his view. He was halfway down the wall toward the stairs when the rifle cracked. No. It actually boomed in the enclosed space, and a shower of woodchips erupted from the log nearest his head. He hit the floor, his heart pounding into his mouth and his bladder pulsing instinctively, threatening involuntary incontinence.

"Welcome, Jason. I've been waiting for you. That was a 3.06 round with a steel tip. It went six inches into the wood beside your head."

It was Mark's voice.

Jason said nothing. *He couldn't say anything.*

"I know where you are. I've had a bead on you since you left the bedroom and I'll nail you if you budge one inch from where you are now."

He paused, then spoke again with a deliberate cadence. "Get rid of your gun. Uncock it first and drop it over the edge of the railing. Then you'll get up very slowly and come down the stairs with your hands over your head."

"Go to hell! Mark. You murderer!"

Jason had found his voice and his anger was getting the best of him.

A second round crashed into the railing just to the left of Jason's head and he crawled rapidly backward to cower against the wall.

"I'm warning you, Jason. I've got my Browning automatic here as well and one more little bauble I'm sure you'll appreciate. I'm over by the fireplace under good cover. Take a look this way and see what I toss into the air."

Jason looked and saw a standard issue grenade rise up then fall back.

"A little souvenir that one of my uncles gave me from Nam. I'm sure it still works and we need to replace the loft you're laying on anyway."

Jason looked back at the open bedroom door. He had to make a dash for it. The rifle wasn't accurate at this range and he had to bet that Mark had lied about the Browning.

As if he could read his thoughts, West fired four rounds from the Browning that chinked into the wall in neat line two feet long and only six inches above him.

"I cheated, Jason. I'm actually *off the ground* and I'll cut you down if you run for it. Your choice."

"Why don't you just kill me then. You didn't hesitate to kill Annette."

"Actually, I did, Jason. I liked her a lot. I hesitated a whole year until you forced me into it."

"You scumbag. You killed her for nothing. You know that don't you?"

"Truth be known, I should have killed you from the get go. I thought it would be neater with the car wreck and all. What do they say... *the best laid plans...*"

"You're going to kill me as soon as I stand up so why should I take the chance?"

"Try me, Jason. You forget that I'm a man of imagination. *I* won't be killing you, that's a promise, so toss the gun and come down."

Jason's mind was whirling. He knew his anger was powerful enough to let him kill Mark with his bare hands if he had the opportunity. Up here he didn't. He decided to risk it.

"Ok, here comes the gun," and he uncocked the Smith and Wesson and slid it along the carpet until it tumbled into the void at the edge of the loft and thumped on the floor below.

"I'm standing up," he shouted as he rose, fully expecting to be cut down by his partner.

"Nothing funny. Come down the stairs, hands high," snapped West.

As Jason descended the stairs, he saw Mark West step from off a table that had been pushed into the corner beside the fireplace. He left the rifle standing on the table and had the Browning in his hand trained on Jason. He used the gun to point to a wooden chair standing by a small writing table in front of a set of panoramic bay windows.

West said, "Take it nice and easy and sit down here. You're going to be doing some writing for me."

Jason crossed the floor always calculating how far he was from West who cautiously stayed outside a perimeter that would permit him to get off at least three shots before Jason could rush him.

Jason sat at the table.

"Pick up the pen. You'll be doing your own suicide note, so write nicely if you want your new sweet little wife to be able to read it."

Jason smirked. "Why in God's name would I ever do that?"

"Because you want her to live, dear boy. She's in your home right now, taped to a chair with one of my men beside her. If he doesn't get a text message from me before two p.m. he'll cut your sweet wife's throat... *or did he tell me he'd strangle her?* Dear me, so many, many possibilities... Now write or I'll kill you right now and she goes too in twenty minutes."

Jason's heart sank. His mouth became immediately dry and his guts were churning.

"You're bluffing. She's perfectly safe."

"No, she's not. I was counting on the boys in the van getting you but this was always my failsafe plan. You know me well enough to know I leave nothing to chance."

"The van guys were the backup for Malik?"

West looked puzzled.

"Talking in riddles now? I don't know any *Malik*."

"St Lucia. You telling me you had nothing to do with the boat incident?"

"That was ill-conceived from the get-go but I don't owe you any explanations. Get writing," growled West.

"What harm is there in telling me, now. You're going to kill me in a minute."

"Look, we aren't the only players involved in this thing. I haven't had time to figure it all out yet but I will. One of your people tried to run me off the road last night. At first, I thought it might be you but I got a glimpse of him and it was one of your boys."

"I don't have any *boys* working for me. If someone's after you he's doing it on his own... You've made a pile of enemies. Take your pick."

"Be that as it may, next time your man in the Explorer tries to get to me, he'll buy it, not me. Now... get writing or I'll shoot you bit by bit and bury you under the dog kennels."

West took aim and fired a shot into the floor next to Jason's foot. "The next one goes in your knee."

"What do I write?"

"Use your imagination. Make it short. No hidden messages. Just *goodbye darling. I can't take it anymore*. Something like that."

Jason began to truly despair. How would he get to West? He wrote a sentence then paused. "She'll know this is a fake."

"Who gives a crap. I have to make the cops believe it, not her. They know you were at the funny farm. They'll buy it and I'll skate."

West was moving carefully closer to Jason, his gun trained on him. He seemed to be wanting to see what he wrote.

Jason was waiting for him to come just a little closer then he'd charge him.

He hunched over the pages so West wouldn't be able to see and continued writing.

"I didn't say write a chapter. Three sentences. No more!"

Jason held up the sheet his hand partially obscuring the note.

"How's this?" he said as he stood up.

"Who told you to stand. Sit down... I said sit!"

In front of him the window suddenly shattered and Jason dove for the floor thinking West had fired even though he'd heard no shot. He rolled quickly to one side through the shards of glass and scrambled to his feet. He charged at West.

When he rose, West was already lying face down on the floor, his right hand twitching spasmodically around the grip of the Browning which he still held. Blood was rapidly haloing out from under his head where he lay face down.

Jason hit the floor again and crawled quickly away from the window. Skirting the room he retrieved his revolver and crouched behind a sofa to scan the front of the house where the bullets had come from. Nothing moved for a full three minutes before he cautiously stole forward to kneel beside West.

Turning him over, he counted two entry wounds, one in the left cheek just below the eye and a second midway down his neck. Dead center.

He was shaking but he knew he had to get out of there and back to Amy in less than twenty minutes.

He picked up his revolver, grabbed up the pen and paper and, perfunctorily, wiped down the table top and chair back. Then, still watching the front of the building, he slipped out the side door and ran for the woods. In five minutes, he had made his way back to his car without incident.

When he reached the pavement, Jason gave the BMW all the accelerator it could take as he roared down old Georgia number 3, the wind howling through the shattered back window.

CH047

Amy regained consciousness to find herself bound hand and foot to a wooden chair with duct tape. Her first cold realization was that Randall Smith had died tied to a chair precisely like this.

Her wounded arm was on fire and, looking down, she could see that blood had soaked though the terrycloth of her robe. The side of her head throbbed with every heartbeat and she could feel the cloying presence of more blood on the right side of her neck and under the cloth of the robe on her shoulder. Vaguely, she remembered being flung into a doorframe as she had struggled. It must have happened then.

A wad of paper toweling from the kitchen had been jammed into her mouth. It had become sodden enough with saliva that she could easily compress it with her jaws. The paper of the towel was dangerously fragmenting and she could feel a shard of the stuff hanging over the back of her tongue so that any attempt to swallow forced it back gagging her.

'I could suffocate right here!'

Without realizing it, she had began to cry. It wasn't the pain. She could have dealt with that. It was the insufferable fact of being someone's victim again. Her life had been regularly punctuated with episodes... No, not just episodes, but rather *whole periods*, when she found herself subjected to some male's sadistic whims. The wounds Malik had inflicted hadn't even healed yet and already she was bound and gagged, impotently awaiting the next indignity. What merciless, indifferent god had arbitrarily designated his creatures as victims or torturers from the moment of their creation?

'And what was next?'

She was in the hallway between the kitchen and the living room and could see the whole of the latter. Noise came from the kitchen. A fridge door closing. A pop, then the sizzle of effervescence as a beer can was opened. A shadow appeared on the wall beside and behind her.

"Sorry I had to whack you, lady, but you shouldn't have struggled."

The speaker wasn't visible.

"If you keep quiet I'll take out the gag."

She nodded her head in vigorous assent and immediately felt a large nicotine- smelling finger push into the side of her mouth and pry out most of the wadded up toweling.

"Man, this stuff is crap. It don't stay together worth a damn," he said as he stepped out to where she could see him shaking the sodden paper particles from his finger.

Desperately, she spat out the remaining remnants which had infiltrated the space between jaw and cheek. The welcome flood of saliva she felt pouring from her glands facilitated the task. She licked her lips repeatedly until they remained moist enough to speak.

"Who are you?" she demanded unable to banish the indignation she felt from her tone even though she sensed that angering him wouldn't be in her best interest.

To her surprise, he smiled. "Me? I'm just a guy, lady. Just doing a job... Here, wanna sip... It's your beer anyway," he said holding out the can of Budweiser toward her.

She shook her head and clamped her lips shut, half expecting that he might force it on her.

He withdrew the can. "Suit yourself," he said indifferently, raising the can to his own lips and guzzling what remained of the beer.

Finished, he crushed the can in powerful fingers and nonchalantly flipped it over her head. She heard it hit the floor and slide along.

He wasn't tall, maybe five foot ten at most, but he was wearing a muscle shirt from 'Gold's Gym' and his arms and shoulders were massively muscled giving him the appearance of a big man. He was evidently one of those specimens who lived in a gym and whose veins had been forced by muscle hypertrophy from their normal discrete pathways between muscle groups up to positions just under the skin where they coursed like burrowing worms.

His head was shaven and he had a barbed wire tattoo above his right biceps. A purple tear had been inscribed in red ink at the corner of his left eye. His face might have once been attractive but his nose had been badly broken and poorly set, if set at all.

"You checking me out, sister?" he smirked as she examined him.

"Get a load of this," and, without further hesitation, he stripped off his shirt and began to pose like body-builders do in competition.

"Your old man look anything like me, chickey?"

She didn't answer and, unwisely, she didn't try to hide the disgust in her eyes either.

He noticed. "Snooty rich bitch, eh? You like your men wimpy and soft so you can push them around, is that it?"

His eyes had taken on a cruel glint and he leaned forward to put his face directly opposite Amy's, his huge hands closing over her taped forearms on the chair. He stared aggressively at her for several moments then easily picked up the chair with her in it and carried it into the living room where he sat her down opposite Jason's black leather recliner.

He stood above her. "What nothing to say, missy?" he chided.

Her heart was pounding against her rib cage like an angry child kicking at a restraining door but she tried to appear calm.

"You can leave now. I don't know your name and I'm willing not to press charges... Leave me tied up if you wish, then I can't follow you or go for help. You can be at the other end of the earth by tomorrow, if you choose."

Her tormenter cupped one elbow in his hand and stroked his chin with his fingers. His lips were pursed and she could readily see he was mocking her even before he spoke.

"Tempting offer little lady, but you're worth big bucks to me. I'll be long gone by tomorrow. You're right about that, but you ain't going to be chasing me away with your threats," and he wagged his head slowly from side to side for emphasis. "You got anything else to offer...?"

She turned her face away from him and felt the terror of a sexual victim begin marching up her parched throat. She'd become adept at recognizing men's intentions in their faces when the sexual beast that lurks in all of them takes over control in the presence of a helpless woman. She scrunched her eyes shut and then felt his fingers at the neck of her robe.

'No, God! No... No more!'

Roughly he parted the robe and her breasts were laid bare.

"Well, lookee here, will ya," he said and she felt the calluses of his hand on the soft skin of her scarred breast, "been letting the mice nibble on your titties, eh?"

"Get your hands off me you disgusting scum!" she spat out as venomously as she could, swiveling her face back around to confront him.

"Oh, goodness me," he minced, drawing back in mock alarm and holding his hands up chest high mimicking the posture of a scolded child, "the nasty lady's going to hurt me if I touch her."

She continued to glare at him.

He laughed and sat down in the recliner opposite her, resting an elbow on the chair arm and his chin on his hand, staring at her. His head was coked to one side studiously.

"You know, chickey... you have beautiful breasts except for the rat bite... What's the rest of you look like, I wonder?"

"Stay away!" she commanded.

He laughed again and lay back in the chair.

As he did so, a second man appeared in the hallway behind his chair. He carried a silenced pistol in his hand which he raised carefully to his lips in a gesture of silence.

She did her best to keep the surprise she felt out of her face and voice.

"If you want to see what I look like, then let me out of the chair," she challenged.

"Sure and you'll put on a show for me, is that it?" he quipped.

"Yeah, that's it. I promise you a show like you'll never see again for the rest of your life."

The second man was now directly behind the chair. Her tormentor leaned forward, hands on knees and, once he'd taken up that position, the pistol came forward too, the muzzle pointing just behind her tormenter's right ear. The gym rat was about to speak, his lips forming a word when the pistol fired twice with the muted sound of raw eggs dropping onto a terrazzo floor.

Curiously, the man's head didn't jerk left under the impact of the bullets as she'd expected nor was there any blood, brain or skull eruption from the other side of his head.

A sudden look of profound surprise burst onto his face as his eyes opened wide and his jaw went slack. He sat still for an instant, the surprise now etched eternally upon his features, then he slowly slumped forward, arms falling outside his knees and his torso folded onto his thighs, as if he had simply suffered a narcolepsy attack.

CH048

Jason's BMW tore down the highway with the tachometer bumping 4500 but his mind was racing faster than his car. His wife might already be dead. Mark's threats had been tied to a twenty minute time limit that had expired while he'd been frantically re-dialing his home number on his cell phone without even the answering machine interrupting the rings.

He'd considered calling the police for help but what would he have said to them? How would he have been able to explain away his wife's danger, his own presence at the hunting lodge or his motive for going there in the first place? If they knew he'd even been on Georgia number 3 near the time of the van's crash they'd question him about that as well.

Luckily, the cruisers had all left the accident scene when he flashed by at over ninety miles an hour. A wrecker's crew had been standing on the shoulder of the road studying the remnants of the van, one man with his hand on his hips and the other tousling his hair under a cap. They'd both jumped sideways instinctively and stared at the idiot who sped past unrestrained in his carelessness by the crumpled evidence of how quickly a vehicle could become a coffin.

Jason was panicking even though he realized the danger of permitting disordered thought at such a moment. His mind was splitting dangerously into two useless elements. One, like a schizophrenic's auditory hallucination, was cursing him for leaving Amy unprotected, while, in another sequestered recess, his vulnerability had wrapped itself into a fetal tuck and was wailing in anticipatory grief at being abandoned once more.

He despised both parts and struggled to banish them by pure force of will as he attended to the task of getting home to Amy.

With stony-faced resolve he kept his eyes riveted to the road and its curves. His limbs moved with the precision of an automaton guiding the BMW along its careening course into the outskirts of Albany.

When he had run the final traffic signal and cut off one last vehicle in a blare of horns and screeching brakes, he lurched around the corner into his subdivision with the BMW jack-hammering over speed bumps.

The cul-de-sac in which he lived was protected by two huge live oaks whose branches hung low over the entrance like modesty curtains in a seventeenth century boudoir. He peered anxiously through them as he made a tire-squealing charge into the dead-end street.

No other vehicle but his old Cherokee was in sight.

Bouncing over the curb as it cut the corner into the drive, the car lurched to a stop and he flung open his door. Hitting the grass of the lawn running, he felt his feet slide dangerously sideways and he dipped his left arm low to catch himself if he lost his footing. His right hand, clutching his .38, was flung high in the air to offset the momentum of his slide. He came solidly upright as his foot found purchase on the cement walkway leading to the front door which was slightly ajar.

He took the porch steps in a single leap and lowered his left shoulder as he hit the door without slowing. He wanted to be fifteen feet into the room before he needed to deal with anyone who might be holding a gun on his wife. The door slammed against the wall with the sound of shattering glass and he spun to the right to absorb the shock of the collision and still keep running. Ducking into a semi-crouch as he moved, he scanned the hallway then the living room to his left until he flattened himself protectively against a wall, his gun outstretched before him in both hands.

Amy had been sitting on the carpet beside his black recliner. She screamed when he burst through the door and was in the act of scrambling behind the recliner when she recognized him.

"Oh, Jason," she gasped, "Thank God you're here!"

She was no longer showing any fear but Jason moved away from the wall and swung his gun to cover the hallway from the kitchen, nonetheless.

"They're gone. It's alright," she said.

He looked at her as she knelt on the floor, hair still damp from a shower and her knees protruding from the cloth of the robe folded under her.

She raised her arms to him and he went quickly toward her dropping his gun on the carpet as he, too, fell to his knees.

Her eyes were red-rimmed and brimming. Falling into his embrace, she nestled her face into his shoulder and began to silently sob, her body vibrating in his arms while she poured out her relief in tears. Her hands clutched and re-clutched convulsively against his back as if she needed the repeated tactile reassurance that he was really present and not simply a hallucination in a day already overfull of unbelievable horror.

For several minutes, they said nothing. Jason caressed her hair and surveyed the room. Across from the recliner beside which they knelt, a kitchen chair was turned on its side. Bands of duct tape circled its armrests and front legs. Two other pieces of the same tape, wadded into irregular balls, lay alongside the chair.

Over Amy's shoulder, he could see linear indentations in the carpet where it appeared the recliner had been positioned before it had apparently been moved. The pile of the carpet in the immediate area of the marks was tousled and appeared to be wet as if someone had recently been scrubbing it.

"What happened?" he asked solicitously without attempting to move her off his shoulder. "Can you talk about it, darling?"

She sniffed audibly twice to clear her tears and then raised her face from his shoulder but kept her eyes downcast and didn't look at him when she spoke. "Not here, Jason," she shuddered.

"Let's go out to the pool and away from this room," he suggested.

He stood and helped her to her feet. When she started walking, the limp caused by the pain from her flank wound that had almost disappeared since returning from St. Lucia was back. Like the dazed victim of a car crashed, still awash in the shock of the inconceivable, she leaned on his arm as if she were incapable of negotiating the path through the house to the patio.

When they had reached the kitchen, she shifted her hand from his arm and leaned on the table.

"Jason, there's blood on this robe... Could you get me something to slip on from the bedroom. I'd like to get it off."

She was looking at him and forcing a reassuring smile. "I'll be fine until you get back."

He found a black silk robe with a Chinese motif embroidered on the front panel in her closet and hurried back to her side. The terrycloth robe lay on the floor around her ankles and he could see her trying to tug a blood-stained and sodden bandage over her wrist and hand.

"Let me get that," he said and slid it carefully off her hand which trembled visibly until she placed it again on the table's edge.

"I'm going to re-bandage your arm and your side. Try to stand here for just a few more minutes, darling."

"The bandages are on the floor," she said jerking her chin in the direction of the counter where the phone receiver lay amidst the rolls of gauze and tape she'd been getting when she was attacked.

"Yes, I saw them," he said as he gathered up the material he would need and rejoined her to examine her wounds. "The stitches are still in place. I'm surprised the arm bled like it seems it did," he commented absently as he began winding the gauze around her arm.

She snorted feebly and there was irony was in her tone when she spoke. "If you'd seen him twisting it behind my back you'd understand why it bled."

"I'm sorry, Amy. I didn't mean to minimize. I was just talking to keep myself from cursing out loud about all this."

She touched him gently on the shoulder with her other hand. "I understand. Me too."

The dressing of the wounds was quickly finished and Jason helped her into the Chinese robe. She tried to fasten the ties but she swayed and her hands simply fumbled inefficiently with the cloth.

"I'll do that."

"Can't even do up my own robe... These last few days have taken it out on me, Jason... I feel like an old woman..."

"And you still look like a princess," he added when her voice faltered. "Here, let me carry you like you deserve."

She didn't protest and, taking her into his arms on the side opposite her wounds, he made his way across the kitchen through the open patio doors and out beside the pool.

A shimmering orb in the western sky, the sun, like an angry incandescent eye, glared at the earth causing them both to squint against its reflected glare on the pool's surface. Jason sought refuge from its assault under the shade of the bamboo stand that housed the nest of the mad mockingbird he'd jousted with weeks before.

The bird's young had been hatched and raised and now the only noise emanating from the thicket was the low-toned ticking of bamboo stalks jostling each other in the afternoon breeze.

He set her carefully into a pool chair and adjusted the reclining back until her face and torso were well within the protection of the bamboo's shadow. He pulled up a second chair and sat at her side leaning over to stroke her hair as she stared up at the flittering bamboo leaves above them.

"It was horrible, Jason... And, then it just got worse."

He sat in silence.

"The first man was a skinhead, I think. He had tattoos all over and a face that had obviously been beaten on more than once. He tied me to the kitchen chair and threatened me."

"Did he say who sent him?"

"No. I tried to get tough with him, threaten him, but it didn't work."

"Did he hurt you?"

"Well, he manhandled me at first. Bent my arm behind my back and knocked my head into the wall while we struggled."

Jason's face darkened as she continued.

"He was going to hurt me sexually. I'm sure of that but he never got the chance."

She shook her head and pursed her lips at the recollection.

"How did you escape him?"

"I didn't. He'd had me captive for only about twenty minutes or so. Brigham had called from St. Lucia and I was on the phone with him when I guess this guy cut the line. Next thing I know he was playing hacky-sack with me and then I'm trussed up *again*. He had wadded up a paper towel in my mouth and I almost choked on it."

Amy had been attempting to minimize her travails as she'd watched Jason's countenance turn thunderous. She didn't want *any* male anger around her and his growing rage made her irrationally uneasy.

"Jason, please try to listen without broadcasting your anger on your face. Everything is over now and there is nothing you can do. You don't know what it does to me to see you furious like that." She was pleading with him.

He drew a deep breath and let it out in an audible rush. He then began to knead his eyes with his fingertips, hiding the rest of his face behind his palms. His head was shaking slowly in disbelief.

"I'm sorry, sweetheart. Last thing I want to do is upset you anymore. I can't believe all the crap you've gone through these past few days. I'll do my best... How's this?" and he unconvincingly forced a closed-lip smile onto his face

"Better than the thunderclouds anyway," she replied.

"So, if you didn't escape the skinhead, what happened?"

"What happened is even more unbelievable than being mugged in my own kitchen. Every time I think of it, I have to shake my head to convince myself it really took place."

He continued to restrain himself, his lopsided half-smile still pasted artificially on his face.

"A second guy... In some ways a lot scarier than the skinhead... sneaks up behind him with a silenced pistol."

"How'd he get in the house. Didn't the alarm system go off with either of them?"

"You might as well not have an alarm system, Jason. They both walked right in like the place had a real estate 'open house' sign on the lawn."

"That's incredible."

"That's nothing. If you thinks *that*'s incredible, it gets a lot worse," Amy continued.

"The second guy, who is a least fifty and real paunchy, just puts the pistol behind the first guy's ear and shoots him twice... Pam.! Pam.!... Not a word."

"He didn't say anything before he shot him?"

"Nothing. I thought he was just going to threaten him then tie him up or something but he just shot him with what must have been a .22 because the bullets stayed inside his skull."

"Did the killer look Italian?" asked Jason

Amy pursed her lips in thought for a moment before answering.

"Not like any Italians I know, at least none I remember for the moment."

"Could you describe him?"

"Well, he was older, past middle age, like I said, and fat. His face was pocked marked like he used to be an acne farm as a kid. And he talked funny."

"Talked funny like an accent?" Jason asked.

"No. He didn't have an accent, he just spoke like he had marbles in his mouth and couldn't open it properly to enunciate without dropping them. He wore one of those tasteless expensive suits that shine like they've been ironed by accident."

"Anything else?"

"Not that I remember... No, wait… He smelled like garlic. I smelled it when he bent over me to cut off the tape... And his hair... it was so greasy I could see the scalp through the comb lines like he'd wiped it down with olive oil on purpose."

"Amy, Italians don't put olive oil on their hair,"

"I mean something like olive oil. Now that we're talking about it, I remember there was a young Italian doctor I worked with once and he had the same kind of oily hair. It used to stain the back of his lab coat at the neck."

"I think I know who sent the second man," said Jason. "Did he hurt you?"

"No. That's what was so macabre about the whole scenario. He'd come prepared to kill someone and, then as soon as he did, he pulled a plastic drop cloth from his pocket and spread it on the dead man's knees to catch the blood that was starting to drip from the guy's head wound and his nose."

"A drop cloth?" Jason repeated incredulously.

"Well, a piece of plastic anyway. Then he takes out a white garbage bag and slides it over the man's head and ties it off. And, all the while, he's apologizing to me in his gravely voice about getting a few drops of blood on the carpet. It blew my mind! This killer thinks nothing of murdering someone but he seems full of regret about getting blood on the carpet... It makes no sense, Jason? Can you explain it to me?"

"If he's who I think he is, he's a hired assassin. Killing people is a job for him just like medicine is for us."

"He didn't even seem angry with the guy he killed. I mean, *he never even knew him... Never even spoke to him*! It gives me the chills just to realize that people like him exist in the same world I do."

"He's not in *our* world, Amy. In our world people have to be insane to kill someone. He comes from another world where everything is turned on its head."

"Oh, he was real, Jason, and *right here in our world*. I watched him and another young guy who came in to help him move the body. The young one even scrubbed the blood out of the carpet. They're here right in the middle of this world which, sometimes, seems like it belongs more to people like them then it does to people like us. And, I'll admit that it scares the hell out of me, even if they saved my life. Where do monsters like them come from?"

"When I said that they weren't from our world, Amy, I meant that we have to act as if they don't exist. If we're forced to search for a psychopath behind the eyes of everyone we meet, we'd be so on edge all the time that life would become unbearable."

"So we just pretend that they don't exist and get on with our lives because most people aren't psychopaths, is that how it works?" she asked.

"Yes, well sort of..." he answered.

"And when one of them surfaces and blows our presumptions all to hell, what do we do, Jason?"

"We cope. We get through it after all the panic and anguish that they cause."

"And just resume believing the lies that we're safe from mutants like them?"

Jason shrugged and managed a half-smile. "What other choice do we have, darling?"

She looked away from his face and appeared to be studying the bamboo leaves above her. She was remembering St. Lucia. "Jason I really want to go back to St. Lucia and just work quietly in the clinic. Couldn't we do something like that?"

"We can certainly talk about it but I've got a big mess here now with TurnerWest... *Mark is dead too.*"

"What?" she exclaimed sitting upright. "How?"

Jason recounted the events at the hunting lodge and told her about the van accident as well.

"So the skinhead was Mark's man?" asked Amy.

"I presume so. Yes."

"Then who were the Italians?"

"They work for a man in Detroit called Gallo."

"Isn't he the lawyer handling your father-in-law's petition?"

"Yes, but he's Mafia as well."

"What are they doing down here killing people?"

"They think whoever is after me might try to harm the children as well, so I guess they intervene wherever and whenever they want," he said, shrugging his shoulders.

Amy ran her hands through her hair and slipped her legs over the sides of the pool chair, straddling it. Looking him clearly in the eyes she said, "Do you realize how crazy all this is, Jason? These guys are helping you today but next week they could be putting plastic bags *over our heads* and apologizing to someone else about *our* blood on the carpet or the bedcovers!"

Despite the obvious pain she was feeling from her wounds, she swung her good leg over the lounge chair and got up and limped out into the sun to stare down into the pool as she attempted to process what she's just learned.

"Amy, I think they killed Mark too, but the police may suspect me."

"That would please your father-in-law. Maybe he had planned it this way," she said.

"No, I don't think the old man hates me that much. He just wants the kids for his wife's sake. He doesn't really give a damn about me."

"As long as you're not a problem for him, you mean, don't you?"

"Frankly, I don't think we're in danger anymore."

"So you believe Mark was behind Malik's attack on us in St. Lucia?" she asked.

"Why not? It fits, doesn't it?"

"Brigham said the money for Malik came from Atlanta. The police may know who sent it in two days."

"Still could be Mark. He uses Atlanta banks," suggested Jason.

"I hope you're right. How do we call off the Italians? I don't think I can get a night's sleep knowing they're around."

"I'll talk to Gallo tomorrow," promised Jason.

"Until you do, I'd like us to take a room in the biggest hotel in town. Something right across from the lobby."

CH049

The phone beeped insistently and Jason rolled over to lift the handset from the cradle. Beside him, Amy slept soundly despite her misgivings of the night before.

"Hello,"

"Could I speak with Dr. Jason Turner, please, this is Dick Kellerman"

"I'm Dr. Turner, Mr. Kellerman. How did you know where to find me?"

"I've been calling your house and office since yesterday with no luck. Your office told me you were in town so I figured you might be in a hotel and I just started calling. I got lucky, I guess."

"Depends on what you want, Mr. Kellerman," responded Jason dryly.

"I work as a producer for 20/20 and I'd like to arrange an interview with you if possible."

"On what subject?" Jason asked cautiously.

"About three weeks ago, we received an anonymous audio tape. Quite startling really as it seemed to contain a forced interview with one Randall Smith whom we later learned was murdered in Albany, a little before we received the tape."

"And how does that concern me?" asked Jason.

"You're mentioned on the tape, doctor, you and several others including a senior executive of Cumberland Health, a Mr. Kleinberg."

"Go on," said Jason who was now sitting up in bed and fumbling in the end table drawer for a pad and something with which to write.

"Well, the tape contains a lot of incriminating accusations against Kleinberg and Smith, and by inference, CHC. We've checked out most of them and they seem to be well-founded but we need to get corroboration from you and your partner, Dr. West."

"Dr. West may not cooperate if I'm right about the allegations. In fact, he's beyond any collaboration, at the moment," said Jason.

"He may not indeed, but what about you?"

"Why can't you research and air your story without my interview? You have this tape."

"I'm afraid we can't use it. It's been decided that the tape contains Smith's actual murder and our executives believe it would be tasteless to use it. Besides, unless I miss my guess, it will probably be sequestered as evidence in a murder investigation, in fact as evidence in about three or four official investigations."

Jason pondered a moment. "I'd have to think it over," he said. "I'd need legal advice."

"You're under no suspicion as far as we're concerned, Dr. Turner."

"Of course," replied Jason, "but I'm a cautious man."

"When do you think you could give me an answer?" asked Kellerman.

"A few days at least."

"Then may I call you Friday? At home or the office?"

"Friday afternoon at home," said Jason.

"Thank you for your time, Doctor and I apologize for the disturbance."

* * *

Jason had been mulling over the 20/20 call for a good fifteen minutes before he decided to contact Gallo. Amy was right about the Italians, allies today, they could be enemies tomorrow. The 20/20 connection might just give him some leverage. It was nine fifteen and Amy was still sleeping. Gallo's number appeared on his palm pilot screen and he dialed it.

"Gallo and Costanza, attorneys at law," a female voice singsonged.

"Mr. Gallo, please. Dr. Jason Turner calling."

"Mr. Gallo's in a conference, sir. May I take a message?"

"I think he'd appreciate being interrupted. I'm going to have to insist you tell him who's calling, Miss."

"Please hold, doctor."

She went off the line and was replaced by a Sicilian guitar and accordion duet which lasted only a minute before her voice returned.

"Dr. Turner, Mr. Gallo has asked me to have you give him a number that is not your home, your office or your cell. He'll call you back in twenty minutes."

Jason gave her the number of the hotel and said, "Ask him to call me back in five minutes. I'm already at this number."

"Very well, doctor. I'm sure that will be fine," and she hung up.

Precisely five minutes later, Gallo called and Jason snatched up the receiver in mid-ring not wishing to awaken Amy who stirred and turned over but remained asleep.

"Good morning, Dr. Turner. Have you taken up residence at the Howard Johnson now?"

"Just for the night. Our carpet at home needed a little cleaning," answered Jason sarcastically.

"What can I do for you?"

"What you can do is precisely *nothing more.* You've absolutely done enough, thank you."

"You're welcome," replied Gallo without any discernible emotion in his voice.

"I mean it, Gallo. Things are finished now."

"You seem to forget, doctor, that we've been doing business together because our interests coincided for a period of time. We aren't blood brothers." There was aggression in his tone that caused Jason concern.

"Is that a threat, Mr. Gallo?" he tried to respond with an equal amount of weight in his voice.

"Not at all, but there are still some mutual matters that remain unresolved and we're on the same side in only one of them."

"And what one is that?"

"The fishing trip to St. Lucia was a bit of a problem, I understand," said the lawyer.

"I don't get your meaning."

"I think you still have someone out there who'd like to see you and your new wife dead."

"Mark's already out of the picture, thanks to you," said Jason.

"*I had nothing to do with Mark West's death.*"

"That's the official line and I understand that," said Jason, "but I don't believe you."

"You're free to believe what you choose, doctor, but you run the risk of proceeding on false assumptions."

"Then, who did kill Mark?"

"I've already told you that there are several parties involved," repeated Gallo.

"20/20 just called me this morning."

Jason listened carefully for any indication that his implied threat had been understood.

"And?..." was all he got back.

"They want an interview."

"I'm not surprised. Are you?" asked Gallo.

Jason decided to ignore the question.

"You have no concern about what I might say?" queried Jason.

"You say what you wish, doctor. I've nothing to do with you outside of your father-in-law's custody action, which by the way will resume actively next week."

Jason's anger broke through, "We had an agreement," he snapped.

"An agreement to suspend any action on the case before the courts as long as the children were in danger. In my opinion, that danger has passed and we'll be proceeding where we left off," said Gallo.

Jason had hoped that Gallo, would have been intimidated by the potential of being named on 20/20 but he now realized that the lawyer had been more than circumspect in his dealings and nothing could be traced to him. In fact, on the surface of things, Jason was a more likely suspect in the deaths of Smith and Mark than some faceless mob hit man. If he even mentioned the mafia connection publicly he'd be suspected of inventing implausible explanations at best.

He was deflated. "Then, I guess we have nothing more to say to each other, Mr. Gallo."

"See you in court, doctor."

When Jason hung up the phone, his shoulders slumped. He was sitting on the edge of the bed and he ran his hands through his hair and sighed. Amy's hand touched his shoulder and then the bed moved as she pulled herself up and leaned against his back kissing him gently on the neck.

"How long have you been awake?" he asked without turning around.

"I heard most of that conversation with Gallo. You look down. Bad news?"

"Before I called Gallo, 20/20 called me about Smith and the whole CHC thing. They wanted an interview. I thought I could use it as leverage with Gallo to get his men out of here and maybe even win some ground in the custody thing."

He blew out his cheeks and let his breath exhale noisily while he flipped open the fingers of his right hand symbolic of an exploding balloon.

"But no luck."

"And the court case?" she pursued.

"It's on again as of next week," he responded feebly.

"Does that mean you'll be going to Detroit?"

She slid her arms over his shoulders running the fingers of her hands down through the hair on his chest.

"Not right away. TurnerWest business and the police here will take precedence but, as soon as I can get away, I've got to have one last try at talking old man McLean out of his custody initiative."

"Do you really think there's much hope of that?"

"No, but putting the kids through a courtroom scene and the pain of seeing a fight between me and their grandparents is worth at least my best effort. I've got to call them tonight."

"What about 20/20?" asked Amy.

"Think I really have no choice about that. It's the means of blowing CHC out of the water and they deserve to pay for what they've done. I can't pass that up. Besides, I'm considering a suit against them for damages to TurnerWest. The investigation will bring up so much dirt that they'll settle in a minute and then quitting medicine here and moving to St. Lucia is a realistic possibility."

"Oh, Jason, if only it could happen that way," she enthused.

"There's still a lot to sort out, Amy. There's the kids'custody to resolve and then Gallo also implied that Malik may have been hired by someone other than Mark.

"Then who tried to kill us?" she asked.

"I believe that Mark *was* involved with Malik. He as much as admitted it to me. What I don't know is who killed Mark?"

CH050

The flight from Atlanta had been filled with his rehearsals of what he would say to his children and his fearful anticipation of the inevitable confrontation with his parents-in-law... particularly, the judge.

Now, as he drove along the lakeshore approaching the McLean mansion, he continued to rehearse. However, like an addled playwright, his mental dialogue was never the same from one draft to the next. He truly didn't know what to say to influence the McLeans which didn't bode well for a process that appeared to be proceeding irrevocably toward a confrontation in court.

He was paralyzed by indecision.

His hands began to sweat and his pulse accelerated. He needed more time, more preparation, more persuasive arguments... more of everything but trepidation. Ahead to the right, he saw an oval of pavement placed next to the lake as a scenic outlook for tourists and others wishing to enjoy the magnificent vista. He braked and pulled right, snuggling the rented Buick up to the curb inside the confines of a yellow painted rectangle. He sat for a couple of minutes but quickly found the air conditioning hum and the confines of the car irritating.

He shut off the engine and got out to stand hesitantly on a small sidewalk, faced with yet another decision, even though it was as simple as deciding whether to turn right to one of the benches or left to sit upon the grass.

Despite the rapid denouement to his problems in Georgia, his life still seemed to be inundated with decisions, large and small, important and mundane, endlessly demanding his attention. He felt as if he were standing at the bottom of a deep narrow cement form holding a shovel and looking up above him at a patch of sky while a metal chute was spewing tons of cement down to where he stood. Without respite, he was forced to shovel and distribute… knowing that the moment he slackened his efforts, the concrete would begin to bury him... slowly but inexorably.

He turned left on pure impulse and found a level spot, large enough to sit upon comfortably, on the gentle slope leading to the water's edge. Wearily, he knelt, then got down on all fours and finally, sat down drawing up his knees which he encircled with his arms. The grass was soft and fragrant and a light breeze mixed its pastoral perfume with an ample measure of lake scent producing a pleasant olfactory slurry that he drew in through his nostrils, as deeply as he could. The benevolent effect of the incidental deep breathing shunted relaxation into his tense limbs and he sighed audibly, his eyes shut to reality.

If only he could pass the rest of his life here on this spot of grass, answering to no one, passive and empty of care. If only his responsibility could be shorn from him by some benevolent deity, who, looking down and surveying the interminable turmoil of his existence, finally said... "*Enough*"*!* If only his children and parents-in-law could look into his heart and see the total lack of malice, the bountiful stores of affection, the infinite longing for peace, and say ... "*We understand*". If only he could stand back as a spectator to the events of his life, viewing the sum total of all his decisions, actions and errors, all laid out before him, and honestly say ... "*I did my best*".

He inhaled again pulling deep into his lungs all that was fresh and good and clean from the lake, the breeze, the grass. And he held the breath... allowing its soothing magic to leach into his bloodstream for distribution to every cell... and he held it, held it, held it until he could hold it no longer. He felt a tear upon his cheek, warm, wet, unbidden… and knew it came from the unconscious realization... hard and flinty and cold... that, despite the lake, and nature and its influence, '*if only's*' didn't count in life... Not in his life, nor in the lives of others.

He opened his eyes and blinked at the blinding glitter of a billion sun shards, shattered and shimmering, as far as he could see, upon the shifting turquoise surface of the lake. Almost at his feet, the languid lapping of water against shore created an indolent tempo where hiatus, not stroke, marked the measure.

He willed his mind to slowly decrescendo from the recent effervescence of his worries on the road and, for a long while, he thought of nothing, closing his eyes again and becoming part of a basalt boulder on a beach in St. Lucia.

Eventually however, thoughts intruded upon his transitory bliss.

In what units did you measure '*the best interest of a child*', the affection of grandparents, the love of a father? How did you package the '*arrangements*' that would govern a child's time with those who demanded a share commensurate with their blood ties and the amount of attachment they were deemed by a court to deserve? At what point did a parent show more proof of love by backing away from, rather than by wading into, the fray and battling for a portion of a child's heart? Who had the innate right to decide how a family would be configured?... The child?... Those who struggled over the child?... And, when no one could agree, what was the likelihood that the court would be just as incapable of justly decreeing how things would be?

At least for now, here, quiet on the shore of the lake, Jason's mind was calm and clear enough to formulate the questions, but the relative tranquility of the moment did nothing to provide him with answers.

The fact that such an immensely important, elemental decision... *With whom should a child live?...* would be decided by an institution that did not even possess the capacity to love, gave rise to a tremor of anxiety that reverberated deep within him. He was slowly becoming convinced that, however this custody conflict ended, there would be more tragedy than relief for all concerned.

Was there another way? There had to be, but what was it?

He clasped the sides of his head in his hands and squeezed, as if the gentle pressure might miraculously chase the solution from its hiding place in his brain.

When it didn't work, he wasn't surprised and he lowered his eyes, surveyed the impressive vista of Lake Michigan one last time, then heaved himself up from his spot on the grass and turned back toward the Buick.

* * *

Jason was ushered along the final hallway and watched, with more than a little surprise, as the butler stopped and indicated the doorway to the solarium.

"Mistress McLean is waiting for you, sir."

"Thank you," he mumbled as he stepped across the threshold. He had expected convocation to an audience in the austere surroundings of the judge's study.

From a slight distance, he heard a voice...

"Jason?"

The speaker was hidden from his view by a veritable jungle of vegetation. The voice seemed to have come from beyond the verdant bulk of two massive banana trees that dominated a central square bordered by a red brick pathway.

He recognized the voice as that of Mary McLean, but hesitated before using her first name.

"Yes, Mary... It's Jason."

Then, pausing while he bent his head and searched the greenery for her, he asked, "Where are you?"

"Buried over here behind my bananas, dear... Either path will do... Just fray yourself a passage and push through... I have something to share with you."

Her voice was devoid of any tension and he was struck, for the first time, at how much she sounded like Annette. The realization was disconcerting for reasons he could not identify at the moment.

As he looked about his surroundings, he was struck by the fact that all the plants were tropical. The air trapped within the towering glass walls was redolent with plant whispers and the perfume of generous cascading blooms. A profusion of purple, 'king's mantle', drooping under the munificence of its own blossoms' weight clung to a window-side trellis. Its brilliant trailers hung across the pathway to the left and he hesitated to push through such beauty fearing the damage his passage could create.

To the right, a burgeoning geyser of 'elephant ears' sprang from the earth and also partially occluded the pathway. Hidden among the leaves around him were at least a dozen birds, judging by the flitting and chirping he could hear.

There should have been at least a *recording* of the raucous screech of a Macaw to complete the tropical scene. Perhaps, he'd make the suggestion. Above him, the retractable roof of the solarium had been withdrawn until only a screen impeded the autumn sunlight as it streamed down upon the upturned faces of the plants.

He chose the path to the right and lifted aside the elephant ears which swished back into place behind him like curtains in some mystical sultan's apartments.

A flash of yellow, too pale to be the work of nature, was visible ahead and to his left.

Mary McLean spoke again. "Keep coming. I'm at the front wall. You've one more small section of the path to negotiate and you'll be here."

He picked his way carefully through the plants and stopped quietly behind her where she sat on a small concrete bench barely large enough for two. Her hair, which had once been the lustrous copper hue of her daughter's, was still full and luxuriant. Its silver-gray mass had been caught up in a French twist and held with a clip at the back of her head. He supposed the clasp was to keep it from falling into her work-field while she tended to her plants. On the bench beside her, lay a silver gardener's trowel on top of a pair of soiled white work gloves.

He wasn't certain why, but on impulse, he placed his hand lightly on her shoulder before he spoke. "Mary."

She reached up and covered his hand with one of her own, without turning to face him, then lifted it off her shoulder and guided him across in front of her to the other half of the bench. She didn't speak but patted the space beside her with her free hand.

He pushed the gloves and trowel to the very end of the bench and sat tentatively. None of this was happening as he had imagined.

When he was seated, she spoke. Aren't they just magnificent?"

Following her gaze, he realized that she was looking out through the glass wall of the solarium and down across the lawn to the swimming pool.

The day was warm, unusually so for the season, and everything was awash in brilliant sunlight. He saw his daughter Caroline's head appear hesitantly at the top of a fairly high slide close beside a diving board. At first, she was extremely slow at sliding her hands up the silver frame at the top of the steps, as if she were intimidated by the height, and twice she stopped her slow progress to turn half-way round and swat at someone behind her.

Then a second head appeared at the top of the ladder just as she jumped lithely onto the slide and streaked down to skid across four feet of water on her buttocks before disappearing with a splash below the surface. Michael fearlessly dove headfirst onto the slide and was only a few feet behind his sister when he splashed into the pool.

His son surfaced first, spewing water and shaking his head. He was searching for his sister who had cleverly swum underwater well past the point where he had bobbed up. Jason could see her stroking below the surface toward the shallow end of the pool. Bursting from the water to a standing position, she quickly spied her brother behind her and, raising her hands above her head, she ran toward the stairs. He could barely hear her delighted shriek drifting in through the top of the solarium.

Michael pursued her with knife-clean strokes that ate up the distance between them. He swam with none of the wasted energy and purposeless splashing of a child... '*he swims like a man already*', thought Jason and something tightened around his windpipe and caused him to swallow... His son, his little Michael was growing up.

The boy reached the stairway running, just missing his sister's leg with a final lunge over the last three feet of water. She danced away, turned to mock him for a short second, before she was scampering along the side of the pool casting glances over her shoulder and springing in a neat dive into the pool just before Michael reached her. He stopped short, his hands on his hips and waited for her to surface. Gesticulating, Jason could tell from his body language that he was complaining about something.

Caroline thumbed her nose at him and he dove in after her. The chase was on again.

"He's such a well coordinated boy and he worked so hard at his swimming lessons this summer. He only needed a few before he was swimming better than the teacher," said Mary.

His mother-in-law had been laughing delightedly at the children's antics.

"You know, Jason, he swims almost as well as you do," and she looked kindly toward him and lifted his hand to set it between hers in her lap.

He was nonplussed. "Mary, when did you ever see me swim?"

"Did you think that, on the few occasions you visited us at Mackinac, only you and Annette were up and about before six am? You both used to swim together each morning, then sit on the dock and watch the sun rise. And I, not dissimilar to this afternoon, would hide myself on the patio behind the big Tamarac and spy on you. You don't know the joy that simply watching my children brings me."

Her voice grew husky and she turned her face back to the children but not before he saw a tear glimmering along her lower eyelid. She squeezed his hand.

"He already swims better than I do Mary..." *'and he looks so happy and carefree,'* he added, silently.

"You're being modest, Jason. He's no match for you yet, but within a few years," and they both fell silent and watched the children playing.

When she spoke again, Mary's voice was more somber.

"Jason, I chased Angus away to Mackinac when you called and told us you were coming. He didn't understand why I didn't want him here, but I trust that you might. Please listen carefully and don't interrupt me because I'm afraid that I might dissolve into tears at any point and that wouldn't be fair to you, or useful to me. Will you listen, *please?*"

And she looked up at him much as Annette had done on the few occasions that weighty matters had been topics of discussion between them.

"Of course, I will, Mary," was all he said.

"Thank you." And she began.

"You need to know that *I* am convinced that you love your children like life itself. Annette and I often spoke of how you were so much better a father to them than Angus had been to her. It was one of her more profound childhood sorrows that she never seemed able to hold her father's interest like her brother Colin could."

"I believe that it was because of *her* desire to catch her father's eye and garner some of his attention, that her love of daring and risk-taking behavior started. He disapproved of the hand gliding, the skydiving, boat racing and all the rest and they often argued about his disapproval. But that disapproval, and the arguments it generated at least brought them together."

"I'm telling you this to let you know that Annette loved you because you allowed her to do the scary little things that had become such bad habits by the time you two met. You gave her much of what she couldn't get from her father. So, in you, and, with you, she closed a circle that had remained open all her life until then. She wanted desperately for me to *love* you too, and, you know, seeing you through her eyes, listening to the hundreds of anecdotes on those summer evenings at Mackinac that she would tell me, her eyes sparkling with affection for you, *I did come to love you.* But it was a vicarious love, using Annette as the medium that joined us."

She let go of his hands and fumbled in a pocket of the yellow sundress for a bunched up Kleenex with which she dabbed her eyes. She turned and smiled sweetly.

"These tears don't count, dear. I'm still alright," she said and patted his hand.

She continued. "These two wonderful children are composed of Annette and you, yet, hidden deep within the portion of them that arises from my sweet Annette... is *Mary Agnes Stuart McLean.* I am in there too. So you see, I love you, I love her and all that exists in my love for them."

"You loved Annette, and she was part of me. You love the children and Annette and I are all part of them as well... So, I ask myself, how, oh, how could we ever turn upon each other in anger because of all this love? If we lowered ourselves to such mean behavior, it would bring great dishonor to the memory of our dear Annette. Angus, however, doesn't see it that way."

She paused and her voice lost some of its feminine gentleness.

"He's a man of flint and steel with a head as hard and solid as the largest chunk of granite in the walls of that castle he so loves. But he loves me, and if he thought I was in danger, he would draw a blade across the throat of whomever he believed to be threatening me. Now, I would never do anything like that, nor could I take any satisfaction from the fact that he might do it, unbidden, on my behalf. Do you believe me, son?" and she squeezed his hand again and looked deeply into his eyes searching for confirmation that he did.

Her gaze was filled with genuine affection for him.

A tsunami of emotion came crashing over Jason.

When she spoke the word '*son*' it was like a door suddenly opening upon an ocean of unconscious, pent-up, longing and pain. He felt as if his composure was about to disintegrate but he drew a deep shuddering breath and summoned the reserve to disguise his disarray. A visceral trembling had begun within him and, at that moment, he could as easily have flown as spoken. The best he could manage was to nod his head affirmatively.

"Thank you. It's important for me to know you clearly understand that I will have no part in the malice or the legal custody proceedings that Angus has initiated. I will die before I would ever permit my children to be laid upon that legal altar at which my husband has worshiped all his life. I have never defied him but I'm convinced that this is the time to do so, if it comes to that."

It was Jason's turn to mumble a muted, "Thank you."

"Now, please let me dither on for a short while more, Jason, as my story is not yet finished."

She looked past him with her soft gray eyes to something or someone far away. For a moment, she was silent and lost in thought. Then she smiled, came back to him, and began again.

"There is another chapter and its purpose is to help you better understand me. We cannot remain strangers, for I know what Annette would say. I am a dinosaur, as much out of place in this modern world of ours as the monsters from the steamy eons of our past. And, *I am* so out of place, because I am *only a mother*... nothing else... just a mother. Women like me no longer exist. This past of mine began some forty years ago when I first felt the stirrings of life, here," and she raised their hands together to lay them against her lower abdomen, "And nothing in my existence has been the same since."

"I bore my two lovely children who lived and two more who never drew but a single breath, God bless their little souls, and I did it with joy and thanksgiving. I never felt the pain of giving birth... Can you believe that, son? And I held them in my arms and nourished them from my very breasts. I could not have been happier."

There were tears streaming down her cheeks but her voice was full and firm and he recognized them as tears of joy.

"We were dirt poor then because he was in law school still, but it didn't matter. Money is not an essential element of happiness, as naïve as that notion may seem. What I didn't possess, was completely eclipsed by what I did have... my dear sweet children."

Abruptly, a flash of guilt flitted across her features.

"I love my husband, please understand that, and I am convinced that Angus and God... and me as well, all wish that I could love him more. But my children were flesh of my flesh, blood of my blood and although it is considered the worst failure in this topsy-turvy world of ours that adores individualism, I lost myself in them... I lived *through* them. And when,"... her voice broke and her delicate frame began to tremble with emotion.

Jason instinctively placed his arm around her shoulders and drew her to him, caressing her hair to comfort her.

She resumed, "And when they died... Mary Agnes Stuart McLean... *died, too.*"

She was silent except for her sobbing, the tissue clutched in whitened knuckles, tears falling freely upon her clasped hands.

"And then, as I walked like a specter along the corridors of this huge empty monument to money," and she waved a hand dismissively in the general direction of the mansion. "I prayed that God would take me home, as well, for I had no desire to remain in this world alone."

She smiled at him through her tears, turning her face up in mild embarrassment. "You see, dear Jason, I'm really not much good alone. But then you called and said the children were coming and I rose from my affliction as literally as Lazarus walked out of the tomb."

She paused and they both continued looking at each other in silence.

Jason was experiencing a sudden upwelling of affection for this kind gracious woman and he began to regret the years during which they had stood on either side of Annette as strangers.

She broke the silence. "Look at my hands and wrists, Jason and tell me what you see?" and she held out her hands toward him, fingers spread.

He had to examine them only for a moment, as his trained eyes quickly detected the fusiform swelling of the joints, the arthritic nodes at her furthest knuckles, the abnormal prominence of the wrist bones.

"Arthritis," he said.

"Yes, arthritis. And, at night, these hands *and* knees *and* ankles *and* shoulders," she laughed softly and briefly, "In fact, Jason, this whole moth-eaten skeleton *used* to ache and throb until peaceful sleep was no more than a distant memory. But they no longer ache because I've discovered a cure for this and for all my other ills as well."

There was now a twinkle in her eyes.

"Intrigued, doctor?"

"Yes, of course, Mary. What have you found?" he queried.

"Each evening," and her voice had become suddenly somber again, "after the children and I have read our scriptures and they have fallen asleep, I steal back into the bedroom of one or the other of them… Let me simply say that I am convinced angels stand guard over our little ones at night because there is an atmosphere of peace and serenity that falls over the rooms of children when they close their eyes..."

She finished her brief aside.

"I slip down quietly onto the floor beside their beds. Occasionally, I sit but, more often, I kneel and I place my head on the edge of the bed beside them and listen to their breathing. Sometimes, I've fallen asleep there but I've always been able to awaken and steal away without being detected."

"And what is the treatment... for the arthritis, I mean?" asked Jason.

"Well, dear boy, that's it. Just what I've told you! It's a gift from God to mothers. You've seen it work before. Think back to Annette and the children... or even further back to your own young life with your mother. A child falls and scrapes his knees... There's a bit of blood and a lot of stinging but he wants to get back to his play, so he brings his pain to his mother. He might be crying, or he might be trying to be brave but *he's had enough of this pain.* And what does mother do? Why, she looks at the wound, then at the face of the child, tear-streaked and grimacing... and she kisses him and *whoosh...* Just like magic... the pain is gone!"

Jason smiled, leaned over and gave her a little kiss on the forehead.

"The story isn't over... The secret," and she lowered her voice conspiratorially and turned her mouth up to his ear, "is that this gift from God is *reciprocal...* When the mother touches the child, *her pain flees as well.* And there you have it... No more arthritic pain."

They both laughed and she stood up pulling on his hand.

"Give me a hug, son, for you truly are my son, my only son now, and then you go and join the children. They've been missing you terribly. I'll stay here hidden away among my plants for all the reasons I've already explained."

She threw her frail arms around him and clung for longer than Jason ever remembered being just hugged, since he was a child. When she finally released him, she turned him around and pushed him gently down the red brick path.

* * *

Mary had been right about the children missing him. He'd only taken a few steps off the patio onto the grass in the direction of the pool when Michael spied him.

He literally sprang to his feet and began to yell, "Dad! Dad!... Caroline, Dad's here!" and then he fairly tore up the hill hitting his father's chest at top speed and clamping his arms around him while still yelling, "Dad! Dad!"

After a minute of ferocious hugs and a kiss on both of his son's cheeks, they walked toward the pool where Caroline was modestly fastening a towel around her waist before walking demurely to meet them.

He enfolded her in his arms, smelling her mother in her hair and whispered, "I'm so happy to be back with you. I'm sorry it took so terribly long."

She whispered back.

"It was awful, daddy... We really thought you might die. I cried a lot but God heard me."

Michael hovered around them excitedly, then interrupted.

"Ok, Caroline, let him go. We've got to tell him about our plan."

Five minutes later, all three were huddled like conspirators in a circle of three pool chairs. Michael was bubbling over with excitement but he turned to his older sister. "You tell him Caroline... you speak better than me."

"Ok, princess. Tell me," encouraged Jason.

"It's pretty simple, Dad, but it's the best we could come up with. Promise not to make your mind up right away..."

"Unless you agree," interjected Michael, "You can say it's ok, right away if you want."

Caroline's expression betrayed the trepidation she was feeling.

"Dad, now that mom is gone and grandma and grandpa Angus are up here. We think it would be a good idea if we all moved here to Detroit."

She watched his face expectantly.

"Well, dad, could we? There's a real neat house next door. It's almost as nice as grandma Mary's and *it's for sale*!" enthused Michael.

Jason was carried away by thc suggestion. It had never occurred to him. Could it be the solution he'd been praying for?

"But my job is down in Albany, kids, and, with Mr. West gone now, I'm still responsible for a lot of doctors. It's how I earn my living."

"But we're your responsibility too, dad and we're up here... and we *like* it here," piped up Michael.

Jason was thoughtful.

Caroline added.

"And all our family's here, dad. If we lived next door, we could see grandma Mary, *every day.*"

'And she could see you every night,' thought Jason.

Michael spoke again.

"You can sell a business, dad, but you can't buy a family. You could get a job up here as a doctor. When it gets cold in the wintertime, I'll bet there are even more sick people in Michigan than in Georgia."

Jason reached over and tousled his son's hair then pulled the children up against him into another big hug.

CH051

The phone rang and Amy ran to it. It had to be Jason calling from Detroit. "Hello," she said a little breathlessly.

"Hi, sweetheart, how are you doing?" he answered.

"Fine, except that I'm not with you and that always leaves me a little diminished."

"Are you sitting down?" he asked.

"Should I be?" she answered suspiciously.

"I think so."

"Ok, well now I am. What is it?"

"I've been offered a position in Bangladesh."

"*In Bangladesh*," she repeated with obvious surprise.

"I'd be the medical director of a hospital for lepers."

"A hospital for *lepers*...?" she echoed

"Yes, but it would only be for ten years, and then, I think we'd be transferred to Africa someplace," he said soberly... "How are you taking all this?"

"Sitting down," she said flatly.

"It's what I've always wanted to do... Sort of giving something back." He continued. "You don't know how much satisfaction I got from working in that little clinic in St. Lucia and in Bangladesh we'd be needed even more!"

"I can understand that, darling, but I don't remember you ever talking to me about it."

"It's important to me, Amy," he was almost wheedling.

Three beats of silence hummed over the line before she answered. "Darling if it means that much to you, then it's alright with me," she said, reassuringly.

"You mean, you don't mind moving to Bangladesh to a *leper colony*?"

"I thought it was a hospital?"

"Yes, sorry, I meant hospital."

"Jason, if that's where your heart takes you... If that's what you need... I'm your wife and I'll always be at your side. Is that what you needed to hear?"

"Absolutely," he responded.

"Well, when do we leave?" asked Amy. "Luckily, my stuff is still in storage."

"One more thing, darling..."

"Yes..."

"If I don't get approval for the Bangladesh thing," and he paused.

"Yes...?"

"Or if it falls through, at the last moment... How would you feel about moving to Grosse Point, just outside of Detroit?"

There was a long pregnant silence.

Then…

"Jason Turner!!"

Epilogue

It's a mongoose, Michael. Leave the poor creature alone. It's frightened of you."

"I just want to see it again, grandma... I won't hurt him." And he continued to poke the small stick into the burrow where the animal had disappeared.

"Michael Turner, you get back over here and sit down. We're in the middle of our geography lesson. If you don't obey young man, I'll tell your father and there will be no fishing trip tomorrow."

"Aw, grandma..." and pouting, he returned to his chair beneath the huge mango tree which shaded the spot where he and his sister did their lessons everyday with their grandmother.

The family had already been in St Lucia for two months and was due to return home to Detroit next month. No one seemed enthusiastic about the upcoming departure, however. The villa they were staying in was a rental but already it was beginning to feel like a second home.

Amy and Jason volunteered every morning at the little clinic down the road and some family adventure occupied each afternoon. Tomorrow, it would be a fishing trip on the 'Saucy Lady' which Dr. Landry had purchased for a song after the death of her captain.

Mary McLean had accompanied, then home-schooled the children and did not seem to miss her husband, the judge, who called her every evening without fail.

Jason had sold his interest in TurnerWest to the firm's physicians for five million dollars and so he had the time and the means to decide if, or how he intended to interface with medicine in the future. He truly enjoyed the work at the clinic which he had assisted with funds to upgrade the building and the equipment.

The home they had purchased in Detroit was next door to the grandparents' house and the children had continued their daily contact with their grandmother. In fact, the children's lives were so entwined with their grandmother's that they could not have contemplated a separation. Hence, grandma had accompanied them to St. Lucia when Jason had decided that he needed time to consider what the future could hold for them all.

Mary and Amy got along well. In fact, Mary seemed to see many of the traits Amy possessed in common with her daughter and this had drawn them easily together.

Angus McLean had relaxed his opposition to Jason when he learned that the children would be moving next door. He still retained a stiff formality in his dealings with Amy but he was softening slowly. He hadn't come to St. Lucia "because I've never spent that long under any other man's roof and I'm not about to begin now".

The fears that Gallo had expressed about continuing danger from unidentified enemies seemed groundless. However, to coverall the bases, his men had made it clear to Amy's ex-husband, Riley Davis, that any attempt to interfere with the new family could have deadly consequences. It had been months now that Gallo had been out of the picture as the legal custody proceeding had been dropped and the CHC affair had been settled.

The 20/20 expose had been televised and Jason had been a part of it. Following the humiliation and the monetary losses associated with the scandal, CHC had settled a suit by TurnerWest out of court, providing most of the money the firm's doctors required to finance Jason's buyout.

Kleinberg was convicted of conspiracy to commit murder and was serving a ten year sentence in a federal prison.

Just this month, Jason had received a package from Nicaragua. It was a letter from Cal and a picture of him at the charity clinic he had founded in a slum on the outskirts of Manaugua, Nicaragua. His wife Gloria and his children were at his side, the Albany mansion having been sold.

In his letter, Cal never admitted to any participation in the events in Albany following his disappearance, but there was one photo in the envelope which showed Jason's BMW in the woods near the West's hunting lodge.

It was enough to answer many questions.

"Medicine is nothing but stories..."

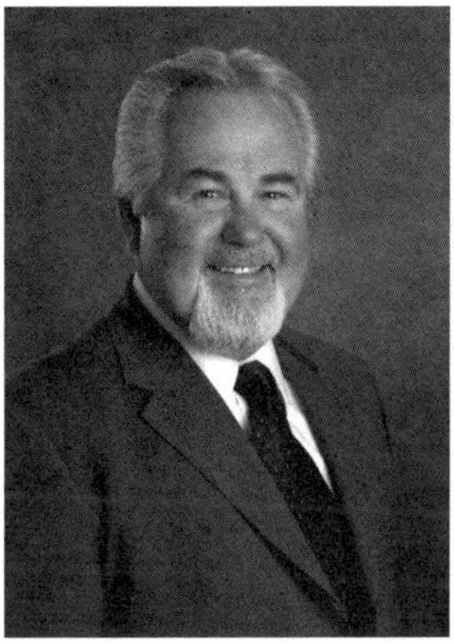

About the Author

J. **Frederic Templeman, MD** is a primary care physician, board certified in both Canada and the US with over twenty years of clinical experience. Dr. Templeman, who entered medical school at age 36, had previously had a successful career in the Canadian diplomatic corps during which he was posted to third world countries in the western hemisphere and was involved in Canadian foreign aid projects. Since becoming a physician, Dr. Templeman has led groups of students and medical volunteers back to the areas where he was previously posted and to other locations where volunteer medical services are needed.

Dr. Templeman is the President of a Utah-based research firm, Phytoceutical Research, LLC. He is also a board member of several research companies active in the field of Natural Products. He believes that excellence in research and in the production of products is essential, if botanical products are to be accepted as nutritional interventions in standard medicine.

As a pioneering advocate of nutritional intervention in standard medical care, Dr. Templeman is sought worldwide as a lecturer and, last year, spoke to thousands of people on three continents.

Dr. Templeman enjoys writing and has written extensively on the medicinal benefits of supplementation with botanical products. 'Covered Lives' is his second novel.

Dr. Templeman, the father of ten children, resides in Utah with his wife Michele.